W9-CAB-771

Yoga, Karma, and Rebirth

Yoga, Karma, and Rebirth

A Brief History and Philosophy

Stephen H. Phillips

COLUMBIA UNIVERSITY PRESS *NEW YORK*

Columbia University Press
Publishers Since 1893
New York Chichester, West Sussex
Copyright © 2009 Columbia University Press
All rights reserved
Library of Congress Cataloging-in-Publication Data
Phillips, Stephen H., 1950–
Yoga, karma, and rebirth : a brief history and philosophy / Stephen H. Phillips.
p. cm.
Includes bibliographical references and index.
ISBN 978-0-231-14484-1 (cloth : alk. paper) — ISBN 978-0-231-14485-8 (pbk.) — ISBN 978-0-231-51947-2 (electronic)
1. Yoga. I. Title.
B132.Y6P48 2009
181'.45—dc22 2008031691
∞
Columbia University Press books are printed on permanent and durable acid-free paper.
This book is printed on paper with recycled content.
Printed in the United States of America
c 10 9 8 7 6 5 4 3 2 1
p 10 9 8 7 6 5 4 3 2 1

Contents

Preface

This book grew out of an upper-division course I developed at the University of Texas at Austin, "Yoga as Philosophy and Practice," and I would like to thank first of all Ellen Briggs Stansell, my teaching assistant for its first three years. Together we discussed all the topics broached here. Concurrently Ellen became a yoga teacher as well as a doctoral candidate, completing a thesis on the *Bhagavad Gita*. Matthew Dasti and Neil Dalal, also graduate students at Texas, made helpful comments, as did my philosophy colleague and fellow yoga student Kathleen Higgins. Matthew helped me select passages from the *Gita* to translate in appendix B. Insights and lots of feedback were provided by my wife, Hope. Kisor Chakrabarti, J. N. Mohanty, and Peter Heehs read portions of early drafts and made solid suggestions. For chapters 2, 3, and 4, the book has benefited from extensive comments by Colin Foote, particularly with regard to Buddhist theories and practices.

Let me thank my yoga teachers, many of whom I have doubtless copied in scripting a yoga class in chapter 1: Brigitte Snyder (best of flow teachers), John Schlorholtz (author of the DVD series *Ageless Yoga*, and my brother-in-law), Peggy Kelly (founder of Austin School of Yoga), Mary Keator, Cary Choate, Jessica Montgomery, Annick Sebbane, Ravyn Abboushi, Genevieve Gilbreath, Larissa Rogers, Jenn Wooten, Charlie Llewellyn, Pam Brewer, Jessica Wozniak, Brienne Brown, Devon Dederich, Jerry Balderas, Enid Baptiste, Kaye Klier, Matt Borer, Rachel Hector, Ana Pilar, Elizabeth

Cafferky, Chuck Hausman ("Kewal"), Dorothee Bethscheider ("Dodo" in Auroville, South India), Kimberley Jones, Esta Herold ("Seva"), Tenille Collard, Jessica Goulding, Jenny Dawson, and Christina Sell. Two of these guru-*ji*s attended my lectures on Indian philosophies at UT and read portions of the book in draft, providing helpful reactions; Ravyn Abboushi and Genevieve Gilbreath thus deserve special acknowledgment—as does Peggy Kelly, dean of Austin yoga teachers, and senior Anusara teacher Christina Sell, who read portions of the *Kularnava Tantra* with me. Tracie Brace, founder of Yoga Rasa, Houston, and Michael Benton ("Mehtab") and friends at Yogayoga, Austin, graciously rewarded a little teaching of Sanskrit on my part by enriching my practice through help as teachers or students, as did dozens more, all of whom I salute with heartfelt thanks.

Chapter 4, first section, written as a presentation at an APA conference, was in large part published in the *Newsletter of the American Philosophical Association* (Fall 2005). Much of chapter 3, second section appears in *The Encyclopedia of Violence, Peace and Conflict*, 2nd edition, ed. Lester Kurtz (Amsterdam: Elsevier, 2008). I also read part of it as the paper, "*Ahimsa* ('Nonharmfulness'): The Vedantic, Buddhist, and Jaina Arguments," Seventeenth International Congress of Vedanta, University of Miami, Oxford, Ohio, September 2007. Ideas on the mind-body problem in particular were developed in connection with efforts by Daniel Bonevac and me to introduce the readings in our *Introduction to World Philosophy* (New York: Oxford University Press, 2009). Much of the second section of chapter 2 was presented at the International Seminar on Understanding Consciousness, Ramakrishna Mission Institute of Culture, Kolkata, January 2008, and will appear in the conference proceedings. The third and fourth sections began as the paper, "The Mind-Body Problem in Three Indian Philosophies," presented at the International Conference on Mind and Consciousness, Indian Institute of Technology, Kharagpur, West Bengal, January 2002, and included in the conference proceedings. Part of chapter 4, third section will appear in the *Jadavpur Journal of Philosophy* (in press) and was read as part of the Sri Aurobindo Annual Lecture Series, Jadavpur University, Kolkata, 2008. Special thanks go to Indrani Sanyal and her colleagues in the Philosophy Department at Jadavpur and to editors and others who have facilitated these papers and publications.

I am especially grateful to Wendy Lochner, Christine Mortlock, Leslie Kriesel, Martin Hinze, Derek Warker, and Milenda Lee at Columbia University Press. Wendy Lochner in particular had a large hand in shaping this book through championing the appendices as well as editing several sections while encouraging me to write for a wide audience.

Yoga, Karma, and Rebirth

om paramatmane namah

Introduction

Setting an Intention (or, Enlivening an Intention Already Set)

agnim ile. . . . I call the fire, ancient priest of the sacrifice, the divine who summons (the divinities), bringing here jewels.
—*Rig Veda* 1.1.1

This is the life energy (*prana*) that radiates out from every being. Knowing this, the knower tends not to excessive disputation. / Playing and relishing in the self (*atman*) with self as his delight, doing works he becomes the best of Brahman knowers.
—*Mundaka Upanishad* 3.1.4

Sumedha: "Surely a buddha I shall be."
—*Jataka* 1.3

Setting himself in a clean place in a steady *asana* (posture, seat) that is neither too high nor too low (to be comfortable), on a cloth, animal skin, or kusha grass, there fixing heart and mind on a single point, working to bring his thought and emotion along with his faculties and organs under control, let him practice yoga for self-purification.
—*Bhagavad Gita* 6.11–12

atha yoga-anushasanam. . . . Now instruction in yoga. Yoga is the stilling of fluctuations of thought and emotion (*chitta*). Then the seer (the conscious being) rests in its true nature. At other times, fluctuations are identified with.
—*Yoga Sutra* 1.1–4

Yoga is the unity (*ekatva*) of one thing with another.
—*Malini-vijayottara Tantra* 4.4.1

The consciousness traditions of ancient India constitute the roots of yoga teaching. Buddhism carried yoga eastward, and all Eastern spiritual traditions—including the martial arts—have common background with the yoga traditions of India. Some have argued that Christianity too is influenced by yoga, perhaps in the figure of Jesus himself. Clearly Sufism is. In India, traditions of yoga practice include or overlap with Vedantic, Jaina, Buddhist, Sikh, Vaishnavite, and Shaivite teachings. These are multidimensional complexes of ideas and culture, and are in large part the origins of yoga training programs that have spread all over the world.

There is, for example, the invocation, dedication, or other ritual beginning of a typical yoga class. This can be as simple as a single outbreath of the chant *om*, which is a mantra or sacred syllable according to very old Upanishads. Upanishads are "secret teachings" composed in Sanskrit, which was the lingua franca of ancient and classical India.[1] Upanishads are the oldest texts in which the word *yoga* is used in our sense, our anglicized "yoga" (some earlier usages carry a different meaning). The meaning and symbolism of *om* is laid out very early in the *Mandukya Upanishad* (c. 500 B.C.E.) and elsewhere: "*Om* —this syllable is all this (universe)" and so on.[2]

There are indications of yoga practice even earlier than the earliest Upanishads. The *Rig Veda* ("Rig" from Sanskrit *rik*, which means "verse"), the oldest text in Sanskrit (c. 1200 B.C.E. or earlier), is a source for yoga teaching, although, to be sure, there are disputes about its meaning. We will survey yoga literature in the last section of chapter 1, setting the Vedas, Upanishads, *Bhagavad Gita*, *Yoga Sutra*, and other yoga texts in chronological order, as we identify the main themes of Yoga philosophy and trace their development up to the modern period. This book will become a first-person defense of a contemporary view that all yoga practitioners and sympathizers can stand behind confidently. But first we will review our Yoga inheritance.

Another example of reverberations of the Indian past in the modern studio is the practice of a teacher's asking everyone to "set an intention" for the class to come, the session of an hour or so of asanas and conscious breathing. Sometimes it is suggested that one might "tune into" or refurbish an intention already formed. Such setting of an intention (*samkalpa* in Sanskrit) and *bhavana* (enlivening an intention already set) are found in the Upanishads in stories of young people going to a guru to learn the truth of the self (*atman*). Because resolve shapes what is possible, much emphasis is placed on intention, *samkalpa*, in yoga traditions—on the idea of what is to be accomplished through yoga practice. Yoga philosophy has long held that practice follows thought, as well as that what we do is what we become. Traditionally, the "thought" here in this mantra is *samkalpa*. Yoga asks us to set our sights high. In the Upanishads, the names of some of the seekers, such as Satyakama in the

Chandogya (c. 800 B.C.E.), "He whose desire is the truth," conform to the theme.

A wonderful dramatization of setting an intention occurs in the earliest texts of Buddhism (c. 300 B.C.E.) in the story of Sumedha and the Buddha's "first vow."[3] Wealthy, well educated, and of high social status in the "town of Amara, a place of beauty and delights," a young man named Sumedha, despite the surrounding splendor and advantages he has in society, comes to the realization, "What misery to be born again, and have the flesh dissolve at death!" And he resolves to find freedom from evil through yoga. Then after years of yogic discipline, Sumedha hears of the arrival in Amara of a buddha (awakened one), Dipankara by name, a person of such radiance, power, and wisdom that throngs gather to strew flowers at his feet. Sumedha joins the crowd, loosening his long, matted hair to form part of the buddha's path. As the Blessed One approaches, our yogin is inspired to want to be like that, setting an intention that, according to Buddhist tradition, remains firm through lifetimes of more moderate practice and progress (the Middle Way)—until he is born Siddhartha Gautama of our age.

Recognizing the sincerity of Sumedha's intention, Dipankara stops and announces, "Surely a buddha you shall be." From his words echoed by the crowd, Sumedha comes to carry with him not only the intention but also a deep confidence. One of the tasks of a Yoga philosophy (Buddhist or another) is to protect such confidence from attack.

Similarly, in the *Bhagavad Gita*, which is of about the same time (c. 300 B.C.E.) as the Jataka tale of Sumedha, it is the sincere aspiration of the character Arjuna that provokes his divine charioteer Krishna to instruct him in yoga and provide a whole worldview to boot (see the introduction to appendix B).

Yoga is more than postures and breath control. It comprises processes of psychological transformation complementing physical development and maintenance of good health. The *Yoga Sutra*, for example, lays out asana and breath control (*pranayama*), but only as practices among other practices, specifically, as two limbs within an "eight-limbed" *ashtanga yoga*. The *ashtanga yoga* of Patanjali includes meditation and right focus as well as ethical and personal constraints (*yama* and *niyama*). One goal of this book is to help yoga teachers and practitioners appreciate the breadth and depth of yoga. Traditionally, yoga is a way the sacred can come into life.

There are of course many kinds of yoga: *hatha* yoga, which targets the body and breath; meditational or *jnana* yoga; *karma* yoga, which is the yoga of action and self-sacrifice; *bhakti* yoga, which is the yoga of devotion and love; tantric yoga aimed at uniting with Shiva/Shakti; Kundalini yoga to open the occult *chakras* or centers of consciousness and awaken the "serpent power" (*kundalini*) to rise in the central channel (*sushumna*); the "eight-limbed" *ashtanga* yoga of the *Yoga Sutra* focused on quieting the mind; the specialized yogas of *japa* (repetition of mantras or sacred syllables); yogic sleep (*yoga nidra*); and so on. The list is long. A second purpose of this book is to chart common and uncommon suppositions of the central manuals of the more prominent types.

Practices of yoga are not only grounded in ancient spiritual traditions but also defended by certain Eastern philosophies. This book, despite the attention to history, is itself a work of Yoga philosophy, extending classical Yoga traditions. As a practitioner, I think of it as yoga for the *buddhi*, for the intellect, or *svadhyaya*, self-study, in the phrase of the *Yoga Sutra* (2.1). The point is to develop intellectual confidence about ideas used in yoga practices. Thus the central goal, beyond sorting and clarifying, is to defend central concepts involved in the practices, especially certain psychological concepts (such as karma and its underpinnings in mental dispositions, *samskara*), as well as pieces of Yoga philosophy from the past.

The phrase "Yoga philosophy" (with a capital Y) is sometimes used by scholars to refer to the views of the *Yoga Sutra* and its commentaries. These views are without question important for this book. But here "Yoga philosophy" is construed much more broadly, and the resources for our own Yoga philosophy include Vedanta and the Upanishads, the little-known school of Nyaya, Buddhism, Jainism, tantra, and other Eastern and now Western philosophies centered on yoga practices. Indeed, as practices of spiritual development from all over the world, including from Western traditions, are by analogy "yogic," so too are philosophies. Thus Rumi's is in our usage a Yoga philosophy. Patanjali's *Yoga Sutra* is mentioned here probably more than any other single instance of yoga literature, and a new translation is appended (appendix C). But my intention is not to defend the philosophy of the *Yoga Sutra*. In general, "Yoga" (with the capital) will designate a framework of ideas about self and reality connected tightly with yoga practices by way of explaining the experiences or abilities to which the practices lead. By this definition, there is much that qualifies as Yogic within classical Eastern and now some modern philosophy with a global audience. The classics of Yoga are, however, mainly Indian: Vedantic, Buddhist, Jaina, Nyaya, and tantric texts as well as the *Yoga Sutra* and its Sanskrit commentaries. Especially from such classic sources, which are mostly in Sanskrit, I try to frame a Yoga philosophy that is not so much new as useful to, in particular, yoga students and teachers. This book is dedicated to everyone who has led or will lead a yoga class, or has begun a serious practice. It is also, to be sure, written for philosophers and students of philosophy—with a global interest.

Chapter 1 opens with a section on the nature of yoga theories, which is followed by a description of a yoga class (what it's like from a first-person point of view) along with some suggestions for yoga teachers and practitioners, and then a section on yoga literature. First-person description shows levels and types of theoretic commitment, although nothing more bold practicewise will be undertaken than what goes by the name of Sun Salutations (along with two varieties of breath control and a couple of mantras).

Chapter 2 takes up a challenge to Yoga theory from scientific materialism and recent work in metaphysics by academic philosophers. Theoretic commitments and options for Yoga are laid out. Yoga philosophic inclusivism is the disjunction of views that together form a spiritual camp, opposed to a collection of views that are materialist. Materialism locates causal power solely in objects, things that are material and only material. Yoga does not, locating our power over ourselves in something subjective, something more than a brain. Yoga philosophy is not limited to any single position on the relation of body to mind or spirit or consciousness, but all Yoga philosophy stands in opposition to certain claims held in common by materialists. Indeed, at the heart of Yoga, I shall argue, is commitment to two-directional causation and possibilities of self-development.

Chapter 3 takes up the psychological concept of karma and explores its metaphysical and, especially, its moral dimensions as well as its importance for yoga practice. Karma constitutes habits and is summed up as character, character built up from below, from choices we make. There is also a special meaning of the word in "karma yoga," which is explained following the *Bhagavad Gita*. The concept of karmic fate is also illuminated, as well as the foundations for the yogic practice of nonharmfulness (*ahimsa*, nonviolence). A view of ecological responsibility flows from a right understanding of karma.

Chapter 4 examines Yogic views of rebirth, sifting superstition from occult psychology. Principal arguments for and against reincarnation are examined. The nature of possible cross-life continuity is of primary interest. The soul-making model of the *Gita* is contrasted with an underappreciated tantric top-down model that posits a status for the individual beyond embodiment and embodiments, as in part manifestations of a larger type of self, not just developments along lines continuous with previous births. In this tantric view, spiritual enlightenment is not such a big deal, being both easy to come by and often secondary to the ends of the Divine Mother for the individual, the compulsions of divine shakti or energy to finite manifestation.

Chapter 5 takes up further ethical and social dimensions of yoga practice along with traditional claims of extraordinary capacities and "powers." What is the point of yoga? What are the legitimate goals? Does yoga have social value? The good of holistic health is explored along with traditional teachings. In our age, can yoga be more than physical exercise? I shall argue in favor of an expansionist program, discussing yoga in life, especially *bhakti* yoga, as well as the yoga of beauty and art along with the theme of psychic transformation. Traditionally, however, extraordinary powers called *siddhi*s, if not to be renounced, are thought best directed to the spiritual (*adhyatmika*). We shall examine the tantric among other answers and attitudes, worldly and otherworldly combinations.

Five appendices present new translations from Sanskrit of classic yoga (and Yoga) texts: the Upanishads, the *Gita*, the *Yoga Sutra*, the *Hatha Yoga Pradipika*, and a few other tantric texts drawn from Kashmiri Shaivism.

As mentioned, I have thought of part of the audience for this book as yoga teachers, teachers of asanas and *pranayama*, who are now perhaps the principal conveyors of Yoga philosophy, and their interested students. To you let me say, please be patient with my tentativeness ("What is true is A *or* B *or* C *or* . . ."). Probably many will feel a need for metaphysical doctrines that are more specific than anything here. But nothing here rules out faith in the power of consciousness beyond that defended here explicitly. Versions of theism are discussed, for example, without endorsement, but definitely without rejection (in the last section of chapter 3 the idea of God's goodness is defended by doctrines of karma and rebirth). The point is to open a Yoga umbrella sheltering a whole family of views and spiritual paths. This attitude is in line with the spirit of inclusivism found in many Yogic texts, including the *Yoga Sutra* itself, which presents alternative methods to achieve the yogic goal.[4] As Yoga philosophers, we have to deny materialism; its causal theses have to be opposed, as explained in chapter 2. But our Yoga philosophy tries as far as possible to be friendly to a broad inheritance of philosophies encouraging yoga. Such inclusivism demands abstraction, and details are inevitably overlooked as our plane, our intellectual *vahana*, rises and we scan a wide expanse. And like a difficult asana, philosophic flights, although

Yogic, are not for every practitioner. The basic idea is, however, entirely simple: we may have confidence in our Yoga inheritance.

Thus our Yoga philosophy not only is inclusivist but also has to be in a sense minimalist: trying to say as much as necessary to support the practices and understand the experiences and abilities they lead to, but not more, especially not more as a matter of strong commitment. This attitude is motivated by the facts of our global times and circumstances and the diversity of belief systems in the Yoga camp. Note that an attractive alternative to minimalism is the relativism or perspectivalism developed by Jaina philosophers, *anekanta-vada*, nonabsolutism. This position will be examined closely at the end of chapter 3, but the gist is to treat all views as having a grain of truth, as right with qualifications. In the Jaina spirit, I find a rough trade-off—though hardly a zero-sum game—between ways of weakening the content of claims, mainly abstraction and alternation, and levels of justified confidence. (Devadatta sees what looks like a snake crawl into the doghouse, but is not entirely sure and says, "I saw *something* [abstraction] crawl into the doghouse. I *think it may be* [less than absolute confidence] a snake.") The genius of the Jainas was to forge a logic of the maybe (*syat*) that, we shall see below, is able to disarm metaphysical conflict, an intellectual *ahimsa*, nonharmfulness. The logic of the maybe has both an epistemic and a metaphysical dimension, and my minimalist strategy, though not the same, is similar.

All this suggests another story from Buddhist tradition and a final reminder about the spirit of Yoga theorizing. The story of Sumedha is from the Pali canon of southern Buddhism, where are also found the "Sermons of the Buddha" that scholars view as the oldest Buddhist texts. In a famous sermon in the *Majjima Nikaya*, the Buddha warns against too much intellectualizing. There are questions that "do not tend to edification," and the Buddha draws analogies to a house on fire and to a man shot with an arrow. Just as one would not discourse on the nature of fire, its composition or source, but would rush to put it out if one's own house were ablaze, and similarly a man shot would not discourse on the nature of the arrow but would pull it out, so we should act to change ourselves and win the highest good, not wasting time in idle talk.[5] But it seems to me—as it has to hundreds of previous yoga (and Yoga) enthusiasts, including hundreds of Buddhist philosophers—that a little theory is needed. Otherwise, we might be discouraged, for example, by the materialists, and miss opportunities that yoga presents. Thus is our attitude pragmatic, humble, and not to claim the final word.

1

Theory and Practice

Principles of Yoga Practice and Types of Yoga Theory

Insofar as yoga practice is a form of bodily movement (and sometimes effortful absence of bodily movement), it does not require much theoretical knowledge. Although yoga is not mere exercise, intellectually it's often only a matter of knowing the meaning of words that refer to basic body parts and motions, like lifting your arms and holding your palms together. A yoga teacher conveys skills, mastery of the body, breath, and so on from his or her own first-person point of view. It's "knowledge how" rather than "knowledge that," like how to ride a bicycle or to swim as opposed to certain facts or laws that obtain. Asanas or postures and the transitions between them in a class require little theoretical knowledge, no knowledge of aerodynamics, for instance, although all movement is governed by aerodynamic laws.

Of course, in yoga practice not every body part needs to be known and identified, only those capable of being moved as targeted in the instructions of the teacher—the left hand, for example, as opposed to the spleen. One of the purposes of doing the posture called Corpse Pose, *shavasana,* is to learn to identify body parts, but not as one would in an anatomy class.[1] The main purpose of the asana is to relax the entire body and psychological system consciously, as you lie flat on your back on the floor without going to sleep. Learning to locate and relax a specific part mentioned is a means to this end and is how the asana is taught to beginners in some traditions: toes, arches, ankles, heels, calves, upper and lower thighs, fingers, hands, arms, shoulders, and (to quote a contemporary teacher) "loosening hip sockets and relaxing the buttocks, moving from the tailbone and relaxing through the lumbar, the thoracic vertebrae, relaxing the back of the neck, and softening the throat, releasing any tension from the muscles of the jaws, lips, and tongue, relaxing the cheeks" [parting the lips and moving the tongue to lie away from the teeth], "feeling the eyeballs grow heavier and softer as they drop down away from the eyelids, the eyelids floating lightly above the eyes as you relax the eyebrows and forehead and make the temples grow soft and hollow, relaxing the scalp and crown of the head."[2] Let me stress that these two are not the same: the ability to identify and move or relax a body part as required to do yoga, and knowing the location and function of an anatomical part, such as the pineal gland, as explained in medical science. The distinction is of enormous importance to Yoga philosophy.

Yoga teachings engage, like a "how-to" book of practical instruction, a first-person point of view as opposed to the externalist, third-person point of view of science. Thus Yoga philosophy has a touchstone in the utility of its ideas for the practices. Medical science does not have the same orientation, and although often scientific hypotheses overlap with Yoga principles, the phenomenology (how they appear or are present to consciousness) of the practices as well as of the experiences to which they lead carries Yoga philosophy into its own special area of psychological theory and, as we shall see, metaphysics.

To move more slowly, let us ask whether knowing the body's anatomy, the bones and muscles, the pulmonary, digestive, and cardiovascular systems, could be of help in yoga practice. Shouldn't the ideal yoga instructor, if not the weekend practitioner, know the body parts and their functions as explained in medicine? The answer is complex, and surely not entirely negative. Some such knowledge could prevent injury in imaginable circumstances (though few get injured in yoga since, unlike in sports, we attend closely to bodily feedback). Nevertheless, Yoga instructors need not be medically trained. The direction of the question is misleading. We should not lose sight of the fact that in yoga practice, as in sports, our intellectual knowledge is in the service of what we are doing.

Consider the illiterate yogin or yogini. Many unschooled in letters have without question thrived, being accomplished in the practices—for instance, the revered Sri Ramakrishna, the nineteenth-century illiterate Bengali mystic and guru of Swami Vivekananda (Vivekananda taught Vedanta to William James, among other achievements, at the Chicago 1893

Congress of World Religions, and translated the *Yoga Sutra*). To be able to pull the shoulder blades down away from the ears and relax them, for example, or to spread the toes requires no scientific knowledge whatsoever.

Let us look at instructions and descriptions of Corpse Pose, *shavasana,* in three current yoga manuals: first one that tries to explain scientifically the relaxation process in the midst of instructions, and then two other, more traditional renditions of instructions for the same asana.

> Relax completely, allowing your body to rest on the floor under the influence of gravity. When you first lie down most of the motor neurons that innervate the skeletal muscles are still firing nerve impulses, but your breathing gradually becomes even and regular, and the number of nerve impulses per second to your muscles starts to drop. If you are an expert in relaxation, within a minute or two the number of nerve impulses to the muscles to your hands and toes goes to zero. Then, within five minutes the motor neuronal input to the muscles of your forearms, arms, legs, and thighs diminishes and also approaches zero. The rhythmical movement of the respiratory diaphragm lulls you into even deeper relaxation, finally minimalizing the nerve impulses to the deep postural muscles of the torso. The connective tissues are not restraining you. Pain is not registered from any part of the body—the posture is entirely comfortable. This is an ideal relaxation.[3]

There are at the very least two referential expressions in this passage that are *not* phenomenological, not identifiable in a yoga practice from the inside, from a first-person point of view: "motor neurons" and "nerve impulses." These are part of a theory, of an explanation, not of instructions telling the yoga student what to do or watch for. If they were pared away, you could be told to do the same thing. The term "respiratory diaphragm" is phenomenological; it can be identified proprioceptively in direct inner feeling and control. But in this passage the diaphragm is mentioned as part of a mechanism that, with this asana, is dissociated from conscious control. In a traditional teaching, in contrast, the diaphragm would not be in such sharp focus, the emphasis being instead on "breath energy," *prana,* sometimes translated "life energy," as will be explained.

Next, two "how-to" presentations of Corpse Pose that are woven into traditional Yoga theories.

In what has become the most popular asana manual in the United States, B.K.S. Iyengar, who has trained yoga teachers in Pune, India, for more than fifty years, quotes, on *shavasana*, three verses from the *Hatha Yoga Pradipika* (*HYP* 1.32, which describes *shavasana*, and then 4.29 and 4.30, which provide occult interpretation) along with another classical text. Having just previously spelled out the physical positioning, Pandit Iyengar provides a translation of the verses along with some commentary. In the ideal Corpse Pose, one draws in the senses into a generic sense awareness (called *pratyahara*), which has no particular objects. This in turn is drawn into the breath or *prana* and then the *prana* into a deeper, essentially blissful consciousness:

> In good relaxation one feels energy flow from the back of the head towards the heels and not the other way around. . . .
>
> [From the *Hatha Yoga Pradipika:*] "The mind is the lord of the Indriyas (the organs of senses); the Prana (the Breath of Life) is the lord of the mind. When the mind is absorbed it is called Moksha (final emancipation, liberation of the soul); when Prana and Manas (the mind) have been absorbed, an undefinable joy ensues."[4]

In Iyengar's usage and translation, "Prana" is not just the breath but an energy that flows in occult cavities and canals, not only the lungs. It animates the physical but also a subtle body. Normally the main pranic energy has an upward buoyancy, but, as the master teacher says, in Corpse Pose one begins to feel flow in the reverse direction. This is an important yogic experience. Deep breathing and *shavasana* help eliminate restlessness, agitation, and "stress," Iyengar says, but getting rid of these in turn is part of a larger process of controlling and harmonizing the "Breath of Life," as he translates *prana*.

Philosophers might expect that this "Prana" is bad theory. But it is clearly more a matter of direct experience than the earlier "motor neurons." The concept may have a theoretic side, but here the word even in the *Hatha Yoga Pradipika*'s expanded sense has concrete meaning for yoga practice and in yogic experience.

Gestalt psychologists and others have taught us about "seeing *as*," about how our beliefs and conventions influence our perceptual language, even basic depictions of that which we perceive. Do you see the faces in the trees, the duck or the rabbit? A doctor will see a hairline fracture in an x-ray if she thinks there is one on other evidence, and not if not. Standing on a cliff overlooking a movie set, the uninformed will see an old western town. But when told it's just a set, a person will suddenly see the façades. Perception is theory-laden. This does not mean that we should be skeptical about tables and chairs, but it might mean that we should be skeptical about "Prana." For theory impinges on even the lowest-level use of names to pick out something of which we are directly aware, and not everyone talks about *prana* as they do about tables and chairs.

However, in yoga it is common to become aware directly, intimately—of objects of which formerly, before the practice, we were unaware. And this is true even though these things or phenomena are parts of ourselves, of our very own bodies or consciousness! Thus, in good faith Iyengar and many others, including myself, say that in yoga we become aware of *prana*—which is at a minimum more than filling and emptying the lungs—phenomenologically. This is perhaps most readily evident in breath and attention being directed and merging at specific spots. In any case, the claim is that pranic energy, which includes but is more than breath, is a matter of as immediate an experience as anyone's own inner feeling of legs and arms.[5]

Before moving on to another traditional explanation of Corpse Pose, let us note that whatever the precise nature of "Prana" in Iyengar's usage, the object of which the yogin or yogini is aware stands outside science. You will not find *prana* mentioned in any medical textbook, no "Breath of Life" as understood by Iyengar or any other traditional yoga master. Though not all agree with Iyengar overall, there is a common phenomenology of *prana*, of "life energy," in yoga *shastra*, the traditional literature that teaches yoga practice and Yoga philosophy.

By reputation the most popular asana manual nowadays in Europe, *Asana Pranayama Mudra Bandha,* by Swami Satyananda Saraswati of the Bihar School of Yoga, provides instructions for Corpse Pose that include a dramatic and even more controversial example of a mysterious but reputedly phenomenological item, i.e., a "spiritual center of consciousness," or chakra. Chakras are crucial to tantric occult psychology. The instructions also include a nicely complementary *un*controversial phenomenon of yogic awareness, *pratyahara* (also mentioned by Iyengar; see above), "pulling the senses back from their objects." We'll take up the uncontroversial first.

> Relax the whole body and stop all physical movement.
>
> Become aware of the natural breath and let it become rhythmic and relaxed.
>
> Begin to count the breaths from number 27. Mentally repeat, "I am breathing in 27, I am breathing out 27. I am breathing in 26, I am breathing out 26," and so on to, back to zero. . . .
>
> Duration: According to time available. In general, the longer the better, although a minute or two is sufficient between asana practices.
>
> Awareness: Physical—first on relaxing the whole body, then on the breath and counting. . . . Spiritual: on ajna chakra [the "third eye," or center of consciousness located between the eyebrows].

Benefits: This asana relaxes the whole psycho-physical system. It should ideally be practiced before sleep, before, during and after asana practice, particularly after dynamic exercises such as surya namaskara [Sun Salutation, an asana series that marries breath and movement]; and when the practitioner feels physically and mentally tired. It develops body awareness. When the body is completely relaxed, awareness of the mind increases, developing pratyahara.[6]

This "pratyahara" is limb number five of the eight-limbed yoga, *ashtanga yoga,* of the *Yoga Sutra,* literally "pulling back." At *YS* 2.54–55, it is spelled out as "the disconnection of the sense organs from their objects as if in imitation of the talent of the *chitta,*[7] 'thought and feeling' (to be still). From that comes supreme control of the sense organs." The *Bhagavad Gita* also has several verses on this (e.g., 6.24–27; see appendix B), as do other yoga manuals, old and new.

Such "*withdrawal* (of the senses from the objects of sense)" is the yogic equivalent of phenomenology as practiced in philosophy, it seems to me. Philosophy students, I think, will naturally like the exercise. Something similar is taught in the tradition of Descartes. It involves paying attention not to the dog that is barking but to the sound of the bark and the "canoid shape" (in the phrase of Bertrand Russell); the smell of the flower, not the flower itself; the "sense data" of colors and so on, taken altogether, multidimensionally, regarded as mere objects of the senses. In classical India as in the West, a presentation dissociated from its objective indication is viewed as having a type of objecthood (*vishayata*) where veridical experience is the same as illusion. The snake that is a rope looks real. In *pratyahara,* the rope that is real looks like an illusion. We witness sense presentations as though their objects were not there, "*pulling back* (the organs of sense)" into a generic "sense mind" (*manas*).

In the yoga studio, a modified *pratyahara* seems all that is possible, since one has to hear and trust the words of the instructor transmitted through the sound of his or her voice. One can, however, close the eyes, as one does normally with at least certain postures, and while practicing breath control, *pranayama,* by itself (as opposed to in conjunction with a flow or sequence of postures). And closing your eyes heightens other capacities, as is traditionally taught. With Corpse Pose, *shavasana*, though, mastery requires *pratyahara,* at least according to Swami Satyananda and other traditional teachers.

Just how to interpret the sense data of yoga will occupy us in the next chapter, on the mind-body problem, where we will look at top-down approaches to the relation of theory and practice. Now, in contrast, let us look at Yoga theories from the bottom up. Through *pratyahara* and other practices, changes occur in experience; there are new phenomena. How should we think about these?

For example, consider the obviously controversial term, "ajna chakra," in the last quote on *shavasana*. I say it is controversial because I presume not everyone is aware of this "center of consciousness." I would guess that among the entire human population, few would report being conscious of anything such. But there are many yogis and yoginis who are committed to its existence as a matter of immediate experience, prototypically a yoga master such as Satyananda in line with a confluence of traditional texts. It is hard to know how to interpret such experiences. But any self-respecting Yoga philosophy has to defend their possibility and their value. Of course, not everything traditionally imputed to the center of consciousness has to be endorsed. But one point of Yoga philosophy is to remove intellectual blocks (*granthi*, *pratibandhaka*) we might have to this or another line of yogic self-development. The *ajna chakra* is traditionally taught as the "third eye," a mystic center of consciousness in a subtle body somehow connected with the center of the forehead, between the eyebrows (see figure 4C). It is traditionally described as luminescent, bluish or camphor white (as seen in inner vision), and comprised of two lobes or petals spanning the body's midline. In Yoga psychology and cosmological theory, the third eye is not itself made of matter but is capable of transmitting spiritual influences on us and our physical selves. Such influences or energies are said to originate in other worlds or planes of being or from a deeper or higher self. Yoga philosophy does not necessarily endorse all of this, but it legitimates intellectual as well as practical exploration of such ideas.[8]

In much the same vein of occult psychology are the *bandha*s of hatha yoga. These, however, are physical contractions, certain muscle tightenings, which are under our direct control. Masters of yoga talk about them as both bodily and spiritual—unlike *ajna chakra,* which is said to be only spiritual and not ordinarily under our direct control. The *bandha*s are, furthermore, much exercised in hatha yoga, especially in advanced practices. They are locks (*bandha* = [psychic] lock) said to enable transition to a sense of energy flow in occult pathways and between or in and out of chakras such as the third eye. Again, unlike chakric centers of occult consciousness, *bandha*s are voluntarily exercised in asana practices as well as in breath control, *pranayama*. One does not have to believe in or be able to identify chakras in order to exercise a *bandha*.

 Ordinarily we do not pay them much if any attention. But we do not "awaken" to their activity. We initiate their activity through conscious engaging or letting go.

There are three *bandhas* prominently referred to in hatha yoga: *mula bandha, uddiyana bandha,* and *jalandhara bandha,* respectively Root Lock, Stomach Lock, and Throat Lock. A fourth, *maha bandha,* the Great Lock, is the simultaneous practice of all three. Let us look again at our three manuals, in reverse order this time, starting with Satyananda explaining the *bandhas* in the tantric psychology of chakras, then Iyengar on Stomach Lock, and finally our contemporary anatomist on Root Lock.

From *Asana Pranayama Mudra Bandha* (see figure 4C for the chakric system that Swami Satyananda mentions and figure 4A for the theory of vital and mental bodies or "sheaths," *kosha*, which he refers to obliquely):

> These three bandhas directly act on the three *granthis* or psychic knots [which block the flow of psychic energy]. . . . The granthis prevent the free flow of prana along sushumna nadi [the central channel of tantric psychology: see figure 4C] and thus impede the awakening of the chakras and the rising of kundalini [psychic energy asleep in the lower chakras].
>
> Brahma granthi is the first knot and . . . when brahma granthi is transcended, the kundalini or primal energy is able to rise beyond mooladhara and swadhisthana [the first two of seven chakras, linked to the base of the spine and the area above the genitals, respectively, which are said to control the survival and sexual instincts] without being pulled back by the attractions and instinctual patterns of the personality.
>
> The second knot is vishnu granthi, associated with manipura and anahata chakras [the next two chakras, at the level of the navel and of the heart, respectively]. . . . Manipura sustains . . . the physical body, governing the digestion and metabolism of food. Anahata sustains . . . the mental body and the energy body. Once vishnu granthi is transcended, energy is drawn from the universe and not from the localised centres within the human being.
>
> The final knot is rudra granthi which is associated with vishuddhi and ajna chakras [the next two chakras, at the level of the throat and in the middle of the forehead, respectively]. Vishuddhi and ajna sustain . . . the intuitive or higher mental body. . . . When rudra granthi is pierced, individuality is dropped, the old ego awareness is left behind and the experience of unmanifest consciousness emerges beyond ajna chakra at sahasrara [the seventh chakra located just above the crown of the head].[9]

From Iyengar's *Light on Yoga:*

Uddiyana means flying up. The process in Uddiyana Bandha is to lift the diaphragm high up the thorax and to pull in the abdominal organs against the back of the spine. It is said that through Uddiyana Bandha the great bird prana is forced to fly up the sushumna nadi, the main channel for the flow of nervous energy, which is situated inside the meru-danda or the spinal column.[10]

From the *Anatomy of Hatha Yoga* by H. David Coulter, quoted earlier:

mula bandha (the root lock) is a gentle contraction of the pelvic diaphragm and the muscles of the urogenital triangle. It . . . seals urogenital energy within the body, controlling and restraining it during breathing exercises and meditation (again, this is a literary rather than a scientific use of the word "energy"). What actually happens is more easily sensed than described, so we'll begin with a series of exercises.[11]

Here such "literary" usages are unavoidable, dare we say? Of course, according to the two traditional teachers, the literary is literal in an experiential sense. But the explanation tying the practices to occult energies and chakras is at least one level of theory higher, or more abstract, than the system of terms used to teach the exercise. Nevertheless, as with breath exercises, there can be little question that these do indeed expand one's sense of bodily energies—Iyengar's "nervous energy" and the like—to the point of developing special yogic "powers" or *siddhis* (a theme and major preoccupation of this book). The difficulty of how to square different interpretations of these phenomena is pretty apparent.

Our contemporary Yoga philosophy cannot avoid the conflict between the tantric and other traditional explanations, on the one hand, and science, on the other. One of many common texts Iyengar and Satyananda share is the *Hatha Yoga Pradipika,* which belongs to the fifteenth century but summarizes and echoes yogic and tantric texts of more than two millennia. In the university setting, the instinctive suspicion would be that the rich tradition of common sources would be responsible for an identical confusion on both gurus' parts, despite the insistences that chakras, etc. are experiential. Let us call this the historicist worry. We shall return to it along with the issue of a partial intersubjectivity in chapter 4 and again in appendix E.[12]

For the present, it is sufficient to note that the conflict is not just about theories, since the one camp takes as experiential what the other rejects as explanatory and wrong. The distinction between the phenomenological and the theoretical applies to traditional Indian theories as much as to anatomical accounts, but no one tries through practices of controlling the breath to master medical science. The theory of the chakras, et cetera, is supposed to be backed up by rather immediate and convincing experience brought about by, or facilitated by, breath control, *bandha* mastery, asanas, and other practices, so experts tell us.

Without worrying about all the intricacies of Yoga psychology at the beginning, I should like to point out to close this section that it is the path of wisdom to give the benefit of the doubt to yogic testimony, like all testimony, especially from experts, about things with which we are unacquainted. This maxim holds for philosophers but is all the more imperative for practitioners. "Innocent until proven guilty" is to be the byword.[13] The alternative, "Guilty until proven innocent," is unworkable, and slightly crazy in the context of ongoing training.

We must trust our teachers. Theories range from the concrete and particular to the abstract and general, and we are not called to believe every bit of Yoga metaphysics or even psychology. However, we should not be mindlessly skeptical of claims just because we personally have not had the experience (yet!). There are of course contexts and subjects, such as God, where we might legitimately be suspicious of the interests of the testifier or guru. Consider, for example, testimony about sexual relations or religious commitment. But we shall not be able to learn very much if we should have to have a very high level of epistemic or justificational confidence in order to pay attention. (Imagine an obnoxious student in the yoga studio questioning the evidence for *prana*. "Just breathe!" my teacher would say.) Indeed, classical Nyaya (a venerable Yoga philosophy that specializes in questions about the acquisition of knowledge) holds that all knowledge from testimony fuses belief with uptake, and that unless there are abnormal conditions, real grounds for doubt, we all naturally accept—as is our right—the information we receive by being told.[14]

In sum, while there may be real and interesting issues for philosophy, including Yoga philosophy, concerning testimony, it is at least not unreasonable to have as policy giving the benefit of the doubt. Some rather reasonable-seeming doubts will be dispelled in later chapters, in particular chapter 2. But as we turn to a description of a contemporary yoga class, please bracket—as one would (appropriately) if one were actually to attend such a class—doubts about the objects and movements mentioned.

There are several styles of yoga class in modern studios. Probably, classes in India classically were simpler than anything now. They were without rubbery "sticky mats," for instance. However, incense may have been used (an uncommon practice now, I gather). In any case, here we shall attend a few minutes of a class of "hatha flow," which can be described as a dancelike meditation comprised of asanas and deep regular breathing, regulating movements by breath and pausing to hold—or to flow through—a series of asanas. We might like to say that all flow classes combine asanas with *pranayama,* but many teachers restrict proper *pranayama* to practices where breath work is the primary focus.[15] There are many such practices that isolate the breath and make it the target of the exercise,[16] and in a flow class awareness includes more than deep, focused breathing. The breathing is nonetheless the soundtrack of the asana sequences, a rhythm and control challenged by the movements and postures.

The most famous flow series practiced traditionally is called *surya namaskara,* Sun Salutations, and practically all flow classes, including Ashtanga or Power Yoga (at least the Ashtanga Primary Series), incorporate a variation of the sequence. Indeed, many "hatha" classes begin with Sun Salutations, in order to warm up. Personally, I find a flow series called Moon Salutations, *chandra namaskara,* equally good for the challenge to the breath and for the *rasa* (delightful relish) of the asana sequence (surely too the Moon is quite deserving of salutations).[17] But *surya namaskara* is the modern vernacular. We shall follow only part of one variation and then skip to the end of the class, which closes with a breath-control exercise and a mantra.

Music is an important feature of many flow classes, although not all teachers use it. The rhythm of the class with or without music is provided by maximal breathing coordinated by "Inhale" and "Exhale" commands from the teacher. But when used, music ideally blends and interweaves with both the collective breath and the level of muscular and emotional intensity (in, for example, facing pain, which changes collectively as well as for the individual as the teacher leads everyone to attend to it properly, to breath into it, as is said). Music can provide a collective emotional and mental object that both fuses class unity and inspires effort. Furthermore, music can facilitate engagement of an emotionally *bhakti* (devotional love) dimension in asana practice, as it has and does in rituals and singing of *bhajans,* devotional songs, in classical and modern

India. Indeed, I daresay no asana teacher, no matter how filled with *bhakti,* can communicate it as well as can music and devotional singing (as performed by Pandit Jasraj, Krishna Das, M. S. Subbulakshmi, Sheila Chandra, Jai Uttal, and others). Music can also be distracting, and no teacher should have to compete with catchy lyrics. For a flow class, a teacher needs to have good timing, but that is a matter of knowing where peoples' breath is, the timing of inhale and exhale commands. Probably for many students music can be distracting, and perhaps should not be used with beginners who need to concentrate on what the teacher is saying. A flow class, however, presupposes asana familarity, so that minute instructions are unnecessary (despite the impression that may be given below).

Among other difficulties in using music is the unfortunate fact that almost any tune can become stale. Not every yoga teacher is a talented DJ. And clearly some music is more appropriate than other, melodious chanting, for example, although the criteria of successful selection are a little elusive (it seems that any style can suffuse a *bhakti* element). In any case, combining music and asana flow to bring up *bhakti* seems legitimately yogic, *bhakti* being a major inheritance from our yoga forebears. Music is not necessary for *bhakti,* of course. In the modern Anusara yoga of John Friend, for example, many teachers try to engage the heart in devotion in asana practice without music. Sun Salutations, Power Yoga, etc., are often done without it. The presentation of Sun Salutations below cannot of course include music along with the teacher's instructions. But occasionally I should like to return to the topic in comments, imagining its use in the class.

Below, meanings of Sanskrit words and historical observations are provided in notes indicated by superscripted numerals (as usual). My voice as pupil (with chattering mind and tape recorder) is square-bracketed, and comments are not in real practice time but rather in the less restricted space of reflection.

The teacher is fictional, perhaps a composite of many with whom I have been privileged to practice. This teacher, however, probably knows more Sanskrit than most. Also, her style may be a tad pedantic and dry, considering that yoga teachers tend to be full of the *rasa*, the delight, of yoga practice. This teacher is expert not only in asanas but also in knowing, by inner sense, lines of pranic energy along which attention may flow in unison with "breath" (in a sense larger than just breathing). Proficiency in yoga flow requires attention (*manas*) to merge with breath in the foreground so that one leads with breath in all movements and changes of direction and body position. Feeling pranic lines and movements is this and more, a peculiar kind of abstraction and disconnection from one's own body in action while paradoxically at the same time identifying with the energy that controls the body. The key is being able to absorb the mind in the effort. An analogy to dance is not accidental. Our ideal teacher gives her instructions between breaths, so to say, never failing to conduct the breathing correctly according to the flow, whether communicating by voice or with her own breath made demonstrative and loud-sounding. Once a rhythm is firmly set, however—with, say, students of intermediate asana ability—our teacher speaks across breaths, in longer sentences. Individual students may have slightly different breath patterns depending on a variety of circumstances, and they are told to try for as full and regular breathing as possible even if that means missing the beat. Everyone's full extension apparently differs slightly from everyone else's. Nevertheless, in fact people bring their breathing back into unison with the class at various points, especially on the teacher's commands.

As a pupil, I have at least one flaw or peculiarity worth mentioning (compare telling the teacher about injuries before class): I try to practice a kind of "sense withdrawal," *pratyahara* (the fifth limb of Patanjali's eight-limbed yoga), by drawing in the vision and closing the eyes (better to attend to the teacher's voice and my own breath and bodily movement), whereas others are (correctly) positioning the gaze, the *drishti,* with eyes open, as called for by a particular asana, or are looking at the teacher for a model to imitate. Of course, mine is not a genuine or entire *pratyahara,* which would require not attending to the words of the teacher but only to the sound of her voice. The point is that the following presentation is oriented around verbal instructions, not visualization, with no modeling by the teacher (with the exception of loud breathing). However, all the asanas about to be mentioned may well best be learned by looking at someone actually demonstrating or from pictures. All good manuals have drawings or photographs. Here I attempt something different.

[Fourteen or fifteen men and women of different ages enter quietly a sunny room with a polished wooden floor and a dais for the instructor, each unrolling a yoga mat (about six by two-and-a-half feet) in a pattern that respects the placement and surrounding space of other students, all facing the front. Some sit cross-legged with hips raised on a blanket or yoga block. Others sit in Hero's Pose, *virasana,* legs folded with the heels under the sit-bones and the knees together, with spine straight. Those sitting in Easy Seat, *sukhasana,* are noticeably a little more slouching, but most also seem to be trying to sit back properly, tucking the chin in with shoulders back. The teacher enters (everyone straightens a little) and puts a CD into a player (the room is equipped with a sound system) so that she can discreetly begin the music after the invocation. She sits about a minute in Lotus Pose, *padmasana,* on the dais. Opening her eyes, she gets up and closes the door, then returns to her cross-legged seat and greets the class.]

Namas te. Let's begin today standing, Mountain Pose, *tadasana,* bringing our hands together, thumbs touching the heart, each fingertip feeling its partner, in *anjali mudra,*[18] chin tucked, feet hips' distance apart and parallel, weight distributed equally in four corners on each foot, the left and right corners of the front of the heels, the little-toe mound and the big-toe mound pressing down on the floor, on the earth, noticing the rebound of energy, shoulders down and back, chest up feeling the thumbs, elbows up and out, lifting through the crown of the head. Rock a little left and right and up and back to feel your balance. The *Gita* says that yoga is balance.[19] Let's begin with three rounds of *om.* We'll take a full inhale and exhale and then inhale to chant. Inhale. Slowly. Fully. Exhale. Inhale to chant.

[Class in unison chants *om* three times, with three full inhales and the chant lasting as long as the exhale. There is a harmony of voices, though a few remain silent and many chant only in low volume. The teacher's individual voice is discernible above or through the collectivity, and she chants clear and long with an audible interval of silence during each inhalation.]

You may begin *ujjayi pranayama.*[20] Breathe through your nose, restricting the glottis, making a sound like the ocean. You should be able to hear your breath and maybe your neighbor's if you listen. Offer your full breaths into the room, giving their sound over to our collective effort. Let's make this class our *puja,* our offering to whatever we think the highest in ourselves or the universe, our best possibilities. Yoga teaches that *puja* makes bridges and crossings. So, breathe to the very top of your lungs and exhale completely, pushing all the air out as you draw the navel in. Try to maintain full and complete breaths while we celebrate with our bodies and hearts.

Bring your hands down to your sides, stretching your fingers and brightening your fingertips, in this variation of Mountain Pose. On an inhale slowly take your arms up, spreading them out wide—be aware of people on either side—to reach the ears, elbows straight but not locked, shoulder blades down the back, *urdhva hastasana,* Raised-Hands Pose. Let's take one breath here. Inhale. Feel yourself connecting heaven and earth. Exhale. Inhale and lean back and lift with your heart. Exhale slowly and just as slowly bring your arms down, completing your exhalation when your hands reach your sides. Two more times. Inhale, arms up. Hold and lean back, tucking your chin and then, if you can, leaning the head back, gracefully, not hurting the neck, extending from the top of the head, joining the palms in offering. Exhale, bringing the hands all the way down. One more time. Inhale up. Hold and lift. Exhale down.

[Doing this leaning back with arms up can have an effect on the emotional center, bringing a smile. A line of energy flows out the fingertips. Imagine also devotional music, a voice singing *gurave,* to the guru, with tremelos on the "vay" sound just as the class is all leaning back the third time. The accompanying awareness can augment effort, make you try harder to bring the arms down very slowly, eyes closed. Sometimes the teacher says, "Feel your heart center, *anahata chakra,* as you gently lean back."

In many religious ceremonies as well as art performances in both traditional and contemporary India, activities commence with saluations to the guru. Feeling gratitude to the guru is traditionally one of the sources of *bhakti.* The "guru" can be the living teacher in front of you; Shiva, the founder of yoga; an intermediary such as Patanjali, the author of the *Yoga Sutra;* or an entire lineage. This is taken up in chapter 5.

The psychology of *puja,* ceremonious worship and offering to a divinity—to make a stab at definition—will, however, not be much addressed. The yogic connection is said to be the maintenance of occult connections—which tantrics would also view as the purpose of asanas. So the *puja* metaphor is appropriate.]

Inhale up to end with an arched back. Exhale and this time swan dive down with straight back, head up but chin tucked, all the way down to the floor, leading with your heart, chest out, joyful, breathing out with control with your stomach muscles, hands to the floor, ankles, or shins. At the next-to-last moment of the exhale, release the head and the neck and then exhale completely. Hold a half count, *kumbhaka,*[21] and breathe slowly in, enjoying the forward bend. Bend your knees as necessary. Let's take another breath here.

Now inhale and lengthen your spine, lifting your chest slightly. Exhale and fold under. Inhale. Raise up again and hold in the gentlest of heart openings and backbends, knees bent if necessary, fingers on the floor. Exhale and release into Standing Forward Fold.

Inhale now with your fingers on your shins or the floor, and straighten your back to look up, leading with the heart. Hold it there for a moment, feel the energy in your breast. Exhale and fold back down, letting your arms hang loosely on the outside of your legs. Hold out just a second, *kumbhaka,* after you push all the stale air and energy out of your nose and top of the head. Push. Feel your crown. Inhale and come all the way up, lean back, elbows by the ears, fingertips touching, trying to feel each vertebra as you come up. Feel your spine or central channel as you just for an instant hold. Feel the upward flow of prana. Exhale and swan dive slowly all the way down, with straight back, chest up, exhaling with control, *uttanasana,* Standing Forward Fold. Inhale and look up, hands to shins, *ardha uttanasana,* half *uttanasana.* Exhale and fold. Good. Beautiful.

Inhale and step the left foot back into a long lunge, right knee bent, thigh perpendicular to the floor, fingertips lightly touching your mat, toes spread pushing into the floor on both feet, heel pushing back, lifted kneecap on the left. Head and heart up. Let's take three breaths here. Feel the line of energy from your left heel to the crown of your head, neck and back in line, making space between the vertebrae. Exhale and push back into Downward-Facing Dog, *adho-mukha shvanasana.* Inhale and step the left foot forward, keep the right foot back, and keep the left thigh perpendicular; looking slightly up, focus on the crown of your head, in the movement leading with your heart and breath. Three breaths. On an exhale, push back into Downward Dog. Five breaths. Feel the energy lines. Move your heels up and down, stretching out slowly your calf muscles, even if you are able to put heels on the floor. Make sure your fingers are spread. Outer rotation in the upper arms. Shoulders down. Inner rotation with the upper thighs. Spread your toes. Check your alignment. Feel your head and neck in line with your spinal column. *Om.*

Now this time let's repeat the series adding Warrior One, *vira bhadrasana* one. Don't worry about the Platonic Form, the perfect pose, but do your best to have the right alignment: forward knee perpendicular so that you can just see your toes, but then gently tilt your head back into a graceful backbend. Okay, starting from Mountain Pose. Inhale up and exhale swan dive down. Inhale and look up. Exhale and step back to Down Dog. Inhale and lift your left leg even with your spine, three-legged Down Dog, toes pointing toward the floor, and exhale to a long lunge, left foot forward. Inhale and swing your arms up to your ears and lean back, Warrior One, lifting your heart. Let's hold here a couple of breaths. Inhale and lift, exhale and swing the leg gracefully back and then on into Downward-Facing Dog. Take a breath. Now the other side. . . .

[On the swan dive down, often I keep my hands together in *anjali mudra* and trace the midline. Since my eyes are closed, this prevents accidentally bumping into somebody, among other virtues.

To pick up the *bhakti* theme, there are occasions when the teacher's encouragement is crucial, when a phrase like "Good, beautiful" feels authentic and inspirational and not routine. Sometimes she talks with enthusiasm about the beauty of the poses we are collectively making, which, she says, she feels privileged to see.

I like the feature of yoga classes that no one is supposed to see you except the teacher—at least, the usual rule is that no one is supposed to look at you. We do nonetheless get a sense of the class working together, doing the same pose, breathing together, feeling lines of energy in the same ways. It's as though each of us is nothing but a universal body and being, individual quirks ignored (or accepted), individual identity gone. Admittedly, this sense is more likely to come at the end of a class than at the beginning, unless the group is advanced.]

On an inhale pass through Plank—the push-up variation of Four-Limbs Pose, *chaturangasana*—arms straight, eyes or insides of the elbows looking out, outer rotation in the upper arms, elbows hugging the ribs, and then exhale into Knees, Chest, and Chin, Eight-Points Bowing, *ashtanga namaskara,* saluting the Earth, the Mother, touching your mat or the floor with feet, knees, palms, chest, and chin. Stay on your toes, not the top of your feet. Hold and then inhale, rolling over your toes into—your choice—Upward-Facing Dog or Cobra. Hold here a few breaths. Don't throw the head back but lift into a gentle backbend in both poses. If you're in Up-Dog, lead with your heart, push the ground with the top of the feet, move gracefully into a backbend of lightest intensity, chin tucked at first and head back last, eyes up. If in Cobra, lying on your stomach, palms on the floor at breast line, elbows in, tops of the feet on the floor, be aware of your little toes and try to push the whole foot evenly into the floor. Work with the legs and the stomach and back muscles; don't push too hard with your hands. Let the breath do the work as you rise slowly with control. Hold and sway up and down a bit with the rhythm of the breath. Lift on an inhale. Pull your shoulder blades down and back on an exhale. Extend your chest. Lower slowly down on an exhale. Let's do this two more times. Inhale up and hold. Take a couple of breaths. Exhale down. Again. Inhale. Exhale. Now everyone inhale and push back, raising your hips, up on your tiptoes, and exhale down into Down-Dog.

In Down-Dog, while you are breathing five full and deep breaths, try engaging a *bandha.* Let's do Stomach Lock, *uddiyana bandha.* Engage it on the exhale, holding the navel in against the backbone and practicing retention, *kumbhaka,* and then release, but still hold the navel back a little when you inhale, slowly. Try a few times.

[For me, Down-Dog, though maybe the most basic pose, clearly will remain imperfect this lifetime. But I try as best I can to follow the instructions. Stomach Lock I find more difficult to get and hold than Throat Lock and also Root Lock, although Root Lock, everyone seems to say, is generally the most difficult to hold for much duration.]

On an inhale, step or jump to the front of your mat, keeping your hands in place, into *ardha uttanasana,* Half Standing-Fold. Exhale into *uttanasana.* Inhale and sweep all the way up into Raised-Hands Pose. Exhale and trace the midline with your hands in prayer position into *anjali mudra.* Take a couple of breaths. Feel your energy. Let's go again, this time with the first lunge on the left side. . . .

[Our class continues in the same pattern, incorporating several further standing poses, then a sequence of seated poses followed by a few on the stomach and then the back, Bridge Pose (*setu bandhasana*), along with Shoulder Stand (*sarvangasana,* All-Limbs Pose), *shirshasana* (Headstand), Fish Pose (*matsyasana*), a few twists and leg lifts, and then finally *shavasana*, Corpse Pose (about which see the previous section). With each change of sequence, standing, sitting, etc., our tuned-in teacher changes the background music appropriately, in part at least according to tempo. In Corpse Pose, we are treated to soft sounds of gently breaking waves and a barely audible ocean roar and then no music, and no music for the breath work and the rest. We pick up with the instructor bringing the class to life, out of Corpse Pose, to sit cross-legged in *sukhasana,* Easy Pose, me with my hips raised by a folded blanket or two (if handy) so that my knees are below my waist and each is supported by a foot or the floor. We are instructed to keep our eyes closed as much as possible as we change positions and to sit quietly for a minute or two, hands in *chin mudra,*[22] and our focus—our choice—on the heart chakra, the forehead chakra, or the crown chakra.]

Let's open our eyes and do a little *pranayama.* We'll do *nadi shodana,* Cleansing the Channels, the left and right channels of breath energy, which begin at the nostrils.[23] Sit in a comfortable pose, with your spine straight and shoulders above your sit-bones.[24] Easy Pose, Hero's Pose, Lotus, and *siddhasana* are some that are recommended. With one hand comfortably in the lap or on the knee in *chin mudra,* place the other hand on the forehead, the forefinger and middle finger gently resting against the middle of the forehead, symbolically activating the third eye, *ajna chakra.* Position the thumb above one nostril and the ring finger joined by the pinkie over the other nostril. Try to keep some peripheral attention on the forehead center as you keep your main focus on the breath. At the beginning of an exhale, close the right nostril and breathe out the left. Pause after all air is expelled. Keeping the right nostril closed, breathe in gently and smoothly through the left nostril. Hold and retain, closing the left nostril. Open the right nostril and exhale slowly and completely with control, trying to balance the inhales and exhales in length as you balance the flow of air through the separate nostrils into the lungs and corresponding pranic energies. Let's do this silently, at your own pace, for three minutes. Begin. [Three minutes pass.] Okay, now stop on an exhalation through the right nostril and breathe normally.

Finally, let's do a *kriya* from the *Hatha Yoga Pradipika*.[25] Just sit quietly if you don't want to try this. We'll attempt to engage all the locks, the *bandha*s, in a certain order and in connection with in-breath, out-breath, and retention. First, tuck your chin and engage Throat Lock (*jalandhara bandha*), on an inhale. Keep it engaged and breathe slowly a couple of breaths. Then on an exhale engage in rapid succession Root Lock (*mula bandha*) and Stomach Lock (*uddiyana bandha*). That is, with Throat Lock in place, do Root Lock, complete exhalation, and finally Stomach Lock. Try a couple of times and then pay attention to the energy flow along your spine or the central channel. Just watch. Breathe normally.

Let's end with one round of the peace mantra, *om shantih shantih shantih*. Recall your intention and resolve to carry it out with you off your yoga mat. Now the mantra. Inhale. Exhale completely. Inhale to chant.

[The class chants beautifully, emphasizing the final syllable, "hee," the visarga (written *ḥ* in the standard transliteration), of the last *shantih*. The session ends with the teacher bowing to everyone from her seat in Lotus Pose and uttering what has come to be the traditional closing, the mantralike greeting, *Namas te,* "Salutations to thee."]

Namas te.[26]

Yoga Literature and Classical Philosophies

The early and classical literature of Yoga theories as well as of yoga practices is in Sanskrit, an Indo-European language akin to Greek. Current speculation has it that Sanskrit-speaking tribes began invading the Indian Subcontinent from the northwest as early as 1500 B.C.E. Or, possibly, tribes speaking early Indo-European languages migrated from India to the West (there is little archeological evidence). In any case, Sanskrit verses known as the Vedas—Revealed Knowledge—were composed over many centuries, and came to be regarded as sacred within an early culture located first near the Indus River (now in Pakistan) and then in the Gangetic plain. Four Vedas are the oldest documents in Sanskrit. Theirs is an archaic, preclassical Sanskrit, just a little less distant from classical Sanskrit (which begins around 500 B.C.E.) as the English of *Beowulf* is from modern English.

Vedic poems and hymns express various themes, some of which are precursors of Yoga doctrines and possibly yoga practices. The earliest usages of the word *yoga,* however, are restricted to the meanings yoking and joining, joining a pair of oxen, for instance, and more abstractly a connection between any two things.[27] The meaning of self-discipline that is continuous with practices of yoga today occurs in "secret doctrines" appended to the Vedas called Upanishads, which are foundational texts for both yoga practice and Yoga philosophy.

In forms of the root *yuj* from which the word *yoga* is derived, our meaning of self-discipline also occurs in Brahmana and Aranyaka literature that was also appended to the Vedic Samhitas or core texts prior to the Upanishads. See figure 1. Both temporal and textual priority in the sense of the sequence of materials as traditionally preserved runs: Veda (Samhita), Brahmana, Aranyaka, and Upanishad, as determined in the first case by academic indology and in the second by Vedic schools.

To be precise, although the word *yoga* is used for a yoke or any connection between two things in the Samhitas and is not reported occurring in our sense of self-discipline, gradually the verbal root *yuj* comes to be used in this way, for example, to restrain or yoke the mind (*manas,* attention).[28] The tantric sense of *yoga* as union, as in union with God or union with the higher self, is a later usage suggested by the content of Upanishadic teachings but not appearing in at least the earliest Upanishads. (See appendix A, *Maitri Upanishad* 6.25, the last Upanishadic verse rendered, for an early usage in the sense of divine "union." There are also certain verses in the *Bhagavad Gita* which at least suggest the sense of a divine "connection" or "oneness.") "Self-discipline" or "spiritual discipline" is the sense common among Upanishads, the *Gita,* the *Yoga Sutra,* and other classic texts—up to the emergence of tantra, where often the sense of self-discipline becomes secondary to that of union.

Now legitimate Upanishads number more than two hundred, but most collections are much smaller. Different sets have been preserved in different recensions and Vedic or Hindu lineages (including some called Yoga Upanishads). Upanishads were apparently gradually appended to Vedic literature, eleven or twelve or thirteen being the oldest, according to indologists, as well as the most important, according to practically everyone.[29] Recensions follow lineages of teachers and pupils whose

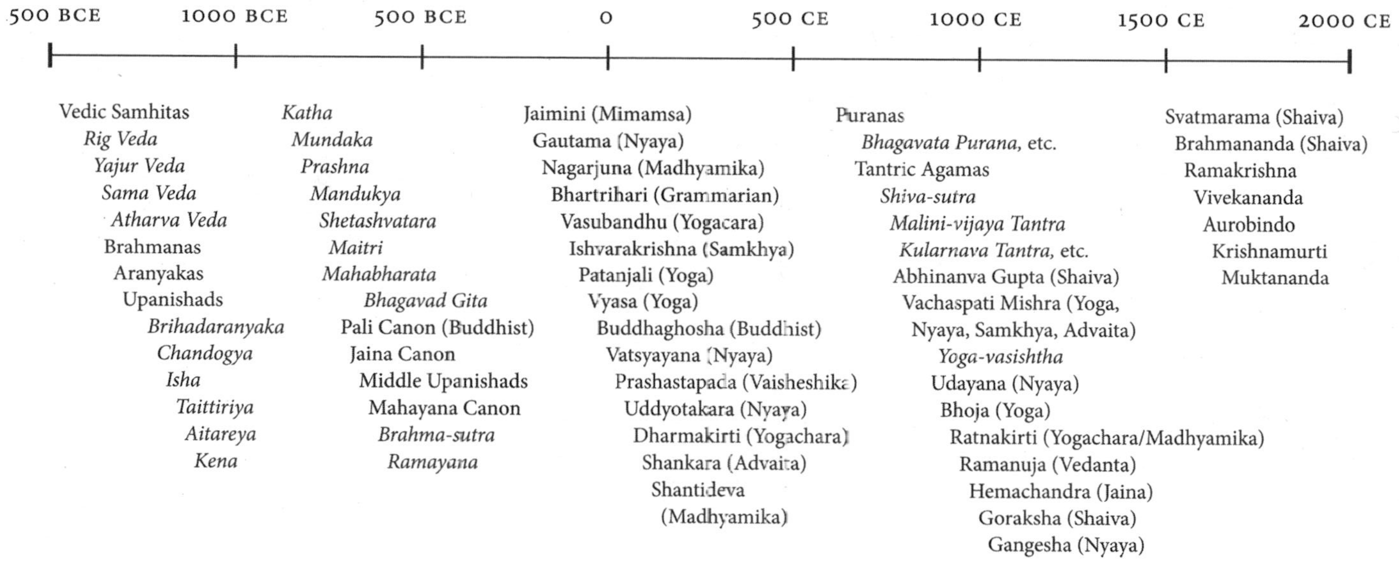

The timeline represents currrent indological opinion which is quite a bit less than certain. Indeed, for the older texts all opinion rests on scanty evidence. For our purposes, the precise dates matter less than order, chronological order, about which there is less dispute. That is to say, whatever is correct about the date of the Vedas, etc., the *Rig Veda* is older than the *Brihadaranyaka Upanishad*. The columns would remain the same if the numbers were altered.

FIGURE 1 Yoga Authors and Literature.*

 religious life early on included rituals employing chants called *mantra* and later broadened to include many forms of yoga in our sense. However, Vedic culture encouraged marriage and family life and practices that contrast with ascetic patterns of life endorsed in some Upanishads, though there are many lines of continuity with Vedic teachings.

Early Upanishads (from 800 to 300 B.C.E.) show most of all a new intelligence that is at once abstract and mystical, free from myth and ritual as well as honed by yoga practice and experience. Prose appears, and Upanishadic poetry is usually discursive, didactic, and less imagistic than that of the Vedas. There is also punning, along with stories that read like jokes. Although argument and elaborations of positions are not nearly as pronounced and professionalized as in later periods of classical thought, even the earliest Upanishads employ self-conscious argumentation, which is rare in the Vedas. Furthermore, much of the reasoning seems self-consciously based on yogic experience. Early Upanishads are above all mystical texts. They are also regarded as revelation, in particular by the classical Vedanta school of philosophy, whose texts stretch from the *Brahma Sutra* (c. 200 B.C.E.) through the classical commentaries of Shankara (c. 700 C.E.), Ramanuja (c. 1050), and others and numerous subcommentaries and other Vedantic literature extending into the modern period.[30]

The Vedanta school takes itself to speak for the Upanishads, but other schools take different attitudes, especially about Upanishadic authority. Most importantly, there are distinct views within the Upanishads themselves about human nature and psychology as well as about reality. Nevertheless, there is a pretty well discernible core message, namely, that there is possible for us a self-discovery—a discovery of a true self or *atman*—which is, or leads to, awareness of the Absolute, Brahman. This state of consciousness is called *brahma-vidya* and deemed our "supreme personal good," *parama-purushartha*, Brahman being the One, God, the fundamental reality. The thesis that Brahman is your self as well as somehow the universe has enormous influence on Yoga philosophy.

See the introduction to appendix A for background to the particular passages translated from the early Upanishads. Concerning the dates of individual Upanishads, the best that can be said is that on the basis of archaisms, quirks of style, and repetitions, scholars identify an oldest group of prose Upanishads along with several later clusters. Much, however, remains controversial, and we should keep in mind that the mainstream classical position (though of course rejected by Buddhists and other groups) is that the Upanishads were "heard" (*shruta*, revealed in yogic experience) immemorially, with no question of chronology. That they speak timelessly may be deemed a genre requirement, an attitude embedded in the Upanishads themselves. Vedantic theists take them to have been uttered by God. Similar genres, such as tantric scriptures (see the introduction to appendix D), which scholars concur are much later than the early Upanishads, are also considered by their advocates to have such a revealed character.

Excluding the early Upanishads, the *Bhagavad Gita* (c. 300 B.C.E.) is the most important early Yogic text, itself seeming to be a little Upanishad inserted into a massive epic poem. The *Gita* is composed in verses that are stylistically continuous with the larger poem, the *Mahabharata*, but the tract is exceptional in its content. This "Song of the Blessed One" is devoted to yoga teaching within a theistic framework. Philosophical in thrust and subject matter, it is not written in the argumentative style of classical philosophy but rather as a yogic teaching, a secret teaching or *upanishad* (as the word is used within the Upanishads themselves and elsewhere), conveyed from guru to student. Krishna, the Blessed One, is the guru in the *Gita*, and lays out several methods of yoga. These will be elaborated later, especially in the third section of chapter 3 and the second of chapter 5, and the *Gita*'s philosophic ideas will engage us throughout.

Table 1 lays out the principal schools and divisions of Yoga philosophy abstractly, independently of the chronologies of the textual traditions, showing certain key commonalities and differences.

TABLE 1

	What is fundamentally real and/or valuable (*sat*)?	How is that reality/value known?
(a) Samkhya	Nature (*prakriti*) and individual conscious beings (*purusha*) whose self-knowledge is the only value	Philosophic "analysis" (*samkhya*); disidentification from personal *prakriti*
(b) Yoga (*Yoga Sutra* and commentaries)	Same as (a) but differentiating humans and the Ishvara (Lord) as well as *chitta* as a distinct form of *prakriti*	Perception (including yogic perception), inference, and testimony
(c) Theistic Vedanta	Brahman (God, Ishvara); transmigrating souls; the universe; right relationship to God the highest value	Testimony and meditation for which there are yogic prerequisites

TABLE 1 continued

	What is fundamentally real and/or valuable (*sat*)?	How is that reality/value known?
(d) Advaita Vedanta	Brahman = *atman* (self), the sole reality	Testimony and nondual experience; removal of obstacles
(e) Jaina	Individual liberation and enlightenment	Character development and yogic experience
(f) Early Buddhist (sermons of the Pali canon, etc.)	*Dharmas* (momentary qualities without bearers); nirvana (a nonmomentary *dharma*)	Nirvana (extinguishing of self-regarding desire)
(g) Madhyamika Buddhist	The Void (*shunyata*, emptiness)	"Not known" as everyday objects are known; removal of obstacles to an already accomplished awakening
(h) Yogachara Buddhist	Buddha nature	Yogic development and experience
(i) Nyaya	Nine types of substance (including transmigrating selves plus the Ishvara) and other categories	Perception (including yogic perception), inference, and testimony
(j) Shaiva	Shiva/Shakti and their self-manifestion	Yogic experience and testimony; *tarka*, metaphysical reasoning
(k) Vaishnava	Ishvara and the Lord's creation or self-manifestation	Meditation, testimony, and godward emotion

CLASSICAL YOGA PHILOSOPHIES

What is the self (*atman*) or person?	What yoga is advocated?	What is the value of yoga?
(a) The everyday person as a false projection of consciousness (*purusha*) into nature	Disidentification; sattvafication of one's personal nature	Self-discovery (discovery of oneself as *purusha*); self-luminous self-experience
(b) Same as (a)	Same as (a) plus the eight-limbed yoga (*ashtanga yoga*), *bhakti*, yogic sleep, and other practices	Same as (a); *kaivalya* (aloneness), self-bliss

TABLE I continued

What is the self (*atman*) or person?	What yoga is advocated?	What is the value of yoga?
(c) An immortal soul (*jiva*) who reincarnates in various bodies (*kosha*) until liberation (*moksha*)	*Bhakti, prapatti* (surrender), development of Godward emotions and *rasa* (spiritual relishing) in life	Comprises an ongoing personal relationship with God full of rapturous delight
(d) A superimposition or projection of self on the nonself (including the "subtle body")	Upanishadic study; meditation, tranquility, and self-control	Preparation for nondual consciousness (which is preexistent)
(e) An immortal soul (*jiva*) who reincarnates until liberation (*moksha*)	Nonharmfulness (*ahimsa*), charity, etc.	Leads to the *summum bonum*
(f) A composite of *dharmas* from the five *skandhas*	The Eightfold Path (right thought, resolve, speech, behavior, livelihood, effort, mindfulness, and meditation)	Leads to the *summum bonum,* nirvana (no self-regarding desire)
(g) Not a good question (the belief that there is a self or person is a spiritual obstacle)	Same as (h), to include development of deconstructive philosophic insight (*prasanga* as *prajna*)	Leads to nirvana and a postnirvana career as a bodhisattva
(h) A continuum (santana) of moments of self-cognizing cognition	The Way of the Bodhisattva	Same as (g)
(i) A combination of an immortal self (*atman*) and a living body	Philosophy as yoga as well as meditation, asana, etc.	Liberation, *moksha,* the *summum bonum*
(j) A genuine self-expression of Shiva/Shakti	A panoply of yogic methods and rituals including the "nonway" together with the ways of Shiva, of the Shakta, and of the minute	Leads to the *summum bonum,* living liberation
(k) Same as (c)	Same as (c)	Same as (c)

*All these schools and traditions value, with qualifications, yogic self-monitoring consciousness along with self-determination and other theses about karma and rebirth. The five questions track important differences. But the chart glides over distinctions within subschools and other nuances. The answers are general and mainstream.

Vedanta is a school of philosophy that derives its name from an epithet for the Upanishads. "Vedanta" means literally the end (*anta*) of the Veda, in both the sense of the sequence of Vedic texts as traditionally preserved and in the sense of the goal or fulfillment of Vedic teaching. Advaita Vedanta is a classical Vedanta subschool that upholds a nonduality (*advaita*) between the individual consciousness and the supreme Brahman ("Thou art That," "I am He"). There is also a second sense of nonduality championed by Advaita: our deepest consciousness is immediate and nondual in the sense of self-illumining (*svayam prakashamana*). These claims are aired in chapter 2.

A second broad division of Vedantic philosophies is the theistic, which holds that Brahman and the individual are in some way distinct though also, in many versions, in some way identical. Theistic Vedanta will also often occupy us.

Then there is Mimamsa, Exegesis, which is Vedanta's sister school focused on the Veda and Brahmanical rituals (as opposed to the Upanishads). Though there are yogic themes among the Exegetes, yoga is not the school's forté (which is philosophy of language), and it will not receive from us much attention. Furthermore, Kumarila (c. 700) and other Mimamsa philosophers reject yogic perception in favor of testimony as the way we comprehend the most important truths as well as *dharma,* the teaching of the way we should live. Endorsement of yogic perception, in contrast, is practically a defining mark of Yoga philosophy.

Buddhism originated a little earlier than the *Gita,* although the earliest Buddhist texts do not predate the *Gita*. The Buddha, who lived in the sixth century B.C.E., preached doctrines similar to the Upanishads and encouraged certain mainstream yoga practices. He rejected, however, what he saw as the imbalances of too much asceticism as well as the Upanishadic doctrines of self, *atman,* and Brahman. He espoused a goal of a supreme personal good, *nirvana,* enlightenment, which is nevertheless comparable to the "Brahman knowledge" of Upanishadic philosophy. Buddhism was socially revolutionary, rejecting caste (as did its sister religion of Jainism; see below).

Like Krishna in the *Gita,* the Buddha-to-be, Gautama Siddhartha of the Shakya clan, was a prince in northern India, or perhaps what is now southern Nepal, in the Gangetic valley. He preached sermons and gave spiritual advice for years after his enlightenment. The oldest texts date to the reign of the Buddhist emperor Ashoka in the third century B.C.E., when an enormous canon sacred to "southern" Buddhism (the Buddhism of Sri Lanka, Burma, Thailand, and elsewhere in Southeast Asia) was compiled. Known mainly in its Pali version, it is sometimes called the

Pali canon. A distinct literature in Sanskrit, much of which was translated into Tibetan and Chinese, belongs to "northern" or Mahayana Buddhism (practiced in Nepal, Tibet, China, Korea, Japan, etc.), though it does not entirely reject the teachings of the southern canon.

Buddhism flourished in India for some seventeen centuries before succumbing to the intolerance of Islamic conquerors. And Buddhism matured in India for some seven or eight centuries before becoming prominent in the courts of China and elsewhere in Asia. Buddhist thinkers were great innovators in many areas of philosophy, including logic, theory of knowledge and justification for what we believe, the assumptions implicit in everyday speech, and causal reasoning. Buddhist yoga coalesces and overlaps with the practice teachings of other schools and movements.

Mahavira, who was roughly contemporary with the Buddha (c. 550 B.C.E.), founded Jainism, another religion and religious philosophy that is concerned with enlightenment and yoga practice, in particular practices connecting with the premier virtue of nonharmfulness, *ahimsa*. Though not historically as prominent as Buddhism, the religion has an extensive literature, and its defenders in the classical period were among the most astute minds.

The formation of the great Hindu or Vedic schools and systems of philosophy (Mimamsa, Vedanta, Samkhya, etc.) occurred at about the same time as the earliest Jaina and Buddhist literature, what we might call the epic period of classical Indian civilization in honor of the massive poem, the *Mahabharata,* of which the *Gita* is a part. Unfortunately, we have little direct record of the debates and efforts of those highly creative intelligences responsible for the wide-ranging explanations—of the world and its ground, of the human in relation to nature and God, of the meaning of existence, as well as of perceptual experience and conventions of everyday life along with, to be sure, yogic abilities and experiences—that make up the six or seven earliest of the major philosophies of classical India, the great schools. The work of the earliest system makers has become inseparable from centuries of later interpretation and advocacy. We know what we know about their formation primarily through their embeddedness in the *Mahabharata* and the earliest Buddhist literature, in particular, the "Third Basket" of the Pali canon, which is centered on metaphysical controversy.

Within the first two centuries of the Common Era, philosophy in India made another quantum leap, this one captured in texts expressly devoted to philosophy and exposition of worldviews. This second jump centered on argument, patterns of argumentation, and the metaissue of what counts as good and bad reasoning. Argument and defense of positions appear in earlier literature, but there is not the attention to details of reasoning—what precisely follows from what and why—that became the obsession by the midst of the classical age. The Yoga philosophies formulated in this period—including that of the *Yoga Sutra* (more about which just below)—are world explanations defended by increasingly intricate strategies.

A pivotal figure in the second revolution was the Buddhist philosopher, Nagarjuna, of the second century C.E. Bent upon establishing that our everyday world, naïvely assumed to be real and captured by the words we use in ordinary discourse, is not in fact real, Nagarjuna won fame as a philosopher because of the penetrating questions he put to all the schools of his time, Buddhist and non-Buddhist, and indeed to much common, nonscholastic opinion.[31]

It was also around the time of Nagarjuna that the sutra texts of the earliest schools appeared in their final forms. The Sanskrit word *sutra* means literally thread, and by extension an aphorism that captures a philosophical tenet in a most succinct statement. The sutra texts are systematic expressions of entire worldviews (*darshana,* world vision), although they are also digests that usually require commentary—probably oral at first—by a guru to students (*shishya*).

Thus much later than the *Gita* is the *Yoga Sutra* (*YS,* c. 400 C.E.) (the subject matter of appendix C). It is written in this new and different style or genre of literature, the sutra collection, threads strung together into a textbook of science, *shastra,* or a handbook for a craft. Though portions of the *YS* probably date way back and are contemporaneous with the *Gita* or even earlier, the final version (what has come down to us) belongs to the period after Nagarjuna. Scholars date the *YS* at about the same time as a similar text, the *Samkhya Karika* (c. 400 C.E.), which presents a similar worldview (a dualism of *purusha,* the conscious being, and *prakriti,* nature, as explained in chapter 2). Further introduction to the *YS* is provided in appendix C.

The Samkhya school is famous for a trenchant metaphysical dualism of nature and consciousness but also for three other teachings that influenced Yoga philosophies. First, there is a disidentification practice theme that relies on dualism, encouragement to pull back into one's true self apart from nature, including one's own nature, one's body, life, and mind. Second, there is emanationism on the part of nature, an evolution of primordial undifferentiated stuff into various forms, principles (*tattva*) or stages of the unfolding of the cosmic display continuing down to the five gross elements, ether, air, fire, water, and earth. The emanationism influenced later tantric conceptions in particular—though tantric principles (*tattva*) are viewed as coming from God (Shiva/Shakti), not an unconscious nature—at least not in the monistic tantra of Abhinava Gupta, which will be our main focus. Third, there is the notion of the subtle body, *linga sharira,* comprised of subtle elements (such as internal sights, sounds, etc., as well as thought and emotion), which is incorporated into tantra but also Vedanta. Early versions of these Samkhya ideas are found in the Upanishads and the *Gita* and in some dualistic tantras as well. But they were only later systematized into a worldview, as explained. In late classical thought, Samkhya was eclipsed by the much greater prominence of Nyaya, or absorbed, as mentioned, into tantric philosophies.

The long-running school of Nyaya philosophy endorses yoga practices and indeed the value of yogic trance, *samadhi,* in much the same fashion as the *YS,* but its fame derives from a hard-headed realism and careful analysis particularly of methods of knowledge. It originated earlier than Nagarjuna, as we know since Nyaya views are among those targeted by the Buddhist dialectician. Nyaya texts span almost two thousand years, with much reflection on yoga and defense of "yogic perception" as a special source of knowledge. The school's primary focus is on knowledge, the means thereto, and right procedures in debate and critical inquiry. Perhaps because of its realist position in metaphysics, it does not enjoy the Yogic reputation of some of its idealist rivals, such as Advaita Vedanta. But Nyaya makes solid recommendations in defense of the reality of the self against materialism as well as other opponents, and in chapter 2 we shall learn much on that score.

Nyaya's root text is the *Nyaya Sutra* (*NyS*), c. 200 C.E., which is also the oldest extant Nyaya text. Commentators elaborated its theses over many centuries, and with Udayana (c. 1000) and Gangesha (c. 1325), a New Nyaya school was launched and solidified. It came to have wide influence throughout the late classical culture, providing in particular the terminology for debates and serious inquiry. Nyaya had a sister school in Vaisheshika (Atomism) that was totally merged into the Nyaya stream by Udayana, and thenceforth had practically no separate literature.

Late Upanishads ("late" according to secular scholarship; see above), the epic poem the *Ramayana,* as well as various minor epics and didactic poems called Puranas contain yogic themes and colorful stories about yogins and yoginis in addition to gods and goddesses, contributing to a rich culture. Some Puranas, the *Bhagavata Purana,* for instance, c. 900 C.E., contain stories of the divine guru Krishna when he was a child; the *Bhagavata* is revered in sects of Vaishnavism as much as any Upanishad. Puranas are nonetheless solidly within what we might call a Vedic or

 Vedantic fold, and in this way differ from another cultural movement of great moment for yoga, tantra, which broke from Vedantic orthodoxy. Here we may also mention the *Yoga Vasishtha,* a long work of more than 25,000 verses also composed about 900 C.E., which combines Buddhist idealist philosophy with themes from Samkhya.

The word *tantra* in Sanskrit can be used for any systematic instruction; a *tantra* is a web or (more literally) woven fabric of belief. It is not the name of a single school of philosophy or yoga practice. Tantra as a movement presupposes Vedanta: texts are called tantras—along with views concerned with yogic experiences, practices, and philosophy—that deny the exclusive right of Vedanta to pronounce on these topics in general and to classify sacred texts in particular. Tantra expanded the base, at a minimum, of yogic and spiritual authority, beyond the Upanishads as "revealed" in yogic experience.

In other words, tantric traditions usually recognize the authority of the Upanishads, etc., but find a greater or more accessible authority in later revelations, the instructions of one's own guru, and personal yogic experience—in reverse order, so it is said, in a notably empiricist temper (per a parallelism argument that is aired in the last section of chapter 4). Among the clusters of features characterizing most if not all tantric views is an emphasis on a feminine divine being or principle, called the Goddess or Shakti, Divine Energy, who secures enlightenment and transformation. Further, not only is *bhoga,* enjoyment, important as part of the goal of yogic practice, but the opposition between *bhoga* and worldly life, on the one hand, and yoga and liberation, *mukti,* on the other, is dissolved on a tantric path: "Enjoyment (*bhoga*) becomes yoga, misbehavior the good deed [or 'art,' *sukrita*], and all of life liberation," says the *Kularnava Tantra* (see appendix D), "for one following the [tantric] Kula Way."

Tantric literature is complex, having emerged in Kashmir and South India at about the same time, clearly by the eighth century C.E., with some texts earlier. But to talk of "emerging" tantra and "novel" practices of yoga and ritual, as scholars do, is to go historically by the standards of the Upanishads, the *Gita,* the *Yoga Sutra,* and Sanskrit literature in general. In truth, who knows how old are the various tantric practices? Some texts say that they, like the Upanishads, reveal the "secret of the Veda," and there are discernible connections with Vedic symbolism. But probably tantra has roots as much in the cultures of people speaking non-Indo-European languages as in the culture of Sanskrit. Perhaps very ancient traditions surface in the Sanskrit of the tantric Agamas, which are the earliest tantric texts (sometimes called instead Tantras, as with the *Malini Vijaya Tantra*, etc.), although as compositions scholars believe they are no earlier than the *Yoga Sutra* (c. 400 C.E.) and many are much later. There are, by the way, more than 700 Agamas and Tantras, by one scholarly count, including texts not only in Sanskrit but also in related languages.[32] When one includes the commentarial and noncommentarial literature, the result is staggering, a broad and complex history of texts and traditions. If then one throws Tibetan (Buddhist tantra, which parallels Hindu tantra) and texts in other non-Indo-European languages into the mix, a series of rebirths would be needed by even the greatest pundit to take them all in. Appendix D, which is devoted to tantric yoga, includes by necessity a small sample, focusing on Kula Tantra and the teaching of the great tantric system maker and synthesizer, Abhinava Gupta, who lived in the tenth century C.E. in Kashmir.

While all tantra is connected to yoga practices, it is not just asanas, breath control, and meditation that are advocated. Indeed, tantra emerged on the classical scene not as something new in doctrine as much as something new in ritual. Classically, tantric practice involved elaborate *puja*s, ceremonies of worship, centered on the Goddess or powerful female divinities or yoginis. These tantric ceremonies, in turn, did not add just new mantras, new ways of mantric recitation, or renewed emphasis on mantra, although this did occur, along with occult gestures (*mudra*) and diagrams (*yantra*), the contemplation of which is said to absorb thought and quieten the mind. Tantra also added new forms of *bhakti* and *karma yoga* (to be elaborated in chapter 3), which are enormously important. But some of the novel practices of tantra, which we may call "transgressional" practices, seem to have offended, for instance, Vedantins, although all late Vedanta shows tantric influence. The most famous, or infamous, of these "immoral" practices involve wine (or *bhang,* which is made from marijuana), meat, and/or sex. Thus does the word "tantra" even in English carry the sense of the illicit and taboo. Personally, I imagine even the so-called Left-Hand rites (compare the connotation of the Latin word for "left," *sinister*) as pretty tame. That tantra emerged against a background of a rather puritanical Vedanta seems a healthy guess (and the transgressional practices directed to the overly self-righteous, not as a palliative to the self-indulgent, as says the *Kularnava Tantra;* see appendix D).

Despite the importance of ritual and practice more generally in the culture of tantra, there are distinctive doctrines running practically throughout all its varieties. Perhaps most notably, there is, as mentioned, belief in a Divine Mother, a cosmic Shakti, Divine Energy, who is cosmologically the active and creative side of Shiva, in Shaiva philosophies the

 Great God, *maha deva*. In Vaishnavism, a similar role is given to Shri or Lakshmi, the feminine side or consort of Vishnu. In Shaiva philosophies, Shiva embraces the omnipresent Brahman—at least according to Abhinava Gupta and company, who will be our main focus. The great tantric master lived in Kashmir at the end of the tenth century (c. 975). He reformulated a Shaiva Siddhanta present in various Agamas that imported the dualism of Samkhya as an interpretative framework (somewhat in the fashion of Patanjali in the case of the *Yoga Sutra*; see chapter 2). Abhinava thus originated a spiritual philosophy of a divine creatrix, a philosophy that is monist yet also world affirmative, as will be explained (in chapter 5 along with appendix D).

Within the classical culture, we may mention finally the more specialized yoga manuals such as the fourteenth-century *Hatha Yoga Pradipika* (*HYP*), which is focused on practices but presupposes many theses of Yoga philosophy and psychology (see appendix E). Like all late yoga texts, the *HYP* draws upon centuries of earlier literature, in this case with admirable conciseness and brevity. It focuses on asanas, *bandha*s, and the breath, along with the benefits of yoga.

The history of modern yoga literature is beyond the scope of this book. The modern era may be defined by a global culture, science and technology, and a global sense of history, but there are modern yogins and yoginis such as Swami Vivekananda (1863–1902), Sri Aurobindo (1872–1950), Swami Muktananda (1908–82), Pandit Iyengar, and Swami Satyananda Saraswati, who write in line with traditional perspectives and to whom I will sometimes refer. There will also be references to modern scholarship, including philosophy and psychology as well as indology. But I shall attempt no overview of trends and tendencies beyond saying that we moderns are the inheritors of all the ancient and classical traditions, and modern Yoga philosophers may be defined as trying, as in this book, to preserve and champion traditional theories—usually in fact with a tilt toward tantra, at least in outlook if not also in name.

2
Yoga and Metaphysics

Yogic Self-Monitoring

All yoga practice and all Yoga philosophy presuppose a monitoring consciousness, though of course details vary with different theories. It is also presupposed that consciously, willfully locating one's attention in the witness produces certain desirable results, such as, most dramatically and uncontroversially, an increased ability to withstand pain. It is also claimed that eventually the practice leads to supernal bliss. Be this as it may, at even a beginner's level it is crucial to learn to observe steadily a bodily sensation without trying to alter it. But it will alter just by being witnessed, normally for the better. Recent philosophic literature has identified several distinct types of consciousness, but Yoga's self-monitoring consciousness is underappreciated.

This type of consciousness might be called self-consciousness, as it is in Sanskrit by its champions, and sometimes in English too, by those who have the Sanskrit tradition in mind. But in the recent academic literature, self-consciousness is usually talked about as the possession of a concept of self or as the ability to use such a concept in thinking about oneself, whereas the self-consciousness that is the concern of Yoga is nonconceptual and independent of thought. In the *Yoga Sutra,* yoga is defined (*YS* 1.2) as the power not to think, and according to all Yoga philosophies as well as yoga studios, humans have the ability to monitor bodily feedback without thinking. Buddhism goes so far as to deny self, but witnessing bodily and psychological movements is at the heart of Buddhist practices. Yoga's self-monitoring consciousness is not a matter of a self-concept.

Indeed, according to the *YS,* our self-concept is the source of our troubles: we identity with thoughts and emotions (*chitta*), a persona that is not us.[1] False identification is an old Upanishadic theme, now commonly identified with the Samkhya school. Samkhya (analysis) proposes careful understanding of one's nature and personality—to include subtle presentations of thoughts and emotions, *chitta*—as the means for self-discovery. This amounts to the self disidentifying with the body and mind. Fluctuations of *chitta* are viewed as part of nature and external to the *purusha,* our true self. All personality is a mask, to be analyzed away as a distraction from consciousness's native state of self-absorption and bliss.[2] According to Yoga (in this usage comprising almost all the classical schools, even the Buddhists who deny an enduring self), the individual conscious being is subject to rebirth, where he or she takes on most literally another persona. In sum, one's true self or consciousness is discovered through achieving a mental silence that allows consciousness to pull back into itself, disidentifying with its changing mind, body, and personality.

In the Upanishads, the term "self-illumining consciousness" is used to describe our essential self. In the *Brihadaranyaka,* it occurs in a passage about transformations of consciousness in dream and mystic trance. A person is said first to dream by his "own light" and then to become "self-illumined," *svayam jyotih.*[3] Light is chosen as an analogy because light illumines itself. A lamp illumining objects other than itself does not require another lamp to be seen. Witness consciousness is said to be able not only to witness other things but also to witness its own witnessing, without, however, doubling.

All the classical Yoga philosophies of India talk about the phenomenon, but the Advaita Vedanta school of Shankara (c. 700 C.E.) gives it the most play metaphysically, putting it at the very center of the Advaita system. As we shall see a little later, Advaita is close to certain Buddhist philosophies here, and although I do not think that either the Advaita or the Buddhist version is tenable, there is a lot to learn for our own Yoga views from these (yogically as well as philosophically) venerable traditions. The central Advaita claim is that this consciousness is "nondual," *advaita,* that it knows itself by being itself, that is, nonreflexively, or at least that it can do so, in a nonintellectual and indeed nonobservational manner. Thus "self-illumining consciousness" seems an appropriate label, capturing what appears to be a consciousness where there is a kind of a self-content.

In other words, Advaitins appear to have in mind a phenomenal consciousness whose content is itself. All Yoga philosophies embrace a version of this, although not all embrace Advaita's. For tantrics, for example, both Buddhist and Hindu, the witness is powerful, over self and others, and a self-determination thesis is, I shall argue, a fundamental Yoga commitment. Advaitins are mysterians or even outright deniers of self-determination. But on the consciousness's self-illumination, the Advaitins have the radical view, which we need to understand if for no other reason than to appreciate the lines of debate.

Advaitins consider the self a "state consciousness," not a "consciousness of," not a transitive consciousness but a, so to say, intransitive one. Thus it is unlike other types of phenomenal consciousness that are transitive, such as awareness of red. Alternatively, it is a "consciousness of" in a sense; it is a consciousness of itself. So here the "consciousness of" relationship has to be understood not as the asymmetrical relation philosophers normally take it to be but rather as something like identity. Note that in the Advaita understanding of this as self-consciousness, "self" is not taken to refer to the body or even the person but only the consciousness that is self-aware.

Contemporary discussions of types of consciousness typically proceed by presenting examples that are analyzed as exhibiting one type in contradistinction with others with which it might be confused. But here, by the admission of distinguished followers of Shankara, the best that can be done is a so-called "indicatory" or ostensive definition. Directions are given where self-illumining consciousness may be found—e.g., the injunction, "Meditate." This is supposed to be like a phenomenal definition of "red" that describes conditions under which one would experience red normally (the color of blood exposed to air). Nevertheless, Advaitins are not elitist, claiming that the conditions under which we would know directly what this is are available to anyone capable of understanding the directions ("Meditate") for consciousness to attend to itself. There is no third-person access to this consciousness, it is said. It does not show itself in action. The gap between this consciousness and everything else makes discourse that seems to be about it problematic, *anirvacaniyatva,* "it is impossible to say."

Despite the self-confessed puzzle about language, classical Advaitins do contrast self-illumining consciousness with other types of consciousness or cognition, *jnana,* presupposing, it would seem, a yogic audience of fellow meditators who know directly, or who could know were they to sit down on their yoga mats, what this consciousness is. But there is also from Shankara and company an identifying argument for self-illumining consciousness, which may or may not be at cross-purposes with the ineffability stance. It is also sometimes called the sublatability argument for the Upanishadic "self," *atman,* as the witness of itself and the subject of all experience. It runs as follows.

Everything dualistically experienced is at risk of being shown illusory through experiential sublation, as a snake appearing can turn out to be a rope. Any cognition and the information it contains could be sublated and shown to be false or nonveridical, except self-illumining consciousness. For, since among conscious states only self-illumining consciousness is not an appearance of one thing in or qualifying another, only in its case is the crucial precondition for sublation not met.[4]

To elaborate, a perceptual illusion can be sublated because a perception presents an object as qualified by or bearing a property. A piece of mother-of-pearl can be mistaken for silver because invariably the perceived object, the real thing in your hand, is taken as being some way or other, that is, as possessing a property. And a property presented may not qualify the object perceived in fact, as in the case of silverhood presented as qualifying what is in fact a piece of mother-of-pearl. Normally, cognition is "qualificative," to render the Sanskrit expression, *vaishishtya;* something *a* is cognized as F, at a minimum. Sublation is an ensuing experience that shows the *a* not to be F.

Self-illumining consciousness is not, however, in this way qualificative. Its nondualistic mode of presentation precludes sublation. It cannot be shown to be nonveridical—unlike all perception and indeed all thinking (remembering, inferring, understanding what someone has said, et cetera), all normal cognition, which is invariably consciousness of the transitive type. Self-illumining consciousness is self-authenticating, at least so Advaitins say to themselves and, it seems, to classical philosophers who were almost invariably concerned with questions about validation no matter what the school or banner under which they philosophized. Interestingly, Advaitins also say that there is no real point to the question about authentication. To itself, self-illumining consciousness stands self-revealed.

I do not intend to pursue the question of the cogency of the sublatability argument. I mention it mainly in the Advaita spirit of trying to get us to recognize such self-awareness. Self-monitoring consciousness is fundamental to all yoga practice and for Yoga philosophy. Self-monitoring consciousness is a bit more than Advaita's self-illumining self, since it not only knows itself in what it monitors, it alters it for the better, bringing integration and wellness. Schools and individuals differ about whether the goal of yoga is self-absorption, as Advaitins seem to think. The phenomenon of self-monitoring consciousness leaves open the question of the best direction of attention. That would be, according to Advaita, consciousness's losing itself in a trance of self-experience to the exclusion of everything else (to frame the possibility rather negatively). This does look to me rather unappealing in comparison with a larger, tantric goal of psychological harmony, about which, of course, there is much more to say. The tantric goal is also, I shall argue, in better consonance with the monitoring nature of yogic consciousness.

Suffice it to say for the present that Advaitins do not put forth the sublatability argument to show that our cognitions and various types of consciousness are unreliable. Advaitins may be illusionists in a sense, but they are mislabeled skeptics. They do not deny epistemic value to sense perception, for example. With their sublatability argument, they would help us yogically, using epistemic terms to distinguish self-illumining consciousness. For Advaitins first and foremost extol the value of self-illumining consciousness, tying it to a supernal bliss (*ananda*). That is, they tie the goal of imperishable bliss as the supreme personal good, the ultimate goal of yoga practice, which is first stated in the Upanishads, to the full realization of self-illumining consciousness. The point of the argument is to encourage people to attend to it, to attend to Yoga's pure witnessing, not the witnessed.[5] We shall see how this connects with both a theoretical minimalism in Yoga philosophy and baseline commitments. Advaita is half right, and there we find a crucial part of the story of Yoga's attitude to science.

Philosophers known by the Advaita label wrote throughout the middle and later periods of classical thought on into the modern period. The resilience of Advaita lies in part in its suitability to be aligned with several distinct theories when it comes to world knowledge, including science. Although there is a mainstream theory of perception, for example, it seems that any hypothesis about the operation of the sense organs and the generation of cognitions through physical processes is compatible with Advaita's central commitment to self-illumining consciousness. Indeed, as mentioned, Advaita appears compatible with all science and externalist theory—except that which proposes to explain self-illumining consciousness itself. More about the exception in a moment.

First, there is no call from the Advaita side to try to explain the world in relation to self-illumining consciousness. For self-illumining consciousness is self-contained and there is nothing to be explained. Furthermore, any such explanation would have to employ terms that are learned through training involving teachers and pupils and the customs of everyday life, whereas self-illumining consciousness is accessible only, so to say, from the inside. This radical internalism can only be ostensibly indicated by speech in the sense explained, not referred to directly. We'll come back to this point about language. What's key is that self-illumining consciousness is in itself nonrelational, whereas an explanation would purport to find a tie between explanandum and explanans. Self-illumining consciousness does not explain anything.

Nor can it be explained. That there is mystery in consciousness revealing diversity, and in the transition from one to the other, is readily admitted by Advaitins. That is to say, why there is both self-illumining consciousness and the worldly display is said to be inexplicable, *anirvacaniya*. More precisely, Advaita does not deny that this consciousness somehow connects with the body and the physical world. There might well be a relation, but it is impossible for us to elaborate. There is an uncloseable gap, not between matter and consciousness, but between our thought about the one and about the other. Here we have a kind of Advaita "mysterianism" on par with the materialist mysterianism that holds that while everything is material, we are constitutionally incapable of understanding how mind reduces to matter. Trying to conceptualize the self-illumining self would be like trying to determine at once the position and momentum of an electron. It cannot be done. Self-illumining consciousness is inaccessible to representation and all third-person point of view. All talk of it is nonliteral, meant to direct a person to the experience.

Yoga theistic philosophers tend to hold self-illumining consciousness as that which we share with God, with Brahman, who as the supreme person in this way knows its/his/her own existence (compare the biblical "I am that I am"). Such theism has just as good credentials in the Upanishads as the Advaita nontheism. The Yoga philosophy of the *Yoga Sutra* largely agrees with the Advaita interpretation, or at least with the Advaita value judgment about self-illumining consciousness. Although Patanjali's philosophy is realist about the objects of sense experience, not "antirealist" like Advaita, all value is placed in the self; nature is intrinsically valueless.

In yoga practices, however, no matter how great the value of the witness to itself, there is always application, always something witnessed. The problem with the Advaita view is not its insistence that consciousness is self-illumining but its ignoring consciousness's other-illumining capabilities. Consciousness is both self- and other-illumining. With respect to the body, it is self-transformative too. Through a combination of identification (sometimes called self-acceptance) and monitoring, yoga practice shows that witnessing brings wellness. Yogic self-monitoring consciousness is transitive in proprioceptive sensation, in developing conscious control, balance, and health. The Advaita tendency to limit the power of consciousness so that it would be able to illumine only itself (everything else being sublatable) does not accord with the evidence.

Nevertheless, there is an asymmetry here between the witnessed and the witnessing that is just the reverse of the asymmetry of materialism (more about which below). Advaita is a spiritual philosophy, without question within the Yoga camp. In all Yoga philosophy, there is a fundamental commitment to the value of self-monitoring consciousness. In finding it basic to what we are up to, Yogins are in solidarity with Advaita, although we depart from the school on the value of the body and the power of yogic self-transformation.

Perhaps the greatest strength of Advaita is that, like much Buddhist teaching, it eschews intellectual argument for advice that runs, "Do this and see for yourself." We don't know why yoga facilitates self-realization, say Advaitins. It appears to work for some, and what's the harm in trying? What we really need, they stress, is simply to know consciousness as it is in itself. Since self-illumining consciousness is what it is and it is already accomplished in our deepest self, yoga practices should be thought of as removing obstacles.[6]

The list of great Advaita philosophers includes several who are expert at dialectics, expert at concocting counterexamples and in general disputing metaphysical theories. Sometimes one can find no motive behind the Advaita refutations beyond a form of delight. And Advaitins typically embrace the science of the day, although there are exceptions. Nevertheless, there are, from the Advaita point of view, theories that overstep the bounds of science and purport to explain self-illumining consciousness itself. Here is where I think all Yoga philosophy should take the Advaita attitude.

I am not so sanguine about the Advaita conception of self-illumination, again because it seems that the self-monitoring has, in the case of the body, power over what it is witnessing. Consider what happens in yoga when you "breathe into" pain. A pain considered at first negatively as simply hurting can be changed into a helpful monitor and even to a pain that is not pain, that feels good and bring wellness and strength. And this is something we can talk about in the most literal and straightforward of terms.

Thus the right Yoga response, it seems to me, is to agree that, as attested in different lineages, a self-absorptive yogic trance is a valuable yogic accomplishment, or ability, but it is hardly the only yogic goal. Self-absorptive yogic trance seems to be psychologically what Advaitins value. And for the person so absorbed, a self-witnessing consciousness may well be *not* related to other things, at least not at the time. Thus it is hard to see how such self-absorption as a live possibility ties up with a fuller self-conception and self-awareness. We may agree with Advaitins on this. But we should part company with them on their unmitigated mysterianism. For consciousness is intimately, bodily relational in yoga, and principles of yoga that specify correlations can be put into words. Consider all the yoga manuals.

In response to similar objections, Advaitins take an epistemological stance: self-illumining consciousness is self-authenticating and, unlike other conscious states and material phenomena, has exclusive access to itself. Thus only it has the right to pronounce on itself. (Of course, about itself it says nothing.)

But whether or not we buy into this or a similar thesis about the authority of self-consciousness to pronounce on itself, clearly consciousness has the right to pronounce not only on itself but also on other things. It is other- as well as self-illumining. Furthermore, it is self-determining and indeed self-transformative. Self-determination is as basic a Yoga thesis as any, and a coherent conception of consciousness as both self-illumining and self-determining is to be desired, denying neither. Advaitins are right that those who would explain consciousness in materialist or externalist terms are trespassers who misrepresent the putative explanandum. Where Yoga departs from Advaita is on the explanans side of theory, with the views that do the explaining. These concern, according to Yoga, the power of consciousness. About the inadequacy of theories that would try to explain self-illumining consciousness in material or "scientific" terms, Yoga and Advaita are in accord.

There are several indications that the radical mysterianism of Advaita is unsatisfactory. Just how do Advaitins know that self-illumining consciousness's relation to other things cannot be verbalized? The idea seems to be that this consciousness's being absorbed exclusively in itself translates into its being explanatorily unavailable. An explanation would be like an unwanted disturbance violating self-illumining consciousness's self-absorbed trance. But how do Advaitins know so much about this inexplicable to be able to explain why it is not explicable? This brings us back to the problem of the language Advaitins use.

Advaitin philosophers draw a distinction between descriptive use of words and the indicatory, as mentioned earlier. The difference is between describing Devadatta's house along with explaining what a house is—say, to a child—and indicating Devadatta's house conversationally by saying that it is the one where some crows pointed to are hovering. The currently hovering crows have nothing to do with what the house is and its proper description. In Sanskrit linguistic philosophy, this is the *visheshana/upalakshana* distinction. It is a distinction between true and pseudo-qualifiers in connection with words used, on the one hand, to pick out something (*a*) by way of a property it really has (F*a*), as opposed to, on the other, words used to direct someone's attention to something (*a*) by means of a thoroughly contingent and accidental relation it has to something else (*b*). It is that something else to which the words refer literally. Advaitins see talk of self-illumining consciousness as a matter of the indicatory, *upalakshana*. There is no way literally to refer to it, since the act of referring is something other than self-illumining consciousness itself. "Speech does not go there," in the words of the *Kena Upanishad*, which are then themselves indicatory.[7]

This move is, however, even considering Advaita's own agenda, unhelpful. In their arguments Advaitins consider themselves to know some true properties of self-illumining consciousness. Why else would they say that it is self-illumining, or nondual, and then reason according to these attributions?

Then to Yoga—which, to repeat, I see as in the service of and responsive to the full panoply of yogic goals and accomplishments, never only to even the fullest realization of self-illumining consciousness—I say, let us expose our necks, committing ourselves to more about consciousness than the possibility and value of self-illumining trance (*samadhi*). Self-monitoring consciousness is not only valuable in itself, as the Advaitins have it, it is valuable instrumentally, in accomplishing health, balance, harmony, self-perfection.

In other words, we may expose our necks without risking much injury in fact, protected by yogic discoveries. The value of consciousness is not only to itself but to our bodies. Yoga practice teaches this lesson to Yoga philosophy. Advaitins seem blinded by the transcendental logic of their sublatability argument to much else of value in what is made available yogically. Nevertheless, as a matter of what one takes to be the last trench behind which lies no option save surrender, the Advaitins, it seems to me, are correct in their (Upanishadic) idea of self-illumining consciousness, which they equate to the (Upanishadic) "self," *atman*.

Yoga on Philosophy's Mind-Body Problem

Many philosophy professionals occupy themselves nowadays with what they call the mind-body problem, how consciousness is related to the body and the brain in particular. There is said to be a hard as well as a soft problem of consciousness. The soft problem is to correlate phenomenal states, such as seeing red or a toothache, with brain states and bodily processes. Great progress in the science of this has occurred just in the last couple of decades. Yoga philosophy views this as the successful specification of necessary but not sufficient conditions in the brain or another body part for the occurrence of whatever physical ability. The soft problem of consciousness will be solved eventually. We shall know how the brain functions. There is no challenge to Yoga philosophy from such developments.

The hard problem of consciousness is to explain why or how material processes result in consciousness or how certain material states or processes can be identical with the thoughts, perceptions, feelings, self-consciousness, etc., we take to be ourselves or to belong to our conscious experience. The hard problem of consciousness presumes a materialist perspective. This presents a certain prejudice against Yoga. For Yoga as a philosophy, whatever its details or traditions, in order to support yoga practices, must make us believe in the power of consciousness, for itself and for its instruments.

In tantric and other non-Advaita traditions, the goal of yoga goes beyond the ideal of realizing a self-illumining consciousness. In the broadest terms, yoga is practiced to promote harmony between whatever is our highest or deepest self or consciousness and mental, emotional, and bodily instruments. Now yogic experience shows, I shall argue, that there is no ultimate separation of mind and matter. Nevertheless, in the current intellectual climate, Yoga philosophy, to defend consciousness and its powers and possibilities, has to insist on a certain division. Yoga has to be dualist—in a sense to be explained—or monist in a different way than materialism is monist, that is to say, spiritually monist, like much Vedanta or Mahayana Buddhism, which though monist, deny that everything is material.

The reigning opinion in universities is, unfortunately, decidedly monist in the materialist sense. In the range of views that dominate professional philosophy, thought and consciousness are considered either in some sense identical to brain states and processes or invariably dependent on them as effects or properties. There is nothing mental or conscious apart from the physical body. Yoga, in sharp contrast, teaches the causal independence of consciousness, its kingship or self-rule, as well as its ability to govern thought, emotion, and the body, indeed all of its various instruments and "sheaths."[8] I shall call this Yoga's self-determination thesis. It stands at the center of Yoga metaphysics. That is to say, central to Yoga is the proposition that we can change ourselves, that our bodies are shaped by karma, by what we do, by exercises and training and self-discipline. Self-determination extends to our emotional and mental bodies as well as our physical "sheath." Consciousness transcends and can make, or shape, its embodiments. Yoga metaphysics— whether dualist or something else—has the responsibility to make the power of consciousness plain.

Antidualist opinion in academic philosophy is carried by arguments first directed against a Western and early modern tradition of viewing consciousness as a substance. Descartes (1596–1650) saw consciousness as a kind of stuff distinct from things physical. But how can consciousness—begins the now standard refutation—be separate from matter? An unbridgeable gulf is unimaginable. If there were an absolute barrier, we could neither perceive physical things nor act in the world. Descartes relied on God to pair up the psychological and the physical. Science, however, admits no supernatural causes. So without God, the connection seems impossible. Modern materialism develops from this insight.

There are of course several competing materialist views, and numerous considerations motivate them.[9] Arguments for one theory and against another occupy the professional journals. On all views, however, explanatory priority rests with the physical in that consciousness is physically caused.[10] "Materialism" is the word I use to capture this common commitment. On all the theories, conscious states are either identical to physical processes or bubble-like effects of physical causes that themselves have no causal power. In other words, consciousness is not only inseparable from the physical body, it is identical to or entirely dependent on physical states. All volition, everything we choose to do, as well as all thought and emotion and indeed self-consciousness, have physical determinants in the brain or another body part.

Materialists are, generally speaking, naturalists. Consciousness may be a bit peculiar as events or properties go, but all subjective as well as objective occurrences belong to a closed physical network, i.e., to the natural world. Consciousness emerges in the evolution of life according to physical, chemical, and biological laws. Yoga's self-determination thesis is, therefore, false, along with much of our common belief about ourselves as knowers and agents.

Yoga denies a supposition common to all materialism, namely, that either an identity or a one-directional causal relationship from body to mind is the truth about consciousness. That is to say, Yoga denies that consciousness is either identical to or the result of physical entities and processes. This is the materialist view boiled down to its essence—albeit a disjunctive essence, two mouthfuls—a *rasa* that is hard for Yoga to stomach, since Yoga is committed to the irreducible reality of consciousness and its power over itself and its instruments. Although there are disputes among Vedantins, Buddhists, Jainas, and other advocates of yoga practices ancient and modern, on all Yoga views at least some consciousness transcends the body and indeed the mind.

According to the new materialists, in contrast, correlations between brain states and processes and conscious states and processes may be extrapolated to deny all such transcendence. Some correlations, such as the severing of the spinal cord and loss of consciousness, are commonly cited in favor of a general connection. However, a dramatic example of a necessary condition is no argument for sufficiency. As mentioned, the soft problem of consciousness is resolvable by identification of necessary conditions for conscious states in the brain and bodily processes. Yoga has no quarrel with this. Our quarrel is with the supposition that things physical could be sufficient for consciousness. You need an unsevered spinal cord to live and breathe and think and feel, but you also need something beyond the bodily instrument.

By definition the mind's receptivity to sensory input and its ability to respond through bodily movement depend on physical processes properly functioning. In other words, we know *a priori* that bodily events, such as visual perception or lifting a limb, depend on the normal functioning of bodily processes. So why should this bit of analytic insight mean that every conscious state correlates with something going on in the brain? Introspectively, yogins report self-consciousness during periods when their brains show practically no activity.[11]

The materialist answer is typically that in such cases science has a project. We may not know yet, but we shall. Science's trajectory is progress. This of course is a convenient attitude toward inconvenient phenomena, such as, to cite another large example, our apparent freedom to move about. The materialist may be taken to presume that any consciousness touted by Yoga would have a physical correlate and exclusively physical causes. After all, what is the alternative? The entirety of this chapter constitutes a response to this challenge and attitude, but here is the gist.

First, Yoga in entering philosophy's mind-body debate inherits rich dualist resources, counterarguments about consciousness that so far have not been answered by materialists. I shall survey a few of these, and give further references.

Second, Yoga metaphysics itself, if it need be dualist, need not be Cartesian, need not endorse a dualism of noninteractive substances. Yoga dualism may or may not find that consciousness is a substance in the sense of a locus or substratum of peculiarly psychological properties, but whatever the precise ontology, Yoga at a minimum will be interactionist, avoiding the mysteries of Cartesian dualism and its noninteractionist progeny.

Yoga need not oppose science, not even brain science, although it must be opposed to causal closure. Brain science reveals necessary conditions, never in themselves sufficient. In classical India, the Nyaya school is famous for making the point. Nyaya, Logic, is a premier dualist philosophy classically allied with Yoga in our broad sense. Nyaya philosophers point out, in the stock example, that a genuine perception of a thorn through the sense of touch requires physical contact between the thorn and a body part, a left toe, for instance. But you do not need the toe to remember the thorn. This is one indication of the transcendence of consciousness.

The Nyaya philosopher definitely would agree with the modern materialist that having a brain is a condition of human consciousness. Cut off the head and the person dies. The particular stream of cognition forming Devadatta's mental life ends with the death of Devadatta, according to Nyaya. This school does not, unlike mainstream Yoga (Vedanta, Buddhism, and so on), recognize an occult or "pranic" body. But Nyaya does recognize that Devadatta the person is a composite of a self and a body and indeed a life. The body is not sufficient for consciousness, since, Nyaya philosophers argue, we see that material things, excepting the living body, are not conscious.

We shall come back to the general topic of causality later in the chapter and also in connection with discussion of karma in chapter 3. Let us move on with the remark that it is not worth disputing the basic anti-Cartesian argument that we are aware of the world that is explained by physics and chemistry and we act and are acted upon by things physical. Cartesian dualism is untenable. But Yoga dualism is different, building from the insights of its Eastern ally, Nyaya.

Four types of causal relationship are recognized by the philosophers of classical Nyaya. Causal capacities are dispositions, *samskara,* which are latent properties, lawful tendencies for something to change under certain circumstances, as captured by conditional statements. For example, water has the disposition to freeze at a certain temperature. The liquid in a glass possesses this property, though its having it is not immediately evident. Similarly, we do not continuously remember our breakfast this morning but can if prompted. Simplifying a bit, we may say that Nyaya finds dispositions of four broad types:[12]

1. Physico-physical dispositions, for example, elasticity, as of a rubber band. (A rubber band is a physical thing both before and after being stretched.)
2. Physico-psychological dispositions, for example, perceptual capacity, the ability to perceive a pot in the stock example. (The sense organs triggered by connection with a physical object of the right type have the ability to generate, for example, the psychological event of awareness of the pot.)[13]
3. Psycho-psychological dispositions, for example, inferential capacity, as sight of smoke on the mountain leads to the occurrent knowledge that there is fire over there. (The self carries the disposition to infer fire from detection of smoke, a disposition acquired by "wide experience" of the connection between smoke and fire.)
4. Psycho-physical dispositions, for example, to effort and action, as wanting the mango on the table leads to the effort and action to pick it up. (The self is the locus of a, let us say, desiderous disposition—*chikirsha* in Sanskrit, desire to do—to such effort and action on the body's part.)

With its self-determination thesis, Yoga is committed to the importance of developing dispositions of types 3 and 4, as will become clear.

The bottom line is that Nyaya's dualism—which is one option for Yoga, so let us say "Yoga dualism"—does not make it impossible to understand mental-physical interaction. There are many obvious correlations, and doubtless many less obvious that remain to be discovered in science or yogic research. Yoga dualism is a thesis that centrally concerns consciousness and self-determination. Consciousness transcends matter and is self-determining or can be. It can reshape its physical sheath, perfect it, bring it into a new harmony with the breath, feeling, and thought. This we find through yoga practice to be the nature of yogic self-monitoring consciousness: that it alters what it monitors, the body, the emotions, thoughts and intentions, whatever it identifies with and nourishes. That is, consciousness changes its embodiments for the better, for health and integration, for what we might call the (tantric theme of) spiritualization of the faculties. In special experiences, consciousness finds it has, or can have, a body of different stuff or energy than the physical (a pranic body, a karmic body, a subtle or astral body, *sukshma sharira*). Always capable of connecting with matter, it can withdraw into itself and, except for the dispositional property to reconnect, be undisturbed by material happenings. This power (called *samyama* in the *Yoga Sutra*) is a foundational fact shaping Yoga metaphysics.

There are laws of self-determination, shown by correlations in the reverse direction from those touted by materialists. These include principles of yoga practice. But Yoga hardly rules out physical dependences. Causal relations run both ways, and mental events are typically the result of a complex collection of factors, some of which are physical and some of which are not. We might add that if consciousness and the body were not at all physically determined, there would be no point to yogic exercises. We do yoga to augment the causal factors that lie on the side of consciousness.

Yoga dualism, in our sense of stressing the power, or potential power, of consciousness, is compatible, it is important to note, with several forms of monism. By sketching a dualist version of Yoga metaphysics (in line with Nyaya), I mean to emphasize the transcendence of consciousness and potentialities of dependence, opposite to the assumptions of materialists. Consciousness can but need not be material. In part it is material in perception of material things and in movements of the physical body. But that it is so in those states is no argument that it cannot exist otherwise.

To sum up our response, then, to the correlations argument of the materialists: Who would not expect (given the truth of Yoga dualism) correlations between brain and mental events? Insofar as the mental events belong to embodied persons, correlations are guaranteed. That there are correlations, however, leaves open the questions of identity and the directionality of the causal relations.

Yoga contends both that consciousness is not identical to the body and that mind-body (or consciousness-body) causality is not one-directional. What we do shapes the body. The physical universe is not causally closed. There are psycho-psychological and psycho-physical dispositions.

The truth of this thesis is rather easy to see. Evidence for it couldn't be closer. For instance, insofar as you and I are moving our eyes as we read (instead of, for example, closing our eyelids), we are right now programming, materially changing, our brains, the physical underpinning of our memories, by reading. Or, if no physical underpinning of memory is required, we are making a psycho-psychological disposition resting in something else, a mind, a subtle body, or a nonmaterial self. But let us suppose that the brain is like a computer, as materialists think. Then each of us is right now chiseling in a property necessary to a later remembering. People who do not do so cannot remember this sentence. Thus we do not have to look at the special feats of yogins to find reverse correlations between mind and brain that refute materialism.[14]

Yoga philosophy admits physical determinations of consciousness but challenges us to recognize our potential. Yoga stresses personal responsibility: we shape our own good selves or personalities and need not be fatalistic or resigned to biological and physical inheritances (yoga as a "makeover" without cosmetics or plastic surgery). There are Yoga perspectives that have us as preparing the way for a larger self to integrate with us, with our ultimate act a surrendering. But on these (*bhakti* and tantra) views too we have to make ourselves ready by mastering the practices, the asanas, the breath control, the meditation, and the rest. What we do to get ready remains essential.

A second prop to anti-Yoga prejudice may be dealt with more briefly. It is motivated by scientific explanations revealing physical identities. That is to say, a "reductionist" argument marshals to the materialist cause scientific successes in explaining things macroscopic by formula, which are taken to govern the microscopic. Consider weather, heat, and crystals. We understand these things by understanding their physics and chemistry. All phenomena, it is then hastily supposed, can be explained by theories that refer only to physical events and entities (niceties about the ontology of numbers, words, theories, etc., being beside the point).

The problem, however, is how to carry out this agenda with consciousness, with thought, feeling, and other mental events, including the meditative experiences of yoga. The fact is that no one has a clue. In the case of weather, the microscopic is both necessary and sufficient for the macroscopic. Mean kinetic energy is identical with heat. Given a certain value for the one, the other will be absolutely fixed. Similarly, if something is H_2O, then it is water. And there is no water that is not H_2O. With this much, Yoga has of course no quarrel: certain physical things and events can be explained reductively in chemical and physical terms without reference to consciousness. The classical Yoga of Patanjali is realist in this sense, and we should have no qualms about admitting physico-physical capacities and processes going on independently of the mind—at least of our minds (the question of the universality of some sort of divine or cosmic mind is another matter). However, Yoga teaches that nothing in the brain ever absolutely fixes the mind—*a fortiori* where "the mind" includes extraordinary states of yogic consciousness. In Yoga we see this, what philosophers call the "explanatory gap," as a corollary to the thesis of the self-determining power of consciousness, its control, or potential control, of its range of instruments (thought, emotion, bodily movement, and so on).

To be sure, how the brain works is now better known. We even have chemical remedies for certain "mental" illnesses. Nevertheless, it must be kept in mind that science presents only correlations between (a) brain or more broadly bodily states or processes and (b) mental phenomena. It does not have a theory about how the latter (b) are *required* by (a) things physical. In other words, neurology and medicine make plain precise dependences of certain conscious states on certain physical processes. When a loud sound goes off near our ears, we hear it, even if our concentration is elsewhere. But we can block out noise, not attend to it, consciously fail to perceive available data. In other words, Yoga grants that the physical factors can predominate in the determination of a mental event. But often the story is different, and never is a physical one by itself sufficient when it comes to conscious states.

The burning question for materialists is why the physical should bring the mental about or require mental events in some other, noncausal fashion. Why should neural firings in the synapses of a brain produce, or even "occasion," consciousness and the life of the mind? This is the explanatory gap talked about in the philosophic literature. It is brought out in a particularly telling fashion by a thought experiment about a possible "zombie."[15]

Imagine an exact physical duplicate of your body that did not have consciousness. (We could also call this the "mannequin" thought experiment.) Clearly we can imagine the artifact without having to imagine that the thing is conscious. So why do you who have the same physical constituents as the zombie have consciousness? Why are you conscious but not the zombie? Why should the state of your body right now bring about your current or subsequent consciousness while the exact same state of the zombie does not engender consciousness? Of course, the Yoga dualist avoids the question because according to us the difference between you and the zombie is the presence in you of consciousness. Consciousness is some sort of basic entity, according to Nyaya and Yoga dualism. Consciousness is irreducibly different from the material body, though it can shape and move a body or (according to monist Yoga philosophies) become one. In explaining the phenomenon of consciousness, there will always be a gap so long as matter is all that is recognized.

The difficulty of the zombie question, and of others bringing out differences between bodies and minds, has spawned incredible ingenuity and dozens of difficult books, without, however, much agreement about proposed solutions. Still, the assumption reigns that mind is somehow equivalent to matter or in itself causally impotent. Isn't this simply prejudice that flies in the face of our abilities? Yoga would urge us to pay attention to ourselves, expand our horizons—perhaps also paying attention to the cogency of dualism![16]

The correlations and reductionist arguments seem to be regarded—however fantastic this may now appear—as the most powerful weapons in the materialist arsenal. There is, however, another argument that is commonly paraded. It derives from the later Wittgenstein, and I shall call it the public-language argument.[17] It too does not challenge the dualism of Yoga. Against the self-determination thesis, it has no force whatsoever.

How could a person identify a subjective occurrence, and thus talk about it, even to herself, without knowing objective, i.e., physical, signs or indications? The basic insight is about a need for public criteria for the applications of words to refer even to subjective events. To talk to herself (silently so that only God or a telepath could eavesdrop), a person has to have words whose application is governed by rules set by convention. If one person can set up a rule and follow it, in principle another can follow it too. How otherwise could anyone keep up with his or her own subjective happenings? In principle, therefore, there can be no "private language." We come to *know* in the sense of "being able to talk about" inward states ("That's a toothache") by learning to recognize behavioral indications, because only bodily behavior has the objectivity—the publicness and accessibility by numerous minds—that makes linguistic conventions possible.

By this demand, it seems that nothing that we could talk about could be unconnected to the physical. And it would seem to follow that nothing transcending the physical should be introduced into the debate about consciousness. However, Yoga dualism is not scathed by the assumption that human beings learn language by learning to recognize public signs. Yoga practices show forms of knowledge and awareness that are not mediated by language. Intellectual position is not the highest prize. This is the core response.

Then with respect to statements of instruction in a yoga class, there are several points to be made. First, the reason there is so much complaint among yogins and other mystics about the difficulty in describing their special experiences is rather obvious. If sentences are in their literal meaning restricted to relations among physical things, then thank God for nonliteral meaning.[18] Through analogy and imagination, mystics do manage to be understood by nonmystics. Why else would there be such a substantial literature? Second, linguistic conventions are developed among master yogins and yoginis, who forge technical terms in connection with special training and meditative experience—for example, the term "chakra" discussed in chapter 1. The technical language of yogic practices is no less an instrument of communication than the special vocabulary of an art, craft, or scientific discipline.

In sum, Yoga does rely on imaginative meaning beyond the range of normal experience. But there is surely a good word to be said in general for imaginative capacities. Our imaginations articulate goals of work. Furthermore, yoga develops its own technical vocabulary to be learned in the course of yoga practice. Therefore, there is no cogent public-language argument that defeats Yoga.

Let us move on to consider Yoga theories of mind-body interaction unencumbered by materialist biases.

Mind-Body Interactive Dualism

In the context of the professional mind-body debate, teachings about yoga practice and experience are dualist in the sense of affirming the integrity of self and consciousness against materialism. Yoga teachings engage a first-person point of view as opposed to an externalist, third-person point of view as in science. We have reviewed positions within the now dominant materialist camp. But there are of course many philosophers who champion such a "how-to" first-person perspective in opposition to materialism. There is thus ready at hand an intellectual alliance, which because focused on errors of materialism perhaps lacks the spirit of yoga practice, but provides philosophically rich resources for Yoga to mine. Existentialism with its emphasis on choice (*we* make choices) and absurdity (science's impersonal view of nature) is perhaps the most prominent among Western dualist schools with which Yoga can make common cause. That is to say, Yoga as an antimaterialist philosophy joins hands with some who couldn't care less about extraordinary capacities and experiences. (Can you picture Jean-Paul Sartre in an asana—*with the pipe?*)

The distinctive feature of Yoga as a dualism is its understanding of mind and body as instruments.[19] The locus of control lies, or potentially lies, in consciousness. The point of all yoga practice is to take a step toward greater psychological harmony, including, to be sure, self-control as in, for example, bodily suppleness and athletic dexterity fostered by yogic self-monitoring consciousness. So, at a minimum, Yoga must be wedded to the value of subjectivity, of being a self, and of exercising control. It has to deny that consciousness is fully determined by matter (*we* determine matter—or a larger self does, on Yoga views where the aim is to unite with a larger self). Yoga, then, is "dualist" in contrast with philosophic materialism. But probably we should say "provisionally dualist" since we want to leave open the question of ties to spiritually monistic views.

This section surveys both the classical Yoga dualism of Patanjali and Nyaya dualism; the former is a close sister of Samkhya dualism, first articulated in certain Upanishads. In other words, dualist philosophies became prominent in India very early and remained so.[20] Patanjali, the author, or more likely compiler/editor, of the *Yoga Sutra,* c. 400 C.E. (see the introduction to appendix C), presents a deeply dualist vision, probably following a Samkhya vogue.[21] Indeed, the *YS*'s dualism is, like that of Samkhya, much more radical than the variety we require. I shall argue that contemporary Yoga dualism should follow Nyaya, which is, of all the classical Indian schools, arguably the closest to common sense. (It also has a long and rich textual history, and is related to *ayurveda,* medicine, and legal texts as well as having much influence in classical aesthetics.) We shall see how Nyaya handles mental-physical correlations in a moment. First let us see what is wrong with the dualism of the *Yoga Sutra* (*YS*).

After defining yoga as mental silence, control of the fluctuations of thought and emotion (*chitta-vritti-nirodha,* "stilling the fluctuations of mentality," *YS* 1.2: see note 7 to chapter 1), Patanjali casts the goal of yoga practice in terms of a radical dualism. There are, one, self (*purusha*) and two, nature (*prakriti*), and though both are real, only the former has value. "Then the seer rests in its true form" (*YS* 1.3), by which is meant (according to all the classical commentators) "rests in itself, self-rapt, unaware of anything other than self, *entirely separate* from nature" (emphasis mine).

There are several problems with this position. Perhaps the worst is that Patanjali's dualism of self and nature is in opposition to his own yogic tradition of *siddhi*s, the extraordinary capacities or powers to which yoga leads, many of which are occult. The ties between yoga practices and *siddhi*s are in my judgment intrinsic, both culturally (in the conventions of designating just certain people yogins and yoginis) and in psychological fact. No one counts as a master yogin or yogini who does not possess *siddhi*s, and all yoga practice helps to develop *siddhi*s at least generically in the sense of self-control. Patanjali, however, seeing self-rapt self-awareness as the sole locus of value (joining Advaitins), places no value in *siddhis*. *YS* 3.37: "Though wonders to ordinary persons [yogic powers] are obstacles to the goal of yoga."[22]

The denial of the value of *siddhi*s presents a problem of textual interpretation. Practically the whole of the *YS*'s chapter 3 (out of a total of four chapters) is concerned with the development of *siddhi*s. In addition to this oddity about the *YS* itself, by setting aside the value of *siddhi*s, Patanjali does violence to yoga tradition.[23] Despite the detailed teachings of chapter 3, our author/editor apparently became concerned exclusively with mystic trance, *samadhi*. On this reading,[24] the man would have compiled the text from sutras that had been formulated generations before him, adding a few framework or metaphysical ideas in accordance with (Samkhya or) his personal sense of consciousness's power to withdraw utterly into itself. There, he seems to think, it can rest content, totally apart from the world.

It may well be that certain yogins have considered this state the single goal of their endeavors. Maybe it's a real possibility, as proposed by Patanjali, who doubtless was an extremely accomplished yogin, a guru worthy of reverence, whatever his merits as a theorist. Probably Patanjali's *samadhi* is the same as the Advaitins' self-illumining consciousness, since both schools claim that the state is blissful beyond imagination. Note, however, that as far as we the unenlightened are concerned, such an idea of "liberated" consciousness—*kaivalya,* aloneness, in Patanjali's term—is pure speculation. The state could not be reported, since reporting requires instruments such as a body and a keyboard.

Furthermore, the *YS*'s dualism is subject to a charge of self-stultification. Such a self-absorbed yogin develops only one of his or her possibilities, being lost to the world. Especially in the light of Yoga's self-determination thesis, this seems a shame. By the power of self-determination I mean to include the ability to enter a self-absorbed *samadhi*, but also potential transformations of body, life, and mind.

Please bear in mind that the criticism that Patanjali teaches a self-stultifying philosophy is not only my opinion but also that of a host of yogic movements in India, belonging to what we may call in general the tantric turn (see below). Embrace of *siddhi*s may be called the tantric refutation of Patanjali's theory.

The mental silence that yoga achieves is not just a state but a power. Patanjali in *YS* 1.3 and elsewhere falls victim to a false dilemma. He says that when the *chitta* becomes quiet the self or true person, *purusha,* rests in its true form. At all other times, he asserts at 1.4, it falsely identifies with *chitta*. However, the self, while self-conscious, can also think if it likes. Ask any yogin, anyone who claims to have the ability to turn off the mind, whether he or she can turn it back on. According to the unacceptably trenchant dualism of Patanjali, in contrast, mentality, *chitta,* is part of nature, *prakriti,* and thus divorced from the self. Since self-awareness apart from nature is the goal, control has to be illusory.

Furthermore, awareness of anything other than self is for Patanjali bad, that is, in comparison with the supremely good trance of self-absorption. He uses the word *kaivalya,* aloneness, for what he sees as the ontological equivalent of *asamprajnata samadhi,* a meditation without prop, i.e., without any content or intentionality other than self-awareness itself, a self-absorption beyond space and time. In this way, the metaphysics of the *YS* is made to tie up with the traditional idea of *mukti* or *moksha,* liberation from suffering and endless rebirth. (But isn't rebirth, generally speaking, a good thing? Would you rather be reborn or totally vanish? More about this in the next two chapters.) In sum, according to the *YS* a self's recovery from other- into self-absorption is the *summum bonum,* the supreme value for a person, *parama purushartha,* the "supreme personal good." But here I say we should line up with tantrism and assume that a larger goal is possible, one not so world-negating, including the proposition that *siddhi*s are good. Tantrics disagree that life is inevitably a matter of suffering, or that its suffering is not worthwhile, not itself instrumentally valuable to a yoga practice that aims at self-perfection.

Patanjali probably inherited many—in all likelihood most—of the approximately two hundred sutras that make up the *YS*. In fact, I think he is responsible only for the text's dualist cast. The *YS* is thematically voluntarist in spite of the dualism of *purusha* and *prakriti* and the world-denying concept of *kaivalya*. These concepts comprise a kind of metaphysical overlay and can be replaced.

Rich psychological veins are there to mine nevertheless, as well as practice concepts of which any Yoga philosophy needs to take stock. Let me underscore that there are invaluable practice concepts from which any yogin or yogini could draw benefit. The *YS* is not the one and only indispensable practice manual, but it clearly ranks among the most seminal, considering centuries of yoga practitioners. And philosophers of all the rival schools know the text. So, despite the untenability of the dualism and Patanjali's impoverished conception of the goal of yoga, the *YS* is an authority for both yoga practices and Yoga philosophy.

The chief cost to yogic sensibilities, honed on the very practices outlined in the sutras, is, as pointed out, the cutting off of one half of Yoga's self-determination thesis, to wit, a denial of consciousness's power, or potential power, over its instruments. Patanjali can make no sense of the healing power of yogic self-monitoring consciousness directed to an injured body part or a pranic blockage. But let us note that Patanjali's metaphysics is also untenable pretty much for the same reasons that Cartesian dualism is untenable: we act in nature and perceive physical objects.

The self's identification with a mind, body, personality, etc., is, according to the *YS*, an illusion. Thus Patanjali aligns himself with world-denying Advaitins who take just one further step to declare the self not only the only value but also the only reality. To be sure, the *YS*'s chapter 4 is comprised of argument directed against idealists, presumably Buddhist idealists, to the effect that nature is real. The main contention is articulated at *YS* 2.22: when a single yogin is liberated everyone else remains bound, and therefore nature must be objective. But if the line separating Patanjali from Buddhist and Advaita illusionists is only on this point, of *prakriti* though renounced continuing in the same old ways for the deluded, it is fair to say he shares their perspective in the crucial point of denigrating normal life. Yoga practice would have no social value, or negative social value, in the loss of an individual to our collective enterprises and culture. Note too that the highest self in Advaita Vedanta seems hardly different from Patanjali's *purusha*, since on both theories there is in enlightenment no awareness of anything other than bliss and self-consciousness.

But, to review, the main problem is that the self does not act on Patanjali's view. Power of will is stripped from consciousness. In accordance with the conception of *kaivalya* and its monolithic value, power is not just renounced but banished as never ever a part of the self. But note that far and away the greater part of the *YS* concerns self-determination, i.e., yogic transformations of body, life, and mind, not just achievement of the highest trance. Indeed, interpreting self-absorbed trance, *asamprajnata samadhi*, as itself a power or a capacity that an accomplished yogin would have, the self-determination thesis can be seen to subsume Patanjali's interest. I repeat that practically a fourth of the text is expressly concerned with *siddhi*s. The power of trance is another *siddhi*.

Finally, let us look at a telling bit of metaphysical reasoning in the *YS*. Quandary occurs about how it could be that the self who practices yoga is not the self who benefits (the former being the illusory image of "self" in nature, the latter the self as it is "in itself," *sva-rupa*). The problem is ingeniously resolved in the proposal (*YS* 2.21) that nature, *prakriti*, is in the service of *purusha*. Nature practices yoga for the purpose of the self's release. Thus nature is teleological; yoga practices serve her highest goal, purification, "sattvafication" of the body, life, and mind, so that the true person, *purusha*, can recover self-awareness and remain forever self-absorbed. However, the idea that not the conscious individual but unconscious matter does anything (including yoga practices) is entirely counterintuitive. Patently it seems proposed out of a sense of system.[25] For *we* practice yoga, not a body, life, or mind mechanically conceived in the fashion of *YS*'s *prakriti*.

In the awakening of chakric centers and other occult phenomena, some yoga teaching has it that we have to wait for a higher part of ourselves that we do not control to take the action for which a person has by yoga practice become "fit" (*adhikari*). In *bhakti yoga* teaching as well as in tantra, we as the yoga practitioners become receivers or objects (as in the expression "*object* of love"). But in such processes of self-integration, clearly what we do counts. We make ourselves fit receptacles of "grace," "shakti," "divine energy," or something else occult. Even the largely theistic Yoga to which these ideas belong is not fatalistic. To be sure, almost all Yoga embraces karma as a causal and moral principle. But karma is misinterpreted as a fatalistic doctrine, as will be shown.

In the final analysis, metaphysics is not Patanjali's talent. As should become ever more plain as we continue, the *YS*'s value lies in its psychological and practice concepts, which can be extracted out of a flawed metaphysics of *kaivalya*.

Fortunately, in classical India and elsewhere hardly all Yoga metaphysics—in our sense—is in accord with the *YS*'s extremism.[26] There are other world-denying views of a supreme good, but, speaking roughly, there occurs a shift in both Hinduism and Buddhism from a world-denying model of enlightenment to a world-affirming one. This is the "tantric turn." It is nicely exemplified in the Buddhist doctrine of the bodhisattva. The saint refuses dissolution of personality in the ultimate bliss of nirvana, that is to say, refuses to enter that utterly transcendent state of consciousness, in order to become instead perfectly embodied and thus a perfect vehicle of compassion. The bodhisattva's six signs, six "perfections" (*paramita*)—generosity, uprightness, energy (joyous effort), patience, concentration, and wisdom—are qualities that make him or her capable of helping everyone achieve the highest good.

A similar idea is present in the *karma yoga* teaching of the *Bhagavad Gita* (elaborated in the third section of chapter 3 and in appendix B). World-affirming Yoga philosophies are hardly rare. In the long history of classical metaphysics in India, Vedantins, Buddhists, Jainas, Tantrics, and others all incorporate yoga practices into life-affirming views that propose different goals than the *YS*'s.

Let us take stock. All Yoga philosophy—and here I include Advaita and theistic Vedanta, Patanjali's dualism, Buddhist philosophies and traditions, etc., practically all the spiritual philosophies of the East sees mind and matter in a dependence relationship that is the reverse of that touted by materialism. Yoga is thus "dualist" by current standards and mainstream sensibilities within academic philosophy. Consciousness comes first in Yoga theory. There are of course interesting details in the different ways mental and bodily phenomena are identified—by Buddhists, tantrics, etc.—some of which we shall look at closely in subsequent sections. But a central commitment in all the views is that consciousness transcends matter, so it need not depend on it. (Not everything is material.) Then in practically all the views, including the dominant strain in the *YS*, it is claimed additionally that consciousness has the power to shape and determine its physical and other embodiments, to control and transform the body, the mind, and the emotions, by the direct action of yoga practices, without external technology, gas engines, electricity, and the like, working on ourselves only.

Yoga asanas, for example, are premised on the power of the mind, or consciousness, to change the body through better connection with *prana,* our breath and life energies, to make it a more supple and reliable instrument. Other yoga practices are to be responsible for changes of consciousness, self-discovery, self-acceptance, and better psychological as well as physical health. Taking aspirin or another drug may relieve a headache, but yoga practices can do the same trick and, more importantly, teach a person how to prevent the affliction in the first place. Physically and mentally therapeutic, the practices are becoming widely embraced by individuals and also in programs of preventive medicine (funded by profit-wise HMOs). Indeed, the practices are fast becoming part of a global culture, no longer restricted to ashrams and meditation halls. The reason, broadly, is that they promote well-being. An adequate Yoga philosophy should explain why this is so—a positive consideration that, it may be argued, pushes Yoga past dualism. This is the topic of the next section. First, I sum up the extent of Yoga's dualist commitment.

Yoga dualism need not be a (Cartesian) division of substances. All that is required is that there be distinctively mental entities and properties such as a self or selves, and not only brains and other material things. In Western terms, Yoga dualism finds its best ally, in my estimation, not in Descartes but in David Hume (1711–76), whose metaphysical minimalism has it that recognizing correlations is theory enough. In classical Indian philosophy, a similar stance is taken by both Buddhists and Nyaya philosophers. Nyaya in particular has what is called a Humean position about causality: we know only *that* entities are related causally (through observation of concurrence), not *why* they are.

Nyaya is not only dualist in the sense of countenancing mental entities, including a self, but also pluralist, finding nine types of property bearer and several types of property as ontological items. An awareness is a psychological property, for example, distinct from physical properties such as colors and shapes that belong to rocks and other things that are made of material atoms. The main point is that Nyaya philosophers formulate causal principles on the basis of correlations without bias about the sorts of things that can be correlated.

For example, sensory connection with an object *a* that possesses a property F is found to be a cause—in the sense of a necessary condition—of a veridical and reliable perceptual awareness with F*a* as its object. An induction is made relating mental entities, e.g., perceptions of such a type, and physical entities, the F-possessing objects that come to be in sensory connection. Correlations are made, similarly, between efforts (which, being goal directed, presuppose cognition) with propositional content and certain physical, i.e., bodily, acts.

Thus Nyaya has an ingenious strategy for the mind-body connection following the motto, "Look for correlations, but don't overinterpret. Be economical." There are causal continuities and processes involving entities that are physical and mental, in one direction through the operation of the sense organs and in the other in guiding action. There is also a third type of cognitive causal relationship, a kind of mind/mind causation exhibited in the causality obtaining between two successive cognitions. This is, by the way, important for meditative accomplishment, according to the *YS* and commentaries, since one wants to be able to battle the firings of distracting *samskara,* subliminal dispositions to desire and remembering, and *maintain* a quiet mind.[27]

A standard objection against Western varieties of dualist interactionism is that they leave the interaction unexplained. Nothing is said about how it is possible that things of such disparate natures interact. Yet to my mind this is a strength. As a philosopher, I can live with Nyaya's Humean skeptical dualism. The mental-physical correlations indicative of yoga progress—"You do this (the mental cause) and that is gained (the physical or mental effect)"—are, I believe, sufficient paradigm for the sorts of research to be encouraged by Yoga theory, if not also for individual pursuits. I shall look at more expansive opinions in the next section.

On the classical Indian scene, there were others who saw intellectual restraint as a strength. The intellectual openness of Advaita Vedanta, the compatibility of Advaita with science, has already been reviewed. There is in Buddhist philosophy a similar position about nirvana and the "emptiness" taken to be revealed in nirvana experience. On these views, which also endorse yoga, we do not know the fundamental nature of the connections of the world and consciousness. The Buddhist Nagarjuna (c. 150 C.E.) is famous for taking a skeptical stance, and interesting discussion of the limitations of mentality occurs in classical sources as well as in a now rather rich secondary literature.[28]

Some great names of Yoga's past—Patanjali, Shankara, and Nagarjuna—may have no interest in Yoga's self-determination thesis (at least as thinkers, as opposed to—wearing different hats—yoga masters teaching practical principles). To try to connect intellectually the world to consciousness through an understanding of powers (*siddhi*s) that flow from its nature as self is to trespass on the unknowable, according to them. But how, then, can so much be known about the unknowable? Our Yoga minimalism avoids such intellectual hubris.[29]

Nevertheless, I can see that a combination of spiritual mysterianism with the Nyaya/Humean causal minimalism may be the path of wisdom: at least there would be room for mental causation and the reverse correlations identified in Yoga psychology, the dependences of body and mind on consciousness. In the context of Yoga, the Nyaya/Humean strategy encourages paying attention to mental causation. This is perhaps the crucial result, potentially the most concrete ramification of the needed shift away from a materialist paradigm for psychological research. Note that, historically, anti-intellectual Advaita and Buddhism have not only encouraged yoga practice but have also maintained a view of rebirth, although it is not any true self that reincarnates, only a karmic aggregate.

Yogic Control and Integration: Spiritual Holism

The dualism just sketched has the merit of protecting philosophers from embarrassment when they try to say something substantial on the relation of consciousness and matter. But more, I think, needs to be said with respect to Yoga's self-determination thesis, at least about the nature of yogic self-monitoring consciousness and about how consciousness can be a cause of physical effects. What is it about consciousness and its embodiments that makes self-determination possible? As pointed out, Yoga philosophy is committed to dependences that run from mind to matter. It should also embrace, I shall argue in chapter 4, karmic continuities of individual identity that stretch past an individual lifetime. (In the context of previous Yoga philosophy, this is hardly a shocking thesis.) Karma is an inheritance of past choices that extends before birth and after death, determining talents and traits in future embodiments as well as in the current lifetime. Emotions affect health, and self-monitoring consciousness leads to wellness, et cetera.

So what makes all this possible, what illumines these mental dependences? And what in general do proponents of Yoga have to say about the metaphysics of self-determination? First note that much has been said, in India and elsewhere, usually in attempts to see the entire world as in some way the result of consciousness. We find self-determination writ large as the dominant theme of whole schools and philosophic movements.

In world-affirming Yoga philosophies, self-determination is tied up with spiritual holism. In the Upanishads, the One, the Absolute, the mystery of Being and Self called Brahman, unites everything. World-affirming Vedanta finds Brahman's consciousness, will, and reality extending everywhere. Or, as in Buddhist philosophy, every event is interconnected, arising interdependently, *pratitya-samutpada,* as claimed by Nagarjuna and practically the whole Mahayana camp. Spiritual holism is key, furthermore, to the interpretation of several important yogic phenomena. That this kind of holism has close ties with Yoga's self-determination thesis will be shown.

I should like to focus on phenomena of psychic integration and their implications for Yoga philosophy. This is admittedly countercurrent, being practically ignored by the entire mind-body industry. But spiritual explanations about ways matter depends on mind are our launching pad. A good example is visualization, e.g., of healthy tissue where there is damaged tissue. This helps it to heal. The consciousness factors of concentration and the summoning up of a healthy image have been shown to correlate with an increase in healing rate.[30] A benefit of Yoga philosophy is being to able to see why this is true. If a person does not believe in the power of a practice, she is unlikely to take it up. An explanation that the self and its attention are intrinsically sacred, healthy, or pure, with the power to pull or attract the body back to its normal state through the exercise is, for example, one way she might be encouraged to extend effort.

Yogic phenomena such as the healing power of visualization—which are special instances of the wellness making of yogic self-monitoring consciousness—suggest holism as well as self-determination in our sense. But many common activities and experiences illustrate the general thesis of self-determination. We don't really need yogic phenomena to show its truth; any voluntary action will do. Just because this is such a wide class, and walking, talking, etc., are so taken for granted, perhaps more useful polemically are extraordinary illustrations of ways matter depends on mind.[31]

Yogic practices and the capacities that are developed by yoga exaggerate or augment everyday dependences that we all know firsthand. For, yoga or no yoga, it seems practically *a priori* that the power of human consciousness is responsible for much of what is human. Yoga metaphysics is a matter of trying to stretch this insight (an asana for the mind) in consonance with the fact that yoga practices show that consciousness could be responsible for more. Bringing the formerly involuntary within the range first of awareness and then of will and control, making it voluntary with awareness and supple, aligned, and healthy, as, for example, with *pranayama,* breath control, is a fundamental Yoga principle. It bears repeating that a good Yoga philosophy would encourage yoga practices by explaining how a reverse dependence is possible (body on mind, or, better, body and mind on consciousness) and why it is good.

One answer is sattvafication, the answer of the *Yoga Sutra:* purification of the nature so that the self can know itself as it really is, namely, separate from nature. This is the *YS*'s theory.[32] Nature is teleological, serving, as Patanjali says, the purpose of the *purusha.*

A different answer connects consciousness with its body or bodies and with nature outside itself. Here the point of yoga is not separation but connection, and consciousness is not in reality separate from everything else but connected, at least potentially. Yoga practices integrate mind, life, body, and whatever spiritual parts we have. Yogic self-monitoring consciousness can be expansive, encompassing all our parts. If this is right, Yoga philosophy should reveal the underpinnings of yogic integration. Consonantly with such holistic phenomena, Yoga philosophy should target connectedness and integration. Thus is there "bottom-up" motivation for a holistic theory showing the possibility of connectedness among parts of ourselves.

There is also a rich inheritance of theory. I propose to examine some of the ideative resources out of which our own holistic Yoga may come. We shall have to be selective, since among spiritual-holism-friendly philosophies are both pantheisms of the West and a broad range of monistic Eastern views, mainly Indian in origin but also Chinese, notably Daoism. This necessary narrowness is unfortunate, for Yoga's alliances are strong. There is also Neoplatonism, Whiteheadean process philosophy, and other views that, though allied in substance with Yoga, cannot be paraded in full dress.[33]

There is good reason, however, to focus on holistic Vedanta. Upanishadic theists can boast of having advocated yoga practices for more than twenty-five centuries, and the Upanishads are Yoga's earliest texts. Holistic theists who hold that the world is the body of God are also important interpreters of the *YS* and other yoga manuals such as the *Bhagavad Gita*. In comparison, a more diminutive holism is recommendable for us, a spiritual holism that stresses large conscious units but perhaps not so large as the Vedantic Brahman. In other words, I plan, after reviewing the full-blown explanations of Vedantic holists, who are theists, to recommend a pared-down version, an open-ended spiritual holism, as our own Yoga philosophy.

Vedantic theism asserts self-determination to be the fundamental relationship between consciousness and matter, God's *maya* (from the root *ma*, to measure or delimit, thus not illusion, as with Advaita), Brahman's making for itself a body in the physical universe.[34] The central theoretic constraint is the antecedent nature of Brahman. This guarantees that everything is interrelated in the self-determinations that create and maintain the universe. Although we have freedom of choice, God's self-monitoring consciousness embraces us and the entire universe. The view is a maximalist theism, which we might for a moment contrast with the minimalist variety endorsed by Nyaya.

Maximalist Vedantic theism is like Platonism in the hands of early Western theists such as Philo and Augustine. In the Indian version, yogic self-integration proceeds from the top, from our big-brother self seeking out us the junior member, the lower brought from above into union, or at least unison and harmony, with a higher self. Nyaya, in contrast, would not presume such a determinate reading, and would reject the idea that such "union" is even possible. Nevertheless, for Nyaya the true self of each of us is—though not God, the *ishvara*—much, much greater than we ordinarily take ourselves to be, the mere living body with a name (see chapters 4 and 5). Each of us is in part a self that is eternal, capable of an unending series of incarnations as well of *moksha*, liberation, which according to much yogic testimony is the supreme personal good. This is hardly a minimalist position. But let us focus on Nyaya's theology, which is clearly a lot more minimal than Vedanta's.

Later Nyaya philosophers infer the existence of God by a causal argument: God is the agent who has brought about things like the earth. But just as Nyaya does not speculate on what makes it possible for mental and physical events to stand as causal factors one for the other, so the school refuses to speculate on the connection between God and the things that, directly or indirectly, God brings about. To be sure, in consonance with the inference to God, Nyaya philosophers attribute omniscience to God as a property needed to bring about the effects whose explanation motivates the positing of an *ishvara*. But the policy is not to specify the nature of a postulated cause more than is required by the explanatory task. Thus Nyaya spokesmen tend not to elaborate, not to speculate on God's nature, and leave it to faith to connect the God required by philosophy to the richer conceptions of revealed traditions.

Theistic Vedantins, in contrast, from Yamuna (c. 700) through tantrics and neo-Vedantins such as Aurobindo (1872–1950), begin with the assumption that the reality of Brahman explains many important details within the worldly display (*prapancha*). For example, emotions are forms of God's delight, *ananda,* flavors or *rasa* enjoyed by Brahman as well as by us, worldly manifestations of an intrinsic nature that is beyond the manifest universe. In this way, theistic Vedantins turn around the materialists' relation of explanans and explanandum: the body is what is to be explained and the nature of consciousness, or Brahman, does the explaining.

Holism is a distinctive feature of Vedantic theism, equivalent to Brahman's all-inclusiveness. How can Brahman become matter? Well, Brahman can do whatever is possible, and what is possible is fixed by what is compatible with Brahman's nature, which Brahman cannot surrender. This guarantees that nothing can lie outside God, that everything is tied up with everything else in being Brahman: *sarvam idam brahma* ("All this is the Brahman").[35]

Brahman's being matter would explain, at the high end, how it is possible that we who are material beings can know ourselves immediately, self-illuminingly, as taught in Advaita and Buddhism. At the low end, it would explain how there can be sensory connections as well as physical transmissions of mental traits. Though it is hard to say how the view would tie up with biology and chemistry, perhaps the holism of Brahman would help explain the emergence of integrated entities that are distinct from aggregates. Biology may eschew final causes in the Aristotelian sense, but the most conservative science recognizes principles of unification that are, let us say, holism-friendly. Water, for example, is a new thing, not anticipated in hydrogen and oxygen atoms. The same is all the more true of organisms. Parts are not pieces. In sum, since matter on this view would be Brahman, material forms can be conscious as well as vehicles of mental determinations and all the emergent phenomena that make up our macro world.

A primary teaching of the *YS* is that through *samyama*, control through conscious identification, instanced in the control we have over our own body's limbs, we can expand the sphere of things subject to volition, as in *pranayama*. Such *siddhi*s as an athlete's being in the zone or (to give just one of the many examples listed in the *YS*) provoking friendship in one's environment through practice of *ahimsa*, nonharmfulness, all seem to flow from *samyama* (friendliness is said to flow from mastery of *ahimsa* at *YS* 2.35). "From *samyama* on X comes *siddhi* Y" is the form of sutras throughout chapter 3. We might also mention craftsmanship and linguistic ability, which are developed through training, through conscious attention to what the Vedantin sees as an extension of the self to mastery of tools as well as of our own bodies and minds. ("Yoga is skill in works," says the *Gita*, *yogah karmasu kaushalam*, 2.50.) Vedantic holism is not shy about the power of yoga, although classically the view is that yoga has to give way to *bhakti* and to receptivity to the action of a higher self.[36]

The problem with theism, whether Vedantic or a Western variety, the conceptual difficulty that above all others has exercised philosophers and motivated atheism, is evil. How, given a loving Creator, can there be such suffering as we witness? It is notoriously difficult to explain evil in all its varieties on theistic premises. This holds true, it seems, even on those views where God is both our highest self and material energy—or perhaps especially on those premises. Personally, I do not think a Vedantic theodicy, a theistic explanation of evil, is beyond reach. A theodicy stressing karma and social justice is broached in the *Bhagavad Gita*, and will be examined in chapter 3. But for present purposes, I wish to take it for granted that it is not easy to explain, e.g., a child's suffering, on the premise that God, or Brahman, is perfect. Appreciating the difficulty helps to motivate a more modest holism and a Yoga philosophy that presents less of a target.

A second motivation for a pared-down holism is Yoga diversity, the plurality of views put forth traditionally to interpret yoga practices and experiences. Minimalism identifies a common core that can be asserted without dispute. The Jaina way of handling diversity while remaining inclusivist will be examined in connection with the ethical teaching of *ahimsa*, nonharmfulness, in chapter 3. This is to adopt the perspectivalism and spiritual relativism called nonabsolutism (*anekanta-vada*). The Jaina view has much in common with a minimalism about to be laid out, since it is a positive perspectivalism that tries to find a grain of truth in every theory—a kind of intellectual *ahimsa* disarming metaphysical contentiousness.

Our nonsystematic or bottom-up version of spiritual holism emphasizes, like theistic Vedanta, possibilities of integration and self-determination not for God but for us. Or, if for God, then that's okay too, in consonance with, though exceeding, our theory. The byword is integration.

In yoga practice, we learn that a little effort at breath control or mental silence produces a feeling of harmony and by objective measures better health. There seems to be a continuum related to the power of consciousness to integrate something into itself, from intuition, thought, desire, and the like at one extreme to the body at the other. There are also the phenomena of surrendering to, in the process of joining, a higher or deeper self. It is difficult to know the limits of this, but the spirit of our bottom-up approach is not to make absolutely fixed pronouncements but to sketch out possibilities to help us believe in ourselves.

Nevertheless, just about everywhere we look we find encouraging analogies. Holism in linguistics stresses a series of significant units whose significance depends upon interrelations among components, the unity of letters in a word, of words in a sentence, and of relevant combinations of sentences in an act of speech. In environmental science, there is species interdependence; in economics, convergence of standard of living through open markets and free trade. Holism about the self in Western philosophy (an example is Plato's tripartite theory[37]), like Yoga, stresses potential harmony among the parts of the being, physical, emotional, and mental. Yoga would add to the list (beyond Plato) the self's spiritual side. But whatever its precise metaphysical theses, Yoga is a philosophy that encourages psychological harmony and transformation directed to greater integration and harmony from the inside.

So I propose that Yoga entertain a position on the mind-body relation similar to what is called neutral monism, in the coinage used to capture the position of William James that the single stuff there is is intrinsically capable of both mental and physical properties.[38] Beyond James, we would see at least in certain units (if not in everything) the disposition further to unify and form complexes with emergent properties that are not explained solely by the constituent parts. This principle could be held to apply even to God, who, like Krishna on some Vaishnava accounts, would seek out souls as much as being sought out by them in *bhakti*. In a less minimal version of metaphysical holism, the view might try to connect with biology, chemistry, and physics by proposing that consciousness emerges from an integration of coarse and subtle elements, from influences ranging from the biological and physical to the cultural and spiritual (*adhyatmika*).

But whether or not we try to reframe science, individual life forms are complex unities, and self-determining human beings are capable of mental and emotional unifications that transcend an individual life. These would be, for instance, unifications with cultural traditions, political movements, and so on, including, through yoga, as taught in the Upanishads, a self that survives death and, normally, reincarnates. Let me dub this view minimalist spiritual holism, or New Yoga for short. In this approach, precisely how high in ascending levels of subjectivity (seventeen, as taught in some forms of tantric Shaivism?) integration might proceed need not be specified.

The strength of dualistic interactionism—upholding of mental causation—is shared by New Yoga. But also it has no quarrel with the thesis that physical events can be causal factors for mental events—the misunderstood truth of materialism. Our position would encourage both brain science and mind-body research in the reverse direction.

The best evidence for all this is the human body and its health. Yogic practices harmonize our parts, thoughts, desires, emotions, breath, self-awareness, and bodily movements, and the result is both a great sense of wellness and its reality. For metaphysical holism, there are also ecology and species interdependences and other considerations that, as suggested, provide buttressing. Everything we do helps to create a new self or person and reverberates throughout the environment.

Unlike materialism, even such minimalist holism as this is not a value-free metaphysics eschewing every kind of final cause. The purposes of human beings both pack causal power and are unifying at a high end, and spiritual unifications in yoga suggest ever greater marvels of complex unities of consciousness. At the low end, our nonsystematic holism would promote hypotheses like that—already suggested by philosophers mindful of the weaknesses of materialism—of a physical-(proto) conscious stuff poised to form unities in atoms, molecules, and indeed organisms.[39]

Everything may be tightly unified in the fashion of the systematic self-determinationism of theistic Vedanta, but the Yoga sketched here is compatible with nontheistic positions, such as the Buddhist and the Jaina. I repeat that whether there is an upper limit to unification need not be decided. We need enough theory to encourage self-development but not so much that we would be required to solve theism's problem of evil or to dictate to physics and biology. And there is at least a grain of truth, it seems to me, in the mysterian view, both the Advaita and materialist versions. The dualism of Nyaya may be all that is defensible philosophically, with "over-beliefs" strictly a matter of faith (but more about this below). At the heart of Yoga is commitment to two-directional causation, possibilities of self-development, and, I should like to add, ecological responsibility (this flows from a right understanding of karma, I shall argue). But beyond providing a useful framework for yogic practices, Yoga need not take a position, at least not inflexibly, on the question of God, Brahman, the Dao, and so on. Yoga philosophy is not theology, and is not an end in itself but is subservient to self-development.[40]

Finally, the difficult question of compatibility with richer systems of religious and spiritual conviction. Just now I mentioned "over-beliefs"—the coinage belongs to William James, who addresses the issue in the great classic, *The Varieties of Religious Experience*.[41] The American pragmatist distrusted what he characterized as the excessively theoretical, grandiose statements of traditional theology and indeed religious institutions. But he found in mysticism and the religious life of individuals much to recommend. He identified a tiny core of justifiable religious doctrine, and encouraged his audience to enlarge upon it insofar as such "over-belief" contributed to an individual's unique inner life.[42] James's philosophic insight is that one knows about one's own over-beliefs that they are not to be displayed in company, that they are idiosyncratic and not publicly justified or justifiable. But James also felt that with this self-consciousness a belief in divine providence, for example, could be important and entirely within a person's rights epistemically.

Should something similar be our attitude to explanations of mind-body relations? Well, no! There are levels of theory. Yogic principles based on mind-body correlations are a middle level of theory, and some are quite concrete and warranted. There is an ideal governing the ways, for example, we work at Downward Dog, *adho-mukha shvanasana*. But that can be interpreted in accord with a range of metaphysical theories. This is the central point. James, in contrast, is talking about the question of God, Brahman, etc., about which Yoga makes no final statement. Alternatively, there is, as mentioned, the Jaina spiritual relativism, which may endorse statements about God, Brahman, and so on, but in full realization that they are justified only "from a perspective" (*naya:* see the end of the second section of chapter 3), that they do not get the highest rating of epistemic confidence.

Particular teachers of yoga—and, more broadly, of spiritual discipline—have framed yogic correlations in widely different terms. What is significant, however, for our purposes is the agreement. Though theologically opposed, Hindus, Buddhists, Jainas, Sikhs, Christians (witness the "prayer of quiet" of Saint Teresa[43]), Muslims, and modern gurus of programs of holistic health proclaim many of the same laws of self-development. My view is that what's really important is to know the psychological rules, the principles governing the yogic *bandha*s, for example, or the opening of chakras as well as the more common practices of asana and breath control. The occult psychological teachings do require a little Yoga metaphysics, but just a little.

To be sure, certain yoga practices have a belief component, or practice intentionality, directed to God—to Shiva, the Divine Mother, Ram, Tara, the Creator, Dao, the Supreme Self, etc. I take it that *bhakti yoga* would not be possible without such intentionality (*vishayata* in Sanskrit, objecthood), directionality of consciousness toward a supreme being. Surely reports of the sacred entering life through yoga are to be taken seriously. To someone steeped in *bhakti,* to recommend a strategy of Jamesean over-belief for the purpose of philosophic legitimacy may seem glibly dismissive. To such sentiment I say that this book is not dismissive by any means, although I do wish to put off most of the discussion of *bhakti* until chapter 5 (but at the end of chapter 3 a theodicy is presented). For the present, only a single observation will have to do, which, though apparently negative, is offered in a (yogic) spirit of intellectual self-discipline.

If the goal of *bhakti* is intimate relation with an unknown *amorant,* a "lover" in an occult but sensuous sense, then who cares about the precise theory of the relationship? Rupa Gosvami (c. 1550) and others in the Vaishnava *bhakti* movement do provide some theory, as we shall see in the final section of chapter 5 on the "spark soul." But it seems to me that all we need is a rough idea and a sense of connectedness to something larger than ourselves whom we can trust to see us through life and death.

Here we find motivation to explore Yogic occult physiology, as we shall in chapters 4 and 5. But here we also find a side of the widespread Hindu doctrine of the *ishta devata,* preferred divinity, that encourages one to worship the god or goddess of her choice. The exaggerated epithets in hymns and poetry can be just that, to wit, appropriate to the medium, and need not be transplanted to philosophy. That the Advaitin Shankara wrote moving *bhakti* poetry makes the case. God belongs to the world of *maya* (illusion), according to the same author when wearing his philosopher's *dhoti.*[44]

Does, then, *bhakti* require that we compromise our best awareness in metaphysics? Clearly not. Buddhists have long differentiated the mindset of disputational philosophy from that of devotion and worship, endorsing both as kinds of yoga.[45] It may well be that it is a better use of time to dance and sing than to argue. Philosophy is notoriously dry, sans *rasa.* But this is then all the more reason not to insist disputationally that others see one's own preferred divinity, *ishta devata,* as the Creator or the one savior.

In *bhakti* something special is known, and the *gopi*s (cowgirls beloved of Krishna), like everyone else in their sandals, are proud of being loved by the Lord. It is interesting that in the *Bhagavata Purana,* when out of pride they become boastful and boistrous, Krishna departs.[46] In both West and East, there are respectable traditions of fideism, operating on the assumption that faith and philosophy are different. In the second section of chapter 5, I shall develop the idea of the indirect spiritual link as key to the thesis that a general idea of God supporting *bhakti* requires only the notion of a mediated relationship. That which stands at the far end of the *bhakti* attitude may remain open-ended conceptually, though at the near end we have intimacy.

The bottom line for us, then, is a dualism in the Nyaya/Humean fashion and the irreducibility of self and consciousness as follows from the truth of the self-determination thesis, and, a little beyond that, minimalist spiritual holism as sketched. Such is the *siddhanta* of New Yoga. Further, given the main lines of previous Yoga philosophy, I feel we should practice thinking about the connections of mind and matter in a more expansive, spiritually monist fashion—all is Brahman, Dao, empty, interdependent. Such an exercise informs but need not determine the position we take. As a Yoga philosopher, I will settle for, in addition to dualist theses about the nonmaterial reality of self and consciousness, a minimal version of spiritual holism. The self can integrate instruments into itself, and there is a continuum in the degree of responsiveness and assimilability among subjectivities, perhaps (*syat*) all the way up to the Absolute. Alternatively, let us embrace a philosophy of the One but in full realization that it is "from a perspective" and not to any high degree objectively warranted.

Such a position may not be inspirational, especially in the couched terms in which it is expressed, but Yoga philosophy need not be carried by rapturous speculation. The practices of yoga promote mental quiet and control, and it seems noisy to insist on the One becoming the Many. In yoga, we want harmony and integration into the highest consciousness to which we have access. Whether that be God, Brahman, emptiness, Dao, or only some larger, more conscious self or continuum—our secret soul, perhaps, that which survives death and reincarnates—need not be decided right now. Though holists in spirit, we are also inclusivists and therefore minimalists (spiritual relativism, as in Jainism, is another option for inclusivists). Such minimalism does not mean that we cannot follow metaphysical flights of imagination sympathetically, as the Jainas teach. Above all, it means that we do not have prejudice against finding chakras in ourselves or other phenomena or pathways relating us to nonphysical beings or forces, especially, we may note, the grace of the theists. Indeed, according to all Yoga philosophy the point is to be open from the bottom up, psychologically or yogically and, I should say, also intellectually as thinkers. So, beyond resistance to reductive materialism and insistence on baseline value for the powers of consciousness, it seems right to have the attitude of the explorer and not the advocate when it comes to the so-called ultimate questions. New Yoga is practice-oriented and faith-neutral.

3
Karma

Dispositions

Despite a widespread interpretation of "karma" as a kind of fatalism, just the opposite is at the heart of the notion: conscious shaping of natural desire, moral responsibility, and freedom. Karma (*karman* in Sanskrit) is a rich concept, having ramifications for ethics, epistemology, and philosophical psychology as well as metaphysics, according to practically all the schools of classical India. Through Buddhism, karma theory is also developed in Tibetan and Chinese philosophy. For our contemporary Yoga, the sense of "karma" in "karma yoga," the yoga of action, is particularly important, since it is central to the *Gita* and other early yogic texts. Karma yoga is the topic of the third section of this chapter. First, I shall pursue the idea's causal and cognitive sides in the broad terms of philosophic psychology. The *Yoga Sutra,* for one, shows less concern for the ethics of karma than for the psychological underpinnings of karma in dispositions, *samskara.*

In the second section, I turn to karma's ethical dimension, looking at karma theory within the context of what philosophers call virtue ethics and the problem of self-development—including yoga practice—which is only one of several duties. Separate duties may possibly conflict. However, in the classical karma teaching, ethical push (What's in it for me to be moral?) is said to converge with ethical pull (What is it about others that makes them worthy of moral treatment?), in that one has special responsibility for and to one's future self. This is perhaps the most important dimension of the karma concept. The best possibility, it is said, is to become an *ahimsika,* one who practices *ahimsa,* nonharmfulness. This is viewed as the highest virtue/duty on some Yoga theories, or as presupposed in what is best and central, as in the Buddhist extolling of compassion and friendliness (*karuna* and *maitri*).

The third section takes up the karma yoga teaching of the *Gita* and its call to disinterested action, and begins to look more closely at the social dimension of karma teaching. In the fourth and final section, karma and rebirth are reviewed as doctrines of moral justice, along with the theistic view that uses them to defend the notion of God's benevolence in the face of evil.

All four sections of the chapter are concerned with the best presentations of karma theory among Yoga philosophers—and indeed try to improve upon them—not with comic-book ideas prevalent in popular culture.[1]

The word *karman* in Sanskrit has multiple meanings. The most basic is action, anything that we do. Ritual action or sacrifice is a second, narrower usage that is picked up in the *Gita*'s karma yoga teaching, as will be explained. For the moment, let us ignore the *Gita*'s sense to focus on the third, habit, broadly understood, probably the most important meaning for Yoga.

Everything we do creates habits. Our karma is comprised of the habits we have acquired. Habits condition desires. We act in certain ways with expectations of the normal fruits. Now desires may be by nature, occurring willy-nilly (though Buddhists, for one, tend to deny that anything is willy-nilly). Habits, however, clearly are our own responsibility, or our culture's,[2] which we assimilate, or not, as individuals. Though habits shape future action, we create them in part through current choice and enactment. We endorse desires and their expressions through choice, making or reaffirming habitual patterns. Karma in the sense of the habits we have acquired determines what we are prone to do. We can make new karma, or new bits of karma, in changing what we are prone to do.

Nevertheless, as used in Yogic texts, Sanskrit *karman* is not the equivalent of "habit" as used in English. *Karman* is, at least in some usages, a collective noun, like "water" in English. We can say that there is a sum total around a single soul or person of bits of karma, and speak of someone's karma as a whole. Unfortunately for translators, we cannot say the same of a person's habits. (The sum of a person's habits could be called her character.) The words "habits" and "karma" are therefore not synonyms. For habits necessarily individuate, like rivers or ruts.

I propose, then, to use "karma" as an English word. Indeed, "karma" *is* an English word, long ago anglicized. In our usage, karma can be spoken of as a generalized line of action ("Murder is bad karma"), but, as mentioned, it can also be summed up. The moral worth of karma both aggregates like buckets of water poured into a tub and individuates with respect to certain acts; for example, a single act of murder has its own karmic repercussions, no matter how good the overall score.[3] The "moral payback" dimension of the theory to be examined in the third and fourth sections relies on both aspects. A particular rebirth depends on the aggregate, according to the mainstream theories, but there are also individual lines of karma, i.e., habits, that are said to continue. It is held that some become so deeply entrenched that they reemerge in the next birth as talents or deep dispositions, as will be discussed. The soul is not a *tabula rasa,* according to Yoga.

A person's habits are maintained subconsciously—Yoga theorists are largely in accord here—through things called traces or dispositions, *samskara,* more literally, that which makes fit, a being-preparedness. These are in part, though not entirely, conditional formulas impressed on the mind or even the brain—let us leave open for the moment their precise location (in the body or bodies we inhabit simultaneously, physical, pranic, mental, etc., according to Vedantic and tantric psychology).

In the simple conception of the *Yoga Sutra* (*YS*), formulas shape "mind-stuff," *chitta,* which also has a vital side,[4] to constitute *samskara.* In other words, mental dispositions have both a mental and a pranic or vital side—the latter an energy vector or coloring characterized as "sattvic," "rajasic," and/or "tamasic," the modes or *gunas* of the psychology of the *YS* as well as of the *Gita* and other texts. The three words represent the traditional theory of natural "strands" of which mind-stuff is composed: *sattva,* intelligence and clarity, *rajas,* passion and energy, and *tamas,* obscurity and inertia. This is a universal and natural inheritance. Specific formations are determined by choice and practice.

Other schools build on these ideas. In Nyaya, for instance, not all *samskara* are psychological. Something with elasticity or impetus, for example, a falling rock, is said to possess *samskara* as a physical property, something like potential energy.[5] Psychological *samskara,* like those that have only physical effects, are not perceived, at least not normally perceived, but rather posited to explain things perceived, like the measles virus that was postulated to explain measles long before it was microscopically identified. These mental dispositions, sometimes called traces or impressions, constitute the subconscious vehicles of karma and are considered causal factors for a range of psychological phenomena, including remembering and any activity guided by what we have learned. Thus karma includes training, and *samskara* are the dispositions we acquire by learning how to do all the things we do, from speaking to asanas.

According to classical philosophers across schools, mental dispositions are formed by perceptions and other cognitive occurrences, including intentions and efforts to act along with actions. Training involves repetition and a kind of circularity, a disposition required to know what to do and the same disposition reinforced by the doing. For example, writing your name requires memory of the name, and the doing of the writing reinforces the memory. The same goes for our ability to recognize something that we have perceived previously ("This is that Devadatta I saw yesterday" is the stock example in classical texts). Thus *samskara*—a very broad idea in the Sanskrit philosophical lexicon—function to maintain both cognitive continuity and bodily skills.

Though *samskara* are theoretic entities, the theory is nevertheless broadly empiricist, much like the empiricism of David Hume's "impressions."[6] A simple version with respect to cognitive occurrences runs: a perception indicating a tree as as a banyan produces a *samskara* that when aroused helps to bring about a remembering, an effort, or another psychological event with the same indication (a banyan tree). Perception is the premier cognitive link with everything known, according to almost all Yoga traditions; yogic perception is an extraordinary knowledge source nonetheless reliable in connecting us to inner realities (see the third section of chapter 4 on the epistemology of yogic perception). Yoga philosophy is therefore empiricist. But not everything we know is a matter of the immediately given. To know objects around us, *samskara*—mental dispositions—make inference and other modes of knowledge, such as testimony, possible. As indicated, these dispositions are themselves known indirectly (that is, by ordinary folk—some yogins can directly perceive *samskara,* according to the *YS* 3.18 and commentaries) by the knowledge source called postulation (*arthapatti*), according to some. According to others, they are known by inference. Again, they are posited to explain memory, expectation, fulfillment, frustration, and other cognitive continuities. Accordingly, there are many types of mental *samskara*.

Beyond this simple theory—and especially concerning the metaphysics of *samskara*—there is quite a lot of diversity of opinion in classical texts. Buddhists conceive of *samskara* as causal continua,[7] whereas Vedic traditions tend to think of them as marks or relational properties, stamps or impressions resting in the self or soul, or in the *chitta*—in any case, in a substance. But practically all contributors to Yoga philosophy—Patanjali and company, Vedantins, Buddhists, Nyaya philosophers, Jainas, tantrics, and others—theorize about subconscious *samskara*. They form psychological bridgework. Whether it be something in this lifetime or something in a previous lifetime that is being remembered currently, we are not directly aware of the vehicles of remembering, and we do not constantly hold before our minds information acquired in the past. Yet the information is retrievable, like patterns or programs in a computer. Dispositions, *samskara*, comprise the storage bank. Some *samskara* are stored in the physical body, but not all. Otherwise, it would be impossible to remember incidents in previous lifetimes or, indeed, have any kind of karmic continuity from one life to the next.

Such mental dispositions are also considered by most of the classical theorists to be vehicles of desire and impulses to act. Our habits have an affective and motivational side. We are born beings of hunger and thirst, sexual desire, who want to survive, and so on. Often we endorse these basic drives when we act. Yoga teaches that in principle will trumps desire, and Jaina traditions in particular show that a person can commit suicide (i.e., bodily suicide, not elimination of the self) by not eating. The motivational and affective side of the theory is perhaps the most interesting. But let us concentrate a little more first on the cognitive side of *samskara* as presupposed in knowledge and action. Here we may again turn to Nyaya.

Veridical cognitions shape the mental vehicles that guide unhesitating effort and action, action that we expect to be in accord with our desires. A person can be lucky and get what she wants guided by a false belief, but, generally speaking, success requires knowledge and knowledge requires beliefs formed by genuine knowledge sources.[8] For example, a perception of a pot forms a disposition to remember it, which, when triggered in an actual remembering, would prompt—given desire to drink—unhesitating effort and action, to fetch the thing. Thus the notion of justified true belief so central to millennia of Western epistemology has much in common with, in classical Indian philosophy, that of *samskara* formed by veridical cognitions that are the results of knowledge sources, perception, and the rest.[9] Our habits include our beliefs, which are maintained by *samskara*.

Note, furthermore, the importance of *samskara* to explain perceptual illusion (as well as other types of cognitive error), what classical Yoga philosophers call pseudo-perception (pseudo-testimony, etc.). For example, a person apparently sees a snake when the thing in front of him is really a rope. We can imagine that from the subject's own perspective the object seems alive. In other words, that the thing is a snake seems to be given perceptually. But at work would be a *samskara* that under normal conditions would prompt a remembering and in the deviant conditions of perceptual error has fused into the current pseudo-perception a snakehood bit of intentionality. (I use here a philosophic term of art to translate the Sanskrit *vishayata,* which is more literally objecthood.) The person's nonveridical cognition has misplaced intentionality (*vishayata*); it presents something (the rope) not as what it is (a snake).[10] This objecthood, this misplaced intentionality or content comes from *samskara.*

Similarly, people perceive a piece of distant sandalwood as fragrant, having actual sense data of the smell though the wood is too far away for connection with the olfactory organ of the body, located in the nose.[11] Such phenomena show dramatically that the mind can retrieve sensory information and project it into current experience. The process is made possible by *samskara,* which make acquired information available later.

Classical Yoga epistemology is dominated by a causal picture, a view of processes that result in veridical cognition, and *samskara*s are important causal factors. The gods and goddesses perceived yogically, for example, in occult experience are considered realities—Buddhism and Buddhist-influenced texts such as the eleventh-century *Yoga-vashishta* aside—and real contact with them viewed as responsible for the experiences. Similarly, *samskara*s play a role in intentional action, whether in the physical universe or other worlds. Cognitions informed by *samskara*s guide action, and conversely we make *samskara*s by what we do. This holds in general. A common biological inheritance is individuated through karma. According to Nyaya's interactive dualism, we carve out individual selves by choices and intentions to do, including choices made in previous lives. We make our own peculiar habits, which are both good and bad, and include, potentially, dispositions—so Yogic texts emphasize—to practice yoga and, indeed, to maintain the practice into the next lifetime—in the famous soul-making conception of the *Gita* (6.40–45; see appendix B)—if we do not reach the goal in this one.

Yoga theists and tantrics have a picture of self-determination that begins with God's emitting the Goddess (*devi, shri*), who gives birth to and nurtures individual determinations that are, to reverse the image, determinations from the top, that is to say, not the result of karma created by us but divine self-determinations. Shiva lets forth Shakti, who manifests herself as us and all the things of the world. This world picture makes karma less important than it is in—to pick just one school—Mimamsa,

Exegesis, the school most devoted to interpretation of the Vedas and therefore to understanding the fundamental principles of language. Mimamsakas see karma as absolutely central to the constitution of the universe, transcending the gods and the goddesses (there is no single supreme person on this view).

But although dismissive of karma by Mimamsaka lights, the tantric view of divine self-determination has plenty of room for determinations we make. Here the creatrix seems a lot like the logos or divine mind of Western theology, and karma fills in the forms. Instead of everything coming up from below and a conception of common karma of the human species and so forth, on this competing conception, certain patterns—like Plato's Forms—would be imposed from the top.[12]

In the *YS*, Patanjali uses the idea of *samskara* to explain the training whereby one becomes capable of sustaining the deepest trance, which is, according to him, the ultimate goal of yoga practice from a psychological perspective. Patanjali's ideal is of a person who does not lose consciousness while asleep and indeed maintains yogic trance, *samadhi*, at all times. This is only possible through the yogin's having created *samadhi* dispositions (*samskara*) from previous days (and indeed previous lives). Then through the attraction of the dualist metaphysics, Patanjali has these special meditational dispositions not only block other *samskara* firings but also, so to say, burn themselves up, self-destruct, leaving no seed (*YS* 1.51). In other passages, the *YS* says that we have to learn not to trigger *samskara* firings as well as not to be distracted by current firings triggered by whatever cause. This is an important theme throughout the text.[13]

In everyday life, many triggers of projection and memory are ordinarily not under our control. So it is easy to see the logic of Patanjali's teaching. In the *YS*, yoga practices are all about acquiring control, the special concern being control of thought and emotion, with the ability to hold quiet mental chatter. Before moving on to the ethical dimensions of the karma conception, let me fill out a bit further, with respect to *samskara*, the picture in the *YS* of the yogin who has perfect control.

In consonance with his or her learning to hold still all fluctuations of mentality (*chitta-vritti-nirodha, YS* 1.2), a yogin learns to be able to check the firings of *samskara*. However, the checking itself is a conscious act, creating or reinforcing a *samskara* of silence. At some point, a last *samskara* firing fires at itself and burns itself up, freeing the consciousness to attend only to consciousness. Note that all the action occurs—in consonance with the faulty metaphysics of dualism discussed in the previous chapter—on the side of nature, *prakriti*. It has nothing, ultimately, to do with what we are, with ourselves as the authors of our acts, even our acts of concentration. The *YS* identifies *kaivalya,* the aloneness of the individual consciousness, with the psychological notion of "seedless trance," *nirbija samadhi* (*YS* 1.51 and 3.8), "trance without any seed [of a *samskara* that would force one back to the waking state]." Ultimately, conscious effort is not what carries one to *kaivalya*. Only *prakriti,* in arising without distorting subliminal "seeds," has the ability to do this.

Different views are presented in Vedanta and still other views in Buddhism. Briefly, on all Yoga philosophies, *samskara* are talked about in connection with being able to sustain concentration and achieve occult powers or *siddhi*s. These in turn connect with conceptions of the goal or goals of yoga, including views about a supreme personal good. Every school's explanation of a *summum bonum* is peculiar to the particular school, and thus *samskara* are thought of ultimately in accordance with preconceived ideas about the fundamental nature of reality.

Abhinava Gupta, for example, a famous tantric of the Kashmiri Shaivite movement who lived around 950 (see the introduction to appendix D), sees the self, the true or highest self, *atman,* as potentially active and as originating *samskara* in primordial creative acts. Divine *samskara* are, in this tantric conception, instantiated in the *mudra*, the gestures, the mantras, the words said, the facial expressions, the postures of the yogin in identification with Shiva in mystic trance (*samadhi*).[14] Psychologically, the picture is of a *tabula rasa* upon which Shiva himself writes, a tablet wiped clean of obfuscating *samskara* by yoga, in which Shiva embeds a divine *samskara,* a seal with magical power to bring those who imitate it, repeat it, or otherwise align with it to taste themselves the sweetness of the trance dance of Shiva's pulsation, *spanda*.

Similarly, in the *Gita* Krishna teaches that Brahman, the Absolute, is active, making *dharma* (patterns of right action) without making karma in some sense, though there is no explicit mention of *samskara*. Whole traditions of Vedantins seem to think that *samskara* make up the body, the subtle body, that is, the *sukshma sharira,* of the transmigrating soul, even though the relation between self-consciousness, or *atman,* and the reincarnating individual is conceived very differently by Advaitins and by Vedantic theists (and the theists themselves hardly agree).

Despite all the diversity of connecting theory, everyone holds that your acts as well as your experiences make up a large part of who you are and who you will be in future births, even though some factors, such as self-awareness, are given from above, being self-determinations, according to some theorists. On all views, dispositions, *samskara,* provide crucial connections in terms of information and tendencies to act.

Buddhists embrace largely these same views, though, as mentioned, Buddhist philosophers see *samskara* as causal continua, in contrast with Hindu or Vedic views (of Vedantins, Nyaya philosophers, etc.) of *samskara* as properties of a self or a substance. Buddhists for their part eschew all notions of enduring substances and thus weave into their psychologies of *samskara* commitments to doctrines of momentariness and "no-self." The question of what survives death will be taken up in chapter 4. There too we shall survey the Buddhist–Nyaya controversy about personal identity (What makes the present person continuous with the person she was in the past?) And we shall revisit translife identity in the very last section of chapter 5.

Finally, a historical note on the ethical dimensions of karma theory. The karma idea first appears in the Upanishads, where the main point seems to be that virtue is its own reward. This holds for this lifetime and our reincarnations. A passage from the *Brihadaranyaka* (c. 800 B.C.E.), 3.2.10:

> "Yajnavalkya," said he [Jaratkarava], "when the voice of a dead man goes into fire, his breath into wind, his eye into the sun, his mind into the moon, his hearing into the quarters of earth, his body into the earth, his soul (*atman*) into space, the hairs of his head into plants, the hairs of his body into trees, and his blood and semen are placed in water, what then becomes of this person (*purusha*)?"
>
> "Artabhaga, my dear, take my hand. We two only will know of this. This is not for us two to speak of in public."
>
> The two went away and deliberated. What they said was *karma*. What they praised was *karma*. Verily, one becomes good by good action, bad by bad action.[15]

Jaratkarava's question targets personal survival, and the answer seems to be that only karma survives. The word used for "person" is *purusha,* which connotes the fully particular individual, whereas the dead man's *atman* ("self" would be a better translation than "soul") is said to merge into ether, *akasha,* translated above as "space." As in the later *Katha Upanishad* (see appendix A), the question of survival concerns the person as an individual, not as the cosmic self, *atman.* Anticipating the Buddhist positions of no-self and karmic continuity, the Upanishad identifies karma as key to a translife personal identity. It is also the most important element in the composite that makes up the living man or woman. Karma can be good or bad, including, presumably, the karma that shapes a subsequent birth: "Verily, one becomes good by good action, bad by bad action."

Thus *samskara* are conceived to underpin an appeal to self-interest that is a foundation of morality. What's wrong with being a thief? Well, your choice to be a thief binds you to being a thief, a karmic pattern that determines what you'll be like tomorrow and next month and next year and in a decade.[16] But the body ages and dies, and strategies to make life as pleasant as possible might prudentially include thievery. Against this, the Upanishadic idea is its rebirth teaching. Imagine determining yourself unendingly, choosing to be a thief not only in this lifetime but into another and endless incarnations. Contrast this with one who acts now compassionately and begins to become forever compassionate. Which would one want to be?

Then there is a second consideration: put crudely, payback, future pain and suffering or future pleasure and happiness. In the Buddhist conception, some karma leads to stable experiences of happiness while other leads to pain, and, unlike in the theistic view where God guarantees the justice of payback, it happens as natural law. Mimamsa has a similar theory. In endless rebirths, not only are you stuck with what you are but also, if you are a legitimate target, watch out, for in beginningless transmigration it's guaranteed, in either this or another body.

Ahimsa, Nonharmfulness

The Upanishadic claim that yoga leads to discovery of a universal self, *atman,* is taken to have ethical implications, in particular that we should practice *ahimsa,* nonharmfulness (also translated "noninjury" and "nonviolence"[17]). Similarly, the ubiquity of sentience in Jaina cosmology and the universal accessibility of nirvana in Buddhism are said to necessitate an ethics of *ahimsa,* according to both classical and modern authorities. And the list of five "social restraints" (*yama*) in the *Yoga Sutra* begins with nonharmfulness (*YS* 2.30: see appendix C). No one can say that only her preferred metaphysics entails *ahimsa,* but each of several positions seems sufficient to justify, motivate, and explain the practice. My own view is that the ethics of Yoga can be constructed independently from Yoga metaphysics. (Buddhists too tend to take this position about the relation between ethics and metaphysics.) But it is instructive to review the ways previous Yoga philosophies have found a relation between the deep nature of ourselves and reality and prescriptions about what we should and should not do. In practically all Yoga philosophies, ethics begins with *ahimsa.*[18]

Yoga and practice of *ahimsa* are said to have, furthermore, a converse side, fearlessness, namely, transcendence of life's evils. We also learn this first in the Upanishads. The *Isha* (c. 500 B.C.E.) makes the connection with yogic self-discovery in a common theme: realization of a cosmic self (*atman*) brings freedom from sorrow. Verse 7: "Those who see all beings as in the self alone / And the self in all beings, henceforth do not recoil (from anything). / For whom all beings are known as just self, / For him how can there be delusion? How can there be grief? / For he sees (everywhere) unity."[19] There is only the single self, the knowledge of which banishes fear and grief.[20] Conversely, we practice *ahimsa,* trying to see others as ourself or having the same self as we.

From the *Gita* (6.32): "Who sees through the lens of likeness to self the same everywhere, Arjuna, whether pleasure and happiness or pain and suffering, that yogin is deemed the very best." The commentary by Shankara (c. 700 C.E., the oldest and most important classical interpreter) takes the words "pain and suffering" to mean the pain and suffering of others, who dislike it just as one dislikes one's own pain and suffering. Similarly with the favorable attitudes of all toward pleasure and happiness. Shankara:

> As to me pleasure is desired, so to all beings with breath pleasure is agreeable. . . . And as what pain or suffering is mine is disagreeable, disliked, in that way for all beings with breath pain and suffering are disliked, disagreeable. So it is explained that one who, seeing the same in all beings, sees through the lens of likeness to self pleasures and pains as similarly regarded by all, well, such a person does not do anything disagreeable to anyone, becoming an *ahimsika,* one who desires no harm—this is the verse's meaning. The one who is in this way an *ahimsika,* firmly settled in a vision of equality, is deemed (i.e., considered) the very best yogin, preeminent among all.[21]

In line with Advaita Vedanta metaphysics, Shankara interprets the self mentioned here and elsewhere in the *Gita* as identical in everyone. The discipline to be practiced to realize it includes seeing others as like oneself. Thus Shankara and hosts of later Vedantic interpreters, including of rival subschools, tie the practices of *ahimsa* to both a yogic goal and a conception of commonality, or identity, of consciousness.

Jainas, like Buddhists, reject Vedanta and the institutions of Hinduism, but not of course yoga practices or *ahimsa.* According to Jaina doctrine, everything is sentient. There is a hierarchy of consciousness, some beings having only a single sense faculty, two, three, and so on. Human beings have eleven sense faculties: five external senses of knowledge and five more of action, along with *manas,* the inner sense, and *buddhi,* rational intelligence. There is a corresponding hierarchy in the prescription of *ahimsa*. Since a goat or a cow has, like us, eleven sense organs (counting *manas* but not *buddhi*), it is not just monks and nuns who should try not to harm such a creature. But, unlike the rest of us, a monk or nun makes effort not to harm anyone in any fashion, for she or he aspires for perfection, or the supreme good, immediately. A householder, in contrast, is not expected to aspire for the supreme good in this lifetime but only for the good karma that will ensure a similarly situated reincarnation. Thus a householder need not practice extreme *ahimsa,* while monks and nuns are enjoined to radical restraint, e.g., wearing masks not to harm even insects.

Within Buddhism, ethical injunctions, although thought of as standing on their own, are at least implicitly supported by a metaphysics of interconnectedness. The doctrine is especially prominent in northern Buddhism or Mahayana—the "Great Vehicle" ("great" because it is to carry all sentient beings to awakening and bliss)—which emerged in approximately the first century B.C.E. and spread throughout northern Asia (Tibet, China, Korea, Japan). In Sanskrit the position is, more precisely, *pratitya-samutpada,* interdependent origination: everything is born under the influence of everything else and influences everything.[22]

Perhaps the most interesting argument for *ahimsa* draws on the idea of likeness of self that we have seen in Shankara's interpretation of the *Gita*, where there is no explicit appeal to self-interest. But prudential reasons are also given. Both types of argument are found throughout the long and expansive history of Indian thought. First the prudential reasoning, which has two parts, a high road and a low road.

The high road is the view that by developing the virtue of *ahimsa* one becomes fit for supreme felicity, the supreme personal good, *parama purushartha*. Every classical view of a *summum bonum* is continuous with every other, the goals conceptualized as self-realization, liberation from rebirth, enlightenment, immortal bliss, nirvana, and so on. Despite the variety, practices of *ahimsa* were and are almost universally considered to have instrumental value for the ultimate good. One must practice *ahimsa* to achieve the best for oneself. Nonharmfulness is yoga.

On the high road the prudential is argued not to be just a matter of self-interest: in seeking the supreme good, concern for self and concern for others coincide. Although the *summum bonum* is personal, it has social value: the liberated (enlightened) act for the benefit of everyone, "to hold together the worlds," in the phrase of the *Gita*. A buddha's career after enlightenment is to serve (*seva*).

The low road relies on the teaching that virtue is its own reward—an

Upanishadic thesis that all Yoga philosophies accept, including, in a modified form, tantrics and Vedantic theists. Each of us is responsible for making ourselves the people we are and will become. This is one side of the truth of karma. Now the best sort of person into which to make oneself, both now and in lives to come, is a person who practices *ahimsa*.

Karma also involves payback or justice. We get what we deserve, whether in this or another incarnation. Thus we should practice nonharmfulness in order to avoid suffering on our own part. The cosmos, in its laws of reincarnation, embodies principles of moral retribution, whether explained, as in Mahayana Buddhism, as due to interconnectedness (*pratitya-samutpada*) or, within Vedantic theism, as God's justice or, in other views, as simply an autonomous and impersonal cosmic force (*adrishta,* the unseen force).

In support of these lines of prudential reasoning, an analogy to expert testimony is drawn. As only an expert craftsperson has the capacity to judge precisely what is good within the domain of the craft, only a person who is himself or herself of good character is an expert on character. Yogins and yoginis practice *ahimsa,* sometimes in extreme forms. These people are the experts, wise about the good. One makes oneself like them by behaving as they do.

Then there is the content of the expert testimony, the words of the yogins and their spokespersons, of Mahavira and the Buddha and Krishna. Of course, as we have seen, a person would not be regarded as an accomplished yogin (at least not genuinely accomplished, a true yogin or yogini) if he or she were not to practice *ahimsa*.[23] Nevertheless, by analogy to any expertise, the circularity is not vicious, so it stands that, as taught by the moral experts, we should practice *ahimsa*.

In a second broad group of arguments, nonharmfulness is defended by an idea of likeness of self, *atman,* as we have seen with Shankara's interpretation of the *Gita*. Jainas, however, probably should be credited for innovating the line of reasoning, which in an old version runs: everything that is conscious hates injury, and the fact that others are like oneself in being conscious and hating injury demands the practices of *ahimsa*. From the *Acharanga Sutra* (c. 350 B.C.E.): "If you say that suffering is pleasing to you, your answer is contradictory to what is self-evident. . . . And just as suffering is painful to you, in the same way it is painful to all animals, living beings, organisms, and sentient beings. [Therefore, one should practice *ahimsa*.]"[24] Respect for others flows from seeing them as like oneself. Other traditions repeat the reasoning more or less explicitly, as in the quote above from Shankara.

The eloquent arguments of the Buddhist philosopher Shantideva (c.

700 C.E.) target compassion, the central Buddhist virtue, not *ahimsa*. Compassion is said to comprise *ahimsa* within a larger concern to eliminate suffering, not just to avoid bringing it about. But the considerations he advances also promote *ahimsa,* and they center on likeness of self or person. Indeed, since there is no nugget of self that endures and suffers, but rather just sufferings—our identities are all fictions, what's important are psychological processes—he reasons that we should be as concerned to eliminate the suffering of others as we are to eliminate our own.[25]

The virtue of *ahimsa* tops the list in the *Yoga Sutra* of (social) "restraints" (*YS* 2.30: nonharmfulness, truth-telling, nonstealing, sexual restraint, and nonpossessiveness are the *yama*s constituting the first limb of the eight-limbed *ashtanga* yoga of Patanjali), and is central in living traditions of yoga practice.[26]

Here is, in sum, profound convergence of moral constraint and self-interest. We must appreciate that nonharmfulness is, first of all, an attitude one is to take toward oneself. In the *Yoga Sutra,* not to mention modern yoga studios, *ahimsa* is tied to *santosha,* self-acceptance (*YS* 2.29–35, 2.42). The idea is not to injure yourself in yoga practice, to "honor the body," even as in the short term the pain of the postures, breath control, or meditation becomes intense. In the studio, *ahimsa* means principally not hurting yourself. One listens and responds to bodily feedback, and learns not to push too hard. The whole advantage of asanas can be lost otherwise. Yoga is a conscious process, learning the body's kinks and patiently straightening them out, or not, depending on bodily signals. Consonantly, the theoretical foundation of a socially oriented *ahimsa*—that since in reality we are one in self or spirit (*atman*), or interconnected, etc., we should practice nonharmfulness—presupposes that *ahimsa* toward oneself is both right and natural.[27]

Nonharmfulness is a principle to apply to oneself, not just to others.[28] But this advice is not merely prudential, for the "pull" of one's future self, the self one is helping to make right now, is, it may be argued, the weightiest of *moral* forces. There is no person to whom one owes greater responsibility, since over others, except in unusual circumstances, one has no comparable power to make and shape what the person is. Pregnant women and parents whose children are very young are, perhaps, exceptions. (The pregnant seem to be the "exception that proves the rule," since a mother-to-be doing yoga shapes for the better [at least] two future selves.) Nevertheless, it is only over ourselves that we have decisive influence, and thus there is a special duty to our own good future self or person. Nonharmfulness applied to oneself provides push to self-development, and, indeed, to yoga practice, which is at minimum a special form of self-development, a kind of prophylactic or immunization to harm. Consonantly, we may note the contemporary movement in medicine to recognize asanas as preventive practice and essential to holistic health.

Interpreters of Yoga philosophy have been perplexed by a corollary to doctrines about self-discipline, namely, that social morality (*dharma*) can be superseded by exigencies of the path.[29] But, coming now to my main argument, it is a mistake to view Yoga ethics so narrowly as to be derived from the notion of a supreme good. In fact, the teaching about the path's potentially superseding customary moral dictates *blocks* deductions of social norms from the conception of a yogic goal. This is apparently hard for some to appreciate. The point is not that there is a Yoga brand of ethics but that Yoga teaches goals that sometimes compete with other-directed duties, like having fun versus doing a chore.[30] Yoga and the duty of self-development carry moral weight, but I should not like to hold that they are the only moral considerations.[31]

Moreover, a common supplement to Yoga self-development teachings is the advice not to disturb the minds of those who are not practitioners by revealing powers and encouraging them prematurely to practice advanced forms of self-discipline. Other consciousnesses are more or less ready for one or another step along a spiritual path, and people vary in the obstacles they face. So, by and large, one should leave others alone. You cannot really do much of anything for them, but you can for yourself.[32]

Interestingly, *ahimsa* was supported by metaphysicians in classical India by argument not so much from a concrete conception of the truly real (though the tactic was tried by some) but from the premise (just now alluded to) that beings are deluded in a variety of fashions and that each consciousness has its own route to freedom.[33] Nonharmfulness means noninterference. Consonantly, in tantric traditions, which view the *summum bonum* as perfection of the individual and not just reabsorption in the One (or dissolution in nirvana, etc.), paths of development—*svadharma,* a person's *own* individual *dharma*—are said to vary. True, the warning is repeated that no one can create a successful à la carte spiritual practice. The mind that is choosing what to include and what to exclude is an obstructed, unenlightened mentality that will often reject something necessary. But the particularity of obstructions and progress explains why gurus give different instructions to different disciples, and helps to uphold a certain pluralism among yogic methods.

It seems, then, that Yoga should encourage a libertarian social ethic, and indeed embrace a value pluralism. (Compare the oft-cited list of four distinct values in Hinduism corresponding to different life stages [*ashrama*] or circumstances: *kama,* pleasure, especially sexual pleasure; *artha*, wealth; *dharma,* familial and community duty; and *moksha,* liberation, the transcendent goal of yoga.) We leave people alone to pursue their own ends, to make their own selves or persons. Self-determination, in the individualist sense, is to be respected. I make me and you you.

This reading is right as far as it goes, but it leaves out the convergence of moral push and pull in karma theory and yogic self-development. Practicing nonharmfulness is good karma, making us better people morally. Not to smoke is a practice required by respect for a future self, the self to whose lung cancer or other illness I may well contribute were I to develop the habit. Looked at this way, not smoking is a duty to self on par with duties not to subject others to harm. A distinction between self-regarding and other-regarding action may be fundamental for law and political philosophy, but in ethics it is more fundamental to see others and self as comparable.[34]

Classical Jaina thinkers appear to practice nonharmfulness even in the controversies of philosophy. The Jaina metaphysical position—called *anekanta-vada,* the doctrine of many-sidedness, the view that no one view (exclusively) is correct, commonly rendered nonabsolutism—has at its methodological heart effort to find a grain of truth in every theory. Although difficult to accomplish, the promise seems in good faith: Jainas enjoy the reputation of being the best historians of ideas among the philosophic authors, at pains to represent fairly a range of positions, whereas polemical misrepresentation is common elsewhere. Furthermore, Jaina metaphysicians do try to synthesize opposed positions. As mentioned in the previous chapter, such relativism/pluralism is an alternative to our New Yoga minimalism as a strategy for maintaining an inclusivist outlook. Inclusivism, in the Jaina view, is a requirement of the yoga of *ahimsa*.

Nonabsolutism, *anekanta-vada*—a positive pluralism of perspectives—is the position that reality is so rich that it makes true, with qualifications, every intellectual stance. Thus the Jaina metaphysics, unlike Buddhist and Nietzschean perspectivalism, is not a form of skepticism but rather a bold promise of reconciliation of apparently opposed points of view. Or, as a skepticism it targets only the exclusivism, or absolutism, that partisans propose for their preferred positions, blind to the truth in their opponents' theories. In other words, Jainas do not set out to challenge even the most general positive claims about the nature of everything or an underlying reality. The point is not to deny but to affirm, to affirm seemingly incompatible perspectives. A special sevenfold logic—called *sapta bhangi,* seven styles (seven combinations of three truth values, truth, fal sity, and indeterminacy), also called *syad-vada,* "maybe-ism"—was developed to facilitate the disarming of controversy. Here are the weapons of intellectual *ahimsa.*

There is a similar metaphilosophical position in Buddhism, the avoiding of extremes, *anta,* advocated by Nagarjuna and his "school of the Middle," Madhyamika. What distinguishes the Buddhist skeptic and the Jaina perspectivalist is that the former rejects, while the latter accepts, the gist of an extreme position. To take a simple example, Jainas argue that Buddhist Yogachara doctrines of momentariness, etc., at the one end and Vedantic doctrines of permanence, etc., on the other are complementary and incomplete without each other, whereas the Madhyamika would reject both as departing from the middle.

The limits to Jaina inclusivism are only practical, but very real nonetheless. Even nonabsolutism is viewed as nonabsolute, subject to the logic of the "maybe," despite opponents' allegations of self-refutation—nonabsolutism as purportedly presenting itself as absolutely true, as the Vedantin Shankara alleges. But there is no self-referential inconsistency in application of perspectivalism to itself, although some modern interpreters, apparently following Shankara, would also label it absolutist.[35] Only an omniscient being would be able to comprehend all viewpoints. There are no true, false, or even indeterminate propositions outside of a framework, a *vada,* a theory or perspective of interlocking beliefs, that is to say, a *naya,* standpoint. And a special logic governs standpoints.

The Jaina *sapta bhangi,* a septad of styles or manners of valuation of truth, is comprised of all combinations of three truth values, truth (+), falsity (−), and indeterminacy (o):[36]

+, −, o, +−, +o, −o, +−o

Because of the three truth values, this has been misinterpreted as a paraconsistent or multivalued logic invented to resolve logical paradoxes and the problem, known to Aristotle, of the indeterminate truth value of some statements about the future, so-called future contingents. But the Jainas' is not a logic of truth-functional connectives. Rather, it is a hermeneutical tool. All truths are truths only from a perspective, but some are true to us and, so far as we know, to everyone. Even if we are not aware of controversy concerning the claim that something *a* is F, this is still only from a perspective, and there may be a perspective in which *a* is not F or in which it cannot be determined whether it is. We presume, without contrary advice, that *a* is F (or that the proposition *p* is true), but we do so fallibilistically—the *syad* in *syad-vada* means that a claim is presumptively true, false, indeterminate, and so on ("may well be _____" is a better translation). No claim is immune from the possibility of error. Nevertheless, some claims, or cognitions, are false, or nonveridical, from our own point of view and every point of view that we know of, and some are indeterminate, *avaktavya,* it is impossible to say. On the classical Indian scene, Advaita Vedanta is the philosophy famous for proposing a third truth value, the inexplicable, *anirvachaniya,* which holds for statements about the relationship of Brahman to the phenomenal display: we cannot know as finite individual knowers what the world looks like from Brahman's viewpoint. Jainas use the category of the indeterminate similarly to classify apparently unanswerable questions.[37]

So what of the combinations of truth, falsity, and indeterminacy, the final four of the septad? In recognizing that a claim can be simultaneously true and false, or another combination, the Jaina view again relativizes to *naya*, standpoints. From some standpoints a claim is true while in others it is false. From our own standpoint, it is true in some standpoints and false in others, and so on. Our own standpoint conditionalizes other standpoints. Thus the Jaina theoreticians would make clear to themselves the tasks before them. For they see reality as making a claim true in the one standpoint and false in the other. Reality is so incredibly rich that it can underlie and give rise to opposed pictures. However, understanding the details in particular cases of controversy is not easy, as shown by the struggles of Haribhadra (c. 750), Hemachandra (c. 1150), and company to actually reconcile contrary views. The sevenfold schema is nevertheless a tool for work in metaphysics, allowing clear categorizing of problems.

Finally, it is worth repeating that the Jaina position is not self-refutational. It may have other weaknesses, but not this, though the point is subtle. A common misinterpretation of the *sapta bhangi* sees it as generating unconditional claims. For example, J. N. Mohanty: "the Jaina developed a method known as *syad-vada,* by which the truths of opposing predications may be synthesized, their one-sided truth claims rejected, and a perfect knowledge of the totality of reality arrived at. Each such predication is conditional, relative to a standpoint, but if that condition is included in the predication, the judgment becomes unconditionally true."[38] This would be like practicing *ahimsa* toward everyone except oneself, a failure that has also been unfairly laid at the feet of Jaina theorists. Jainas do leave open the possibility of omniscience, but to use the seven truth values to try to disarm metaphysical disputes is not to impute to oneself an absolute point of view. Nonharmfulness requires humility.

Philosophy and other forms of intellectual engagement need not be practiced with an intent to produce a "knock-down" argument, giving the lie to the opponent's position and indulging in fallacies of derision. The ethic of the Jainas is to show compassion even to positions really regarded as false. Thus maybe (*syat*) the Socratic method (of trying to show a contradiction in the views of an interlocutor) is not, pedagogically, the best way to train young thinkers. To be sure, Yoga philosophy has not in general followed the Jaina model, but has been insistent upon one or another position as right and others as wrong. Truth treads a narrow path. However, we may regard the minimalism in metaphysics championed in chapter 2 and the alternatives of dualist interactionism and holism explored there as embodying the Jaina spirit. Relativism (positive perspectivalism) and minimalism are brothers and sisters. Again, the main point of Yoga philosophy is to defend possibilities of yoga practice and experience, not a single, absolutely correct theory, the final word. As Nyaya proposes, philosophy is itself a kind of yoga, and like all yoga should be practiced in the spirit of *ahimsa*.

Karma Yoga

Yoga morality begins with nonharmfulness, but it doesn't end there. First, as early as the earliest lists of virtues required of the yogin, exceptions to *ahimsa* have been claimed. Second, service, *seva,* a giving of oneself and what one values to others, becomes crucial to the world-oriented practice called karma yoga.

At the very end of the long prose *Chandogya Upanishad* (c. 800 B.C.E.), we learn that animal sacrifice "at holy places" is excluded from the injunction to practice *ahimsa*. Thus, in a dramatic statement: "he who is harmless (*ahimsant*) toward all beings except at holy places (*tirtha*), he, indeed, who lives thus throughout his length of life, reaches the Brahman world and does not return hither again—yea, he does not return hither again!"[39] Nonharmfulness is not the only value, then, even for the yogin. It can be trumped according to circumstance. (Jainas would disagree by and large, I take it, though they too find other virtues and values—for example, charity—that are possibly in conflict with *ahimsa*.) The question is: What is more important than not harming?

The answer appears to be cosmic harmony, here in the *Chandogya* from the late Vedic age as also practically throughout Yoga literature, a standard answer much elaborated. There are exceptions, significant exceptions perhaps, Samkhya philosophy as well as some lines of Advaita, of Buddhism, etc., that do not deify harmony.[40] But the enormously popular *Gita* has the harmony vision, as do tantrics generally and the yoga teachings of all theistic sects.

From the earliest times, concern for balance among life worlds, mortal and immortal, and prosperity, which depends upon favorable natural forces, appear to have motivated animal sacrifice. Scholar Laurie Patton: "as many Vedic texts and later ritual texts . . . indicate, sacrifice of an animal into the [sacred] fire was part of the ecological balance in the ancient Vedic world; the killing and distribution of the animal was part of a larger understanding of human harmony with natural forces. . . . The gods are given food and return it through their natural bounty; thus, the ecology of sacrificial food production and consumption is the central, guiding metaphor for the survival of earthly and celestial worlds."[41] Over the centuries, animals were used less and less in the rituals of Hinduism, but an ethics of cosmological balance remained in force. That one should strive to perform inner sacrifice, offerings of action to harmony, in order personally to gain equanimity and prosper spiritually was an idea that progressively came to dominate Hindu sensibilities. The trumping power of justice in the political and social spheres can be understood as further manifestations of the harmony motif. Promotion of *ahimsa* in the *Mahabharata,* the epic poem containing the *Bhagavad Gita,* and throughout the Puranas and elsewhere is mitigated by a larger concern for harmony.

The axiological concept is made sharper by taking it as the thesis that worth tracks degree of complex unity.[42] Organic unity is highly complex, and the unity of consciousness evident in human memory, self-consciousness, etc., makes humans more valuable than animals, even those closest to us genetically (compare the Jaina hierarchy of sentience discussed above). Furthermore, the purposes of human beings not only pack causal power but also are potentially unifying beyond the interests of the individual, as we find in the concept of the noble cause or of giving of self for something greater, something extending beyond one's death: family, humanity, works of art. The concept of harmony is not made philosophically sharp in our Yoga inheritance, but this perhaps is an area where we should expect not sharpness but rather a lot of gray. Harmony in any case remains key to understanding the *Gita* and all the more tantric world-affirmativism, as we shall see.

Nowhere is outright tension between yogic *ahimsa* and a larger duty more evident than in the Yoga teachings of the *Bhagavad Gita* (c. 200 B.C.E.). Not only is nonharmfulness preached by Krishna on (of all places) a battlefield, the dialogue between the divine guru and his warrior interlocutor Arjuna is precipitated by the latter taking a step toward an *ahimsa* attitude. Arjuna refuses to go into combat against those he loves. Krishna, the divine teacher, insists he fight. Arjuna declares at the very beginning—in the first chapter (out of eighteen) and the beginning of the second—a sense of sin in killing, even in the name of right rule. Details of plot and some salient passages show Krishna melding *ahimsa* into a theology of cosmic harmony. (See appendix B, the introduction, for the setting and an introduction to the yoga teaching as a whole.)

The attitude Krishna tells Arjuna to take in action, called karma yoga, is the *Gita*'s most striking and original theme, although similar ideas are found in the middle Upanishads (the *Katha* in particular) and in precepts for monks and nuns in both Buddhism and Jainism.[43] The yoga of action (*karma yoga*) is a discipline of acting in a spirit of sacrifice, says Krishna, giving to another without regard for personal benefit.

Apparently any action in principle can be a gift, so long as it is offered with the right feeling and attitude. Specifically, one is to give without concern for oneself. However, the sacrificer is to be confident there is karmic benefit (burning up bad karma and/or making good karma) or transcendence of karmic consequences altogether (nonkarma-making action). Normally, the psychological dispositions one makes through action not only bind but also invite payback into future lifetimes. Only action done as karma yoga, Krishna teaches, avoids moral retribution. Verse 3.9: "Without personal attachment undertake action, Arjuna, for just one purpose, for the purpose of sacrifice. From work undertaken for purposes other than sacrifice, this world is bound to the laws of karma." (See also, in particular, *Gita* 4.21 and 4.22, appendix B.)

Our discussion so far would suggest that at least some forms of yoga are self-directed only. We can even imagine an ardent yogini prone to ignore truly moral duties, who neglects family or profession to master Scorpion Pose. Truly moral duties, an objector might contend, are duties to others, not to one's future self. Should we not aim to develop a more social self and person? As outlined so far, yoga need not be particularly social. Indeed, this seems correct for many practices.

In contrast, the karma yoga teaching of the *Gita* is famously social. The whole point of karma yoga is to forget self-interest through action directed to others' benefit. Furthermore, practically any action or course of action, such as a profession or family activities, would seem to be an avenue for karma yoga practice. After all, Krishna enjoins Arjuna to practice karma yoga in a war, in apparent violation—in an ingenious emplotment—of the yogic principle of *ahimsa*. Arjuna is to kill the opposing warriors and to win the battle, all the while taking a yogic attitude that involves *ahimsa* (*Gita* 10.5, 13.8, 16.2, and 17.14). Yoga can be done in any situation. Yoga is a matter of taking the right attitude in action.

Four senses of the Sanskrit word *karman* are involved in the *Gita*'s conception, two of which we have already reviewed: voluntary action and *samskara* as underlying skills ("Yoga is skill in works," *Gita* 2.50, *yogah karmasu kaushalam*). A third sense, unseen moral force, *adrishta,* will be taken up in the next section on karmic justice. A fourth sense currently in view is sacrifice, *yajna.* The karma yoga teaching of the *Gita* picks up the Upanishadic theme of "cosmicization of the sacrifice."[44]

Sacrifice means giving, giving to the gods that are indwelling in people and things, or to Brahman, the Absolute and origin of the universe who enlivens the gods and is present in every self. What one gives is not necessarily ghee or any other thing into physical fire, but karma, action, presented by a flame of, let us say, self-idealization. One offers the gift into the flame of one's aspiration to be like or with the adored, the beloved, which would be Krishna himself, according to Vaishnavas, whatever be the particular form (god, etc.) of that to which action is offered (*Gita* 9.23–24). The external *puja* or ceremony of offering is taken to symbolize psychological gestures made from the lower to the higher within ourselves—a key idea in tantra (see the "Hymn to the Wheel of Divinities Seated in the Body" by Abhinava Gupta, translated in appendix D) and connected to that of psychic transformation (the subject of the last section of chapter 5).

Thus outlined, yoga can be done in the world, in all kinds of action done for the sake of sacrifice. Yoga becomes *seva*, service. Service promotes cosmic harmony. Thus there would be no incompatibility between *ahimsa* and violence called for in the interest of "holding together the worlds" (*Gita* 3.20), consonant with the Upanishadic exception of animal sacrifice, or, in the immediate case, holding together Arjuna's society. Arjuna is not to intend harm, as part of a yogic attitude, as he works to destroy the opposing warriors, including his own teachers and family, and win the battle. As said by Krishna time and again and confirmed by the circumstances of the conflict, in entering combat Arjuna follows *dharma,* the right path of action, the only action suitable for offering in karma yoga. Service entails an idea of action done for the good of the whole. Karma yoga as perfectly practiced would make all action a beautiful ritual.

The change of consciousness, or attitude, that karma yoga practice involves is supposed to enable an ethical intuition that can transform ordinary action into *dharma,* the right way to live, a kind of divine life. Thus is inaugurated—indulge the conjecture—the "tantric turn" that would marry yoga and the world. The movement is not merely Hindu, although it seems to be launched here in the karma yoga teaching of the *Gita*. Chapter 5 will take up the tantric reconception of the goal or goals of yoga.

To be sure, the *Gita* also embraces the Samkhya theme of disidentification and the elusive "I" (introduced in the Upanishads; see appendix A), which is central in Buddhism. We mistakenly identify ourselves with our personas and psychological processes, which are really constructs of nature having nothing to do with our primordial consciousnesses. Self-monitoring consciousness is somehow mistaken in what it takes to be self. What you are is elusive, changing with your essential ability to identify with instruments such as the body and sense faculties and indeed the mind (the *chitta* of the *Yoga Sutra*). But none of these is really you, nor is it valuable. This is not quite the picture of the *Gita,* however. In karma yoga, you try to disidentify, downplaying your own role, in humility offering your acts as intellectually you know them really to be, namely, not the products of your little self but rather of forces of nature, natural desires in interaction with forces of the mental, vital, and physical universes. The Samkhya of the *Gita* does not find natural objects to be products of delusion or worthless but rather targets false identity.

Furthermore, the *Gita*'s use of the Samkhya theme is incorporated into a larger metaphysical and spiritual vision, a monism, not a dualism like the classical Samkhya of the *Samkhya-karika*. World-changing action is the vehicle of the *Gita*'s karma yoga. Only *dharmic* action is a suitable offering. On this point I disagree with the commentators who say that any action can be done as karma yoga. As a gift to a boyfriend or girlfriend, you do not present something ugly. Here the *Gita*'s karma yoga teaching embraces *bhakti* (an idea developed in chapter 5).

So, we can say that the disidentification theme is present in the *Gita*'s karma yoga teaching but that there is also more to it. Furthermore, it is continuous with tantric ideals of transformation, as I shall show in chapter 5. Some tension between the philosophies of world denial and those of world affirmation is to be expected if the *Gita* is, as I see it, a pivotal and transitional work. Despite the presence of the Samkhya theme, the *Gita* has Brahman, the Absolute, as active, making *dharma,* patterns of right action, including social justice, out there in the world, without making karma. The karma yogin is thought of as a person who can identify with that perspective and thus act without the normal karmic consequences.

Through practice of karma yoga, one self-consciously connects with horizontal and vertical flows of Brahman's own creative energies. The vertical flow is the transcendent sacrifice (see, e.g., *Gita* 4.6 and 4.13). The horizontal comprises the interactions belonging to the separate universes of the separate "sheaths," *kosha:* food and the "food sheath" and the worlds of feelings and thoughts along with one's particular feelings and thoughts, the emotional and mental sheaths (see figure 4A). In different terminology, by karma yoga one opens to a universal *prana* leading to extraordinary powers or *siddhi*s, becoming, in Vedantic language, the Vaishvanara, the "univerally human," which is considered a stage in yogic transformation of consciousness. The tantric turn is all about the formation of a more complex harmony of the divine and the individual.

One of the most striking of the *Gita*'s many striking conceptions concerns reincarnation. If you think the goal of yoga too distant, don't worry, one continues yogic practice into the next lifetime. Arjuna, at *Gita* 6.37, voices this along with the further complaint that if he practices yoga he will be lost to the world, not a success in worldly terms as well as a yogic failure. Krishna replies (*Gita* 6.41–44), "someone [like you describe] fallen from yoga would be born in a household of pure and beautiful people. Or, he would be born just into a family of yogins and yoginis, people of wisdom. . . . There he would recover the purposefulness of his previous life, and would strive, O joy of the Kurus, from that point on toward perfection. For even without trying he would be carried just by the practice in his former birth." This is the yogic soul-making conception of the *Gita*.

The tantric and neo-Vedantin philosopher Aurobindo uses soul making as the lynchpin of his theory of the relation between Brahman and the world.[45] Brahman is in the process of creating materially embodied spiritual individuals who are in part responsible for making themselves across lifetimes. Thus there would be in the material world as a whole a teleological cause, an "attraction of the future," that would be expressed in us in terms of right desire and right effort, i.e., in yoga practices and all their wondrous results. We shall return to this yogic soul-making theory both in the next section and in chapters 4 and 5.

Karmic Justice

Fear of karmic consequence and joy in karmic confidence constitute a second variety of both moral and yogic incentive on most Yoga views.[46] The universe is so arranged that an individual will get her due, if not in this life then in a future one. Karmic justice is a distinct variety of incentive, according to Yoga. The idea is similar to Western religious teachings about heaven and hell as doctrines of moral reward. In this section, I shall examine the slippery concept of *adrishta,* unseen force, which is the name given to the influence of a person's (or a group's) karma on events in the sense of moral retribution, including, most importantly, one's next birth. For obvious reasons, some lines of investigation cannot be closed until I take up theories of rebirth in chapter 4. Here I shall concentrate on matters of ethics, and also, at the end, the theistic problem of evil, against which ideas of karma and rebirth are used to defend the thesis that God is good. The fine points of Yoga views of survival and issues about personal identity will be the focus in chapter 4.

The most widely held picture is that an individual has both a sum of karmic worth and individual lines of karma that attract, like magnets, situations for discharge, karmic cathexis in worldly events causing pleasure and pain in various combinations and flavors. The aggregation depends on moral coefficients added to a total in the case of good karma and subtracted in the case of bad, although the moral worth of some acts stands alone and invites reward or payback independently of the moral worth of the aggregate. The power of karmic vectors to affect events, especially outcomes of enterprises, is considered to be outside or beyond ordinary sensibilities, as is implied in the very word—unseen force, *adrishta*—used in all schools to refer to the causal power of karma's side of justice. This is a fate that can work *apurvaka,* without intermediaries. That is to say, it may bring about a consequence, a bit of bad luck, for instance, in a subsequent birth remotely, without an immediately preceding cause. The classical Indian school of Mimamsa propagated the view that every experience is to some degree, however slight (or overwhelming), influenced by *adrishta.*[47]

The force of *adrishta* is tied to a balance of pleaure and pain, suffering and happiness. That is to say, negative karma is considered paid off, and good karma exhausted, by certain kinds of pain or pleasure. Certain enjoyments and sufferings are, to be sure, deemed themselves sources of good or bad karma. The joke in yoga class is that loosening tight hip joints—a well-known source of torment—pays off bad karma but only if endured with grace. The philosophic point is that the currency of the moral exchange is not merely the moral worth of acts. The workings of karma are complex, and include whole "life lessons," as are captured in the Jataka tales of the Buddha-to-be's previous births (recall the story of Sumedha in the introduction).[48]

Furthermore, on certain Vedantic and tantric and indeed some Buddhist views of an underlying bliss of a true self or no-self state of consciousness, happiness is supposed to be closer to the natural state than pain or suffering, which are deviations. The renunciants' warning that "All is suffering" is not the final word, existence or nonexistence not being so niggardly in happiness and bliss as one might think. Pain and suffering are instrumental—and thus of positive overall value—in leading us to somehow better bliss or to find the bliss at our core. We shall return to this instrumentality thesis in connection with Yogic theism. For the present, the main point is that the workings of karma are typically only part of the picture when it comes to the hedonically positive and negative sides of experience.

Yoga philosophers have also recognized that getting what we want and avoiding what we want to avoid are wellsprings for all our acts. It is all the more true, then, that the precise relations among karma, destiny, and happiness, though presumably lawlike, are not discerned easily. Buddhists in particular are well known for the simplification that with respect to one's own actions one can be sure that cruelty and other evil acts will be avenged (without an agent, an avenger, a judge of the dead), and one will secure good results for oneself by good deeds. The processes remain unknown or even unknowable (except to buddhas, according to Buddhists), but that hardly matters given what we know firsthand about suffering.

Nevertheless, even without its lines very precisely drawn, this picture of moral worth is potentially in tension with the causal picture of *samskara* continuity. Individual patterns of karma—habits and skills—are said to survive and shape the character of the person in his or her next lifetime. The thesis seems crucial to the theory of yogic soul making and is veritably common Yoga opinion, namely, that some habits, values, intentions—karma, in a word—are so deeply entrenched that they reemerge in the next birth as talents or deep dispositions of mental or emotional character.

The problem is that continuity of *samskara* works from moment to moment, without a break, unlike the remote workings of *adrishta*. That the two ideas of karmic force are potentially in conflict can be seen in the notion of Hitler reborn in a nonhuman form subject to constant fear and torture. This may be a righteous image, but since the soul is not a *tabula rasa* according to Yoga, even tremendously positive or negative moral value of the karmic aggregate could not determine a dramatic species crossing, Hitler being reborn as a bat, for instance, or Stalin as a mosquito. What could be continuous between Stalin and an insect? Only a future human being could be shaped by the mental dispositions that are the most important to a human being, I should dare to speculate.

However, it is not just a matter of popular opinion among Hindus, Buddhists, Jainas, etc.; philosophers too hold that there is no guarantee that you cannot take a lower rebirth. Appeals to mental complexity are countered by the consideration that a complex mind can dream or experience itself under simpler forms.[49]

The overall lesson remains the intricacy of karmic laws. The tension between the two ideas of karmic influence leads me to think that by and large, humans are restricted to future human reincarnations. The argument against reincarnation that human population growth has turned up sharply in the last couple of centuries and so there would not be enough human souls to meet the bodily demand can be answered quickly: more souls of higher animals, such as horses and dogs, have perhaps ascended to the human level in recent years than was the rate previously (or maybe heaven or hell are emptying!). In line with our minimalism, all we need say is that an individual who achieves the human level is unlikely to return to an animal incarnation for the very reason that the mental life typical of a human being cannot be continued in the body of a different species. Therefore, it seems reasonable to speculate that the determinant power of the moral worth of karma has to be restricted to birthings by potential mothers within the human species, and of course fathers and others important to an upcoming childhood. Perhaps a karmic sum determines a range of candidate wombs to which are attached likelihoods of future suffering and happiness.

Such speculation is of course pretty airy, since isolating the influence of karma is practically impossible. According to Yoga psychology, we live simultaneously in different bodies or personalities, physical, vital, emotional, mental, and spiritual (see figures 4A, 4B, and 4C). A bad habit for the body, coffee in the morning, for example, may be part of a good mental practice, writing a book, for instance. And not only are there complications concerning types and ranges of pleasures and pains along with the complexity of human action (think of the difference, e.g., between a quick response and a long project), there are further complexities concerning karma itself.

First, it is commonly held that there are interpersonal relations to karma, souls reincarnating in groups, friends and families hanging together through lifetimes—called a "karasse" by novelist Kurt Vonnegut—a group karmically bonded, "soul mates."[50] It's as though the magnetic effect of karma includes drawing together people who have been associated in previous lives. Is there, then, a second type of coefficient qualifying *samskara*? Or is a personal affinity vector somehow contained within *adrishta*? Or are, for example, such ideas as the soul mate or karasse merely wishful thinking, maintained by desire for close affinities to endure beyond death? The evidence for reincarnation is not strong enough to support a very determinate theory and certainly not to support all the popular images.[51]

Second, it is commonly claimed that karma "ripens" according to law; in other words, that *adrishta,* though its consequences are remote, works just at certain times. Temporal factors do seem to be evident in those (evidentially key) instances of people reporting memory of events in previous births. As documented by Ian Stevenson, children of five tend to remember incidents in the life of a previous person when he or she was five, and the same for children of seven, ten, twelve, and so on, years of age, to include, one would suppose, adult rememberings.[52] The law here might be that an act of type A in circumstances C is made probable by karma of type A created in the past, and some sets of circumstances are more probable at certain ages.

The ripening idea also connects with the widely held Yogic theory that one is presented opportunities to change course in life (and to practice yoga) only at specific times. Popularly the idea is expressed in such stories as that in every incarnation, at the age of thirty Devadatta has to overcome a temptation to murder or at age forty meets his guru. Similarly, Siddhartha of our age, says the Pali canon, throws his begging bowl out into the current of the river, where it clinks against the side of the begging bowl thrown by the buddha of the previous epoch, which in turn clinks, gently, the side of a still previous buddha's bowl resting on the bottom.[53] But some popular lore also has it that karmic payback works more rapidly the more developed the individual. We are lucky if we suffer for our sins in the near term, so the idea goes. The image is of bad karma as like a festering sore.

Third, a certain kind of action is said to block, or at least blunt, the retributive force of karma, including acts of atonement (*prayash-chitta*) and auspiciousness (*mangala,* such as chanting *om*).[54] On the *Gita*'s version of the thesis, action in tune with the dharmic (righteous) forces of the universe—or with the action of Brahman itself in the grand sacrifice that maintains the universe—transcends the moral/amoral distinction ("Though acting, the person who sees himself in all beings is not stained [by karma]," *Gita* 5.7, and "He who, depositing actions in [the fire of] Brahman, giving up attachment, acts [in the world], sin does not cling to, like water on a lotus leaf," *Gita* 5.10). Such action creates no *adrishta,* or even wipes out karmic influence altogether. In the *Yoga Sutra*'s conception, a certain kind of meditation creates *samskara* that self-destruct, leaving no karmic residue (*YS* 1.50, 3.9–10). The Buddhist view is that karma operates within samsaric consciousness. Once nirvana is attained and one becomes a high-level bodhisattva, one is incapable of acting in a karma-generating way that would lead back into the unenlightened state. Moreover, claims about certain actions lying outside karmic law occur throughout the perfectionist tradition that emphasizes self-development and the attainment of *siddhis*. Finally, in tantra broadly the yogic soul-making idea is tempered with an inevitable "attraction of the future," to wit, further "manifestation," the ongoing creation of Shakti or Shri.[55] Thus would we be destined to become greater beings than we are now. Therefore, we have to be able to be creative, to make new patterns not bound by karma.

In all these different views, individual will, though itself creating *adrishta* normally, can somehow by force of right effort (or by God's grace provoked by right effort) overcome the influence of *adrishta,* past and present and therefore future. Yoga philosophy is not determinist. In chapter 1, we saw that Yoga denies causal closure in the physical realm. In my judgment, almost all previous Yoga philosophy has it that consciousness and its powers also transcend karma, or can.

Fortunately, in the concept of the bundle of causal conditions sufficient for an effect, *samagri,* classical theorists found a notion well suited to the complexity of karmic consequence. That an event shows karmic justice amounts to the claim that unseen moral force, *adrishta,* counts as a single causal factor bundled into a *samagri,* that is to say, a single factor among many, the bundle being technically what brings about whatever happens.[56] Karmic influence on any particular event may or may not be very great. Yoga has traditionally tended to the view that except in the special circumstances of yogic practice, karmic justice always has at least some small influence.

There are several different psychological versions of karmic justice among classical theorists. Buddhists tend to view karmic justice as tied to the type of contamination of one's perspective that blocks enlightenment. Thus is avoided the need for a divine arbiter of a soul's fate, a referee who determines which souls get the better births the next go-round and which will be born in squalor. Such a naturalistic theory is present in Samkhya and the *Yoga Sutra* and even in some theistic Vedanta, although there is also non-naturalism in some Buddhist schools as well as in more mainstream theistic Vedanta.[57] The differences need not further detain us.

Finally, let us turn to theistic treatments and in particular to ideas explaining how God is not the author of evil. The *Brahma Sutra* of Vedanta has a long section on the problem of theodicy, and the elaboration by the oldest commentator, Shankara, makes plain a mainstream position.[58] Although Shankara is an Advaitin, he takes seriously the theistic teachings of the Upanishads and the *Gita* as meditational aids. Scripture says that Brahman is the source of the world, so since Brahman is unsullied value and bliss, whence evil? How could evil have its source in what is inherently its opposite?

Shankara's explanation is complex, and only the second part is taken over by the more genuine theists. That part, however, remains the centralmost plank on God and evil within the long history of theistic Vedanta. The first part relies on the distinction between Brahman as "without" and "with" "qualities" (or "attributes"), *nirguna* contrasting with *saguna brahman*. According to Shankara, Brahman without qualities is supremely real. Brahman with qualities is talked about in scripture as an aid to meditation. Scripture is like a patient teacher (*guru*), and it is difficult to appreciate that Brahman as supremely real has no qualities. Scripture talks about God, i.e., Brahman with qualities, as preparation to the austere truth—which is that nothing but Brahman without qualities is really real. God too is part of a cosmic illusion due to spiritual ignorance.

Brahman with qualities is God, the Lord and Creator. How then could the Lord, who is perfect—much as in the Western conception—allow evil in the world? Shankara asks this question and moves to the second part of his theodicy, the part that is shared. Here karma as affecting rebirth is the absolutely hinge notion, and the theodicy is a *samskara* version—the Eastern version, we may say, a direct parallel—of the free-will theodicy prominent in Christian philosophy. For not only are we responsible for our karma in making our future births; the Lord is just in arranging the universe so that it embodies principles of karmic justice. Rebirth is fair.

The work of the first part of Shankara's two-part defense is done, in the theistic views, mainly by a sense of gratefulness, it seems to me. God creates many worlds much better than this. But in those worlds I do not exist. Our world is definitely not the best of all possible worlds, but it is a world where I exist. So I am grateful that God in her infinity suffers it.

Alternatively, there is the supposition, which is quite widespread (appearing in Buddhism as well as Shankara's Vedanta), that there is no first creation, that the transmigratory round or universe is beginningless (*anadi-samsara*). Shankara in responding to the objection that at the beginning of the universe there was no good or bad karma denies explicitly that nescience (*avidya*) has a beginning.[59]

Habits, which we have ourselves made and for which we are responsible, the fundamental dispositions of the soul, carry over into and determine the course of a soul's next incarnation. The Lord guides the workings of *adrishta;* unseen force is not blind, according to the theists.[60]

If in this way beyond virtue and vice being their own reward, there is justly payback for bad acts—i.e., beyond the badness of bad habits—and pleasure and happiness for good karma, then God's universe could well be just, at least in the sense required to defend the thesis that God is good and worthy of worship. Thus some of what we see as natural evil would be payback, for which, then, the Lord should not be blamed.[61] And of course some evil, such as pain, has a biological or other instrumental function, without which our world would not be possible. And so the Eastern version of free-will theodicy, coupled with instrumentality considerations, is quite compelling, it seems to me.

In the view of the *bhakti yoga* practitioner, suffering is an opportunity to pay off bad karma. We should be grateful and not generate further bad karma by whining and complaining. Far from disproving the existence of God, suffering is a manifestation of God's love and concern for our welfare. Better to pay off bad karma now than to let it fester, let it blindside us later or in another life. Who cares about it really anyway, since essentially life is delight?

With Shankara the deep question is: Why is there nescience, *avidya,* spiritual ignorance? If Brahman is the supreme reality, our own true self, why is it we are unenlightened? Advaita has no answer to this, it seems. Theistic views struggle with a similar problem: Why, given the possibility of living enlightenment such as Krishna's, are we not all enlightened? The answer, again, is karma. We somehow deserve not to be enlightened. But why does God let us get into such straits? The best answer seems to be that otherwise we would not be who we are and there would not be the opportunities we have for development. Like everything finite, from the gods and goddesses down to a pebble, we have our day in the sun. Gratefulness is the appropriate attitude.

4
Rebirth

Personal Identity

Before the materialist wave broke in the universities, the topic of reincarnation was of considerable interest to philosophy professionals. Pro-arguments by the great nineteenth-century British idealist, J.M.E. McTaggart, were widely discussed. C. J. Ducasse, President of the American Philosophical Association in the 1950s, defended the possibility in a well-crafted work of metaphysics.[1]

Ducasse's theory goes as follows. A human being consists of personality and individuality (a psychic element). Only the latter could survive, Ducasse argues, since there is a physical and bodily component to personality. Individuality, however, is entirely psychological, consisting of "instincts, dispositions, and tendencies" formed by choices and actions in this and previous lives. The American philosopher supposes that psychological processes are developed, or instantiated, across lives, for the sake of proving the possibility of rebirth, he emphasizes, not as an outright assertion as fact. But his sympathies are clear.

Ducasse maintains that if rebirth is to be a real possibility, there must be an interval between death and birth where recollection of past lives is normal. Memory, according to him, underpins the identity of an individual across lives, though (fortunately for the theory) previous lives need not be accessible except in the death-birth interval. Analytic philosophers subsequent to Ducasse have shown through various consciousness fusion and fission thought experiments that memory is insufficient for personal identity.[2] But this is, all told, a minor matter, since there can be no personal identity across lives, as I should like to argue in agreement with Ducasse (and many others who have thought about this). When John Doe dies, the person is gone, only some part of him surviving. Then to avoid what may be called the Leibnizian objection, Ducasse reasons that individuality must help shape personality. Otherwise, as Leibniz writes (quoted by Ducasse), "you might as well say that John died and another, the King of China, was born."[3] So, according to Ducasse, the living person is composed of both a personality, which is contingent upon the circumstances of a particular life, and an individuality, which is more constant across lifetimes.

Let us pause to appreciate Ducasse's method, which is to show the mileage to be got from the requirement that reincarnation make sense. Not only must there be a potentially disembodied individual capable of awareness of previous lives, at least some deep dispositions comprising individuality must influence or determine the personality at certain points in a given lifetime. We can eliminate a lot of nonsense if the reincarnation thesis is to be, in Ducasse's words, a live possibility.

So far, all Yoga philosophies would pretty much agree, since so much is left wide open. The problem with such a general approach is that if we are mindful of our Yoga inheritance, we face unavoidable options and questions Ducasse fails to answer. There are rather concrete Yoga teachings about rebirth that purport to address the facts of the matter, not just possibility. Indeed, taking our cues from Yoga theories, maybe not everything Ducasse alleges really follows from an analysis of the concept of reincarnation on the assumption that it could be real. For example, according to him, individuality would be itself developed, though much more slowly than personality.[4] Now this accords with some yoga traditions such as the conscious reincarnation practices of Tibetan Buddhists as well as the *Gita*'s soul-making theory, broached in the last chapter. We make ourselves with choices over numerous lifetimes. But Ducasse's analysis does not accord very well with two other theories prominent in classical Yoga literature.

A second theory used to maintain translife continuity is Nyaya's view of an individual self—which is the same view, discounting details, as in Samkhya and in the Yoga of the *Yoga Sutra*. Nyaya's essentially disembodied self has nonetheless the practical function of being the locus of psychological properties, including mental-physical dispositions. The self does not develop, on this view, and connections between one life and the next are mainly through the identity of the individual who takes one birth after another according to laws of karma. There are, however, some *samskara* connections that are translife. A child's first voluntary act—to reach for the mother's breast, in the stock example—proves reincarnation, Nyaya philosophers argue. All voluntary action is guided by *samskara*-fed cognition, and the child, *ex hypothesi,* has not formed the *samskara* in the current lifetime.[5] But these *samskara* might be generic and nonindividuating for human beings, and Nyaya philosophers do not elaborate.

I propose to give a full airing to the Nyaya view of the self and personal identity in the context of a famous controversy with Buddhist no-self theory. But let me say from the outset that in the Yoga context the Nyaya picture is, like Ducasse's, not sufficiently rich. In Nyaya we find no talk of a subtle body, a pranic body, the Upanishadic sheaths, and so on, none of the conceptual props of yoga practice that Yoga theorists use to develop views of rebirth. Although there is much metaphysical argument about the self, the school has no occult psychology. About details of translife continuity, Nyaya's minimalism is too extreme (approaching silence!). We are particularly interested in Yoga views that connect practices with ideas about survival, so we need to hear the voices not so much of rational inquiry, as with Nyaya, but of yogic testimony.[6] The *Yoga Sutra,* then, becomes of interest again, not because of the metaphysics of a *purusha* or self but because of its intricate theory of karma and life-spanning *samskara*. None of this is found in Nyaya literature, but the overall metaphysical stances are similar. Both stances seem compatible with soul making, but only in the *YS* is it fleshed out in terms of *samskara,* et cetera.

There is, however, another metaphysical view that is a veritable competitor with soul making. Again, soul making is the idea that continuity is developmental, on analogy to the growth and development in a single lifetime from untrained toddler to accomplished adult. Using Ducasse's terms, according to soul making, personality etches individuality as well as the other way around, with our previous lives shaping what we are now. The competing view is that the psychic individual who survives death is capable of multiple personalities, which are not necessarily continuous with one another, except, perhaps, in the way that an actor has a repertoire and history of roles. The modern medical phenomenon called multiple-personality syndrome is in accord with this way of looking at reincarnation. Some recorded cases are dramatic in the contrasts of personality the living body assumes.[7] In yogic lore, the idea is brought to life in stories of yogis possessing multiple human or animal bodies simultaneously.[8]

In tantric conceptions, individuality emerges in creative self-determination higher in the scale of principles, *tattva,* than the material world and these bodies of ours. The individual is, contra Nyaya, not an absolute: the "I" used by a speaker is elusive (here tantra is indebted to Samkhya), possibly meaning Shiva himself, the ultimate consciousness or self, as well as formations on many lower levels higher than our ordinary consciousness. And, again unlike Nyaya, there are a series of bodily self-determinations (mental, pranic) created by God or the Goddess or the Goddess in league with individuals. The levels of Shiva/Shakti's self-manifestion have our individuality—us souls of humans—linked in complex relationships with a series of bodies up to a deep individual self capable of diverse lifetimes (though itself dependent on the creative action of still higher or deeper levels of consciousness power). Instead of growth, the model is of an unfolding from the top down (again, a Samkhya theme).

There is also a fourth metaphysical position in Yoga on self and personal identity, Buddhist momentariness and no-self theory, which is a stream theory denying that there is an unchanging individual who either develops or self-manifests. I propose in the next section to tie up the metaphysical exploration of this section with psychological models used in yoga practice. First, let us look at a few metaphysical arguments about personal identity with an eye toward the survival possibility.

Indeed, what philosophers both East and West have had to say about personal identity, although typically restricted to this life, has rather obvious relevance for the reincarnation thesis. Are we what survives? Clearly, the ashes of the funeral pyre, the Eastern equivalent of Shakespeare's "food for worms," do not matter. What does matter?

The following list is instructive. Cut down considerably from the eighty-nine items on the original, which is from the Pali tradition of southern Buddhism and the philosopher Buddhaghosha (c. 400 C.E.), it still serves to show the complexity of personal identity. These are, according to the Buddhist, psychological factors falsely identified with, helping to create an unreal "I" that we have to transcend. There is great utility in being able to recognize the types of phenomena you can mistakenly identify with. But at least some of them are also, according to Buddhist reincarnation theory, features or lines of continuity that can survive: "volition, applied-thought, sustained-thought, happiness, interest, energy, life, concentration, faith, mindfulness, conscience, . . . tranquillity of the mental body, tranquillity of consciousness, . . . zeal, resolution, attention," and so on.[9]

Analytic philosophers have brought out what many consider most important to their identities by a variety of thought experiments. Clearly, the mind seems more important than the body, at least any particular body part. We can imagine my brain being replaced by a mechanical brain while I live on, just as with a heart transplant.[10] In a stock example from Nyaya, you need your left big toe to feel a thorn prick in the digit, but you do not need it to remember the incident (including the pain as in that toe). What matters most are lines of psychological continuity. So, within the realm of psychological continuities, the Buddhist list may be considered to present candidate features, although none is essential to our identity, according to Buddhist analysis.

What explains why we should care about our future selves? According to Buddhists, the answer is self-grasping ignorance. Why we should care is explained by causal relationships. In Buddhist analyses, it is false that we are the same person now as previously. Our sense of identity over time is misleading (and worse). Nevertheless, great lamas plot their rebirths, and though caring about what will happen to yourself is for most of us due to ignorance, it is not just common sense but also rational wisdom, given our privileged relationship to our own futures, that we should care about ourselves especially, according to Buddhist and indeed practically all Yoga theories.[11] You can dedicate your yoga practice to another, but the practice shapes yourself, at least foremost and most immediately. Consonantly, theistic Vedanta and Nyaya posit as agents eternal individuals who reincarnate, much like the souls of Platonic and Christian conception in the West.

Eternality of individuals seems, however, a rather maximalist claim. The Buddhist's embracing the Samkhya theme of the elusive "I," of our ability to identify and to disidentify with formations of personality, emotions, thoughts, and so on, has at least a grain of wisdom in it, it seems to me. Nevertheless, the Buddhist stream theory is vigorously and, in the classical context, rather successfully disputed by Nyaya, in particular by Udayana (c. 1000). Note that Abhinava Gupta's tantric view shares features of both, agreeing with the Buddhist about the elusive "I" but also with Nyaya that there is an enduring individual. And in modern philosophy, body and brain theories along with psychological theories look much more like the Buddhist view than like Nyaya.

In a broader context, a soul or consciousness nugget concept as an answer to the personal identity question has been widely jettisoned in modern philosophy. Recently, a reductionist view in many respects similar to the Buddhist no-soul continuum idea, elaborated and defended by Derek Parfit in particular, has had wide play, eliciting a large secondary literature.[12]

REBIRTH

Classically in India, the dispute over personal identity focuses on the gaps, such as deep sleep, as well as psychological continuities, such as remembering. Within Nyaya literature, a specific type of knowledge called recognition is generally taken to be the consideration that carries the day, a kind of knowledge combining perception and memory. The argument is that it would not be possible without an enduring subjectivity.[13] Only the person who experienced Devadatta yesterday could be the person who recognizes him today, since one person does not have another's memories. There is also put forth a cross-modality argument to the effect that only a self can synthesize sensory information received about a single object, a yellow piece of cloth, for instance, from two separate sensory faculties, yellow from the visual faculty and the soft touch of the cloth from the tactile.[14]

On Nyaya's side, a key supporting thesis is that properties have property bearers, also thought of as their locations. Selves and physical things have in common being the bearers of properties, some cross-type, such as dispositional properties, and some type-specific, such as cognition and color. Dispositional properties are inferred, for example a self's capacities of memory and a physical thing's elasticity. In the case of a blue lotus, we perceive both the blue and the flower. We also perceive the color as "nested in" the lotus, so to speak. However, we infer that dispositional properties have possessors.

Much of our everyday speech, *vyavahara,* reflects such a layeredness ontology of properties and property bearers (*dharma* and *dharmin*) through the relations of adjective and noun. And, like David Hume's maxim, "Save the appearances," the principle that *vyavahara* are not to be rejected without good reason is the school's operative rule. Consonantly, perceptions and cognitions of certain other types have as their objects property bearers, or qualificanda, as qualified by properties, or qualifiers, and should be assumed veridical unless shown false. Our cognitive links to objects must be assumed in general true and reliable. Otherwise, the distinction between illusion and veridical experience would make no sense and our efforts would be unsuccessful. Our talk about ourselves shows a layeredness relation between the self and its properties, cognitions, pleasures and pains, emotions, and so on.

Thus, that a self, a pot, and numerous other items endure through change is backed up by our common talk and experience to the effect that we say, for example, that it is the same pot, red now after baking, that formerly was black and this Devadatta we see is that person whom we also saw yesterday, as well as that we ourselves are the same. Then in addition to this presupposition in everyday discourse of our own sameness through change, an analysis of recognition as well as of cross-modality cognition establishes an unchanging self qualified by cognitions as properties.

The Buddhists for their part put forth a stream theory. Causality plays the role of a binder, not a property-bearing self. Everything is in flux, everything is momentary. There are no substances with properties. But so-called properties (*dharma*)—which are really tropes, unique and non-repeating (similarities are "universals" constructed by our minds for practical purposes)—are strung together causally. The current momentary item causes a similar item in the next moment, assuming no drastic change in the surrounding auxiliary causes or circumstances. A seed moment in the granary gives rise to another seed moment that is practically its duplicate, but a seed moment put in the ground with water and warmth gives rise to a sprout moment. Personal identity over time, like thing identity, is to be accounted for by particular lines of causal connection, not by enduring substances.

The chief argument for this ontology—an argument refined by Buddhist philosophers over many centuries—assumes that one thing is identical to another if and only if it has (or can be reduced to) exactly the same powers or properties. Further, to exist is to be causally efficient. So, if a seed has the power of sprout producing, then it is *ipso facto* different from a seed that is not sprout producing. It is not the same seed in the ground as it seems to have been in the granary. Previous moments in a seed stream, so to say, do not have the property of producing the sprout had by the seed moment that actually does the producing. Nothing endures, including us. Everything is always changing. Causality is our word for the regularities.

Nyaya philosophers argue that recognition and cognition across sensory modalities show the inadequacy of the Buddhist stream theory, which is a reductionism departing from everyday *vyavahara* and thus bearing, to begin with, the burden of proof. But the Buddhists claim to have a proof. So let us look a little closer at the first argument and a complaint voiced by the Nyaya philosopher Udayana.[15] If, as the Buddhist proposes, self and personal identity reduce to a series of psychological events held together and ordered causally, the temporal gap between the original experience of Devadatta and the recognition of him now cannot be explained. What happens to the information during the period when there is no awareness of it?

A striking example of the problem is deep sleep, which the Buddhist is forced to view not as an absence of consciousness but rather as a period when the consciousness stream is composed of moments of self-consciousness without object consciousness.[16] It is the lack of object-consciousness that is supposed to account for our inability to remember the nightly occurrence. But Udayana brings out that all remembering presupposes a psychological gap, a period when the information gathered by the original experience is absent from consciousness. On the Nyaya view, it lies latent in the self as the content of a mental disposition. Udayana criticizes the Buddhist on the grounds that such dispositions are excluded by his theory.

Of course, not such discontinuity but rather psychological continuity, as presupposed in the recognition, "This is that Devadatta I saw yesterday," is Nyaya's (and Udayana's) main argument for a selfsame psychological locus, a self. There is also self-perception, as verbalized in such statements as "I am aware of myself looking at the picture" (walking, talking, etc.). But self-perception, in an introspective act, is, like all perceptions, a momentary psychological occurrence and thus incapable of revealing the self's endurance over time, in the Nyaya understanding. But recognition, Nyaya insists, does indeed show, against the Buddhist or anyone, the self's continuity. Devadatta, or anything else that endures, would not be recognized as the object encountered yesterday had the subject who does the recognizing not been the same. The sameness or difference of Devadatta from the one time to the next is not the point. This the stock example is perhaps confusing since with respect to Devadatta the recognition is evidence that he too has endured, like a pot through a change of color. The point is that if I were not the same, I would not recognize Devadatta. If it were not I but some other who had experienced Devadatta—to imagine a change of subject—then only that other and not I would remember him now, that is, genuinely remember. Similarly, genuine recognition of Devadatta presupposes that the recognizer is the same person who had the previous memory-forming Devadatta experience.

Surely this would hold too for Ducasse's death-birth interval. That is to say, if there were recognition of things and events (not only of ourselves, though that would also count) from memories formed in previous lives, then reincarnation would be a warranted assumption. But, to move very fast, interpreting the enduring subjectivity as ourselves, do we have to see it as Nyaya's self? Against Nyaya, I would say no.

Nyaya's Buddhist opponent redirects the force of the recognition argument. So-called recognitive cognition does not show endurance but rather, so the Buddhist claims, only psychological continuity between the earlier and later moments. One moment of I-consciousness is the principal cause of the next; psychological continuity is to be explained causally without Nyaya's cumbersome and misleading posit of self. Every cognition has a subjective and an objective aspect. A moment of Devadatta (as object) experience is followed appropriately in your self-consciousness stream by a moment of Devadatta remembering. The information in both is fused in a moment of recognition. Mental dispositions, like everything else, are momentary, though one moment imparts its selfsame information to the next. The moment is *samskara* impregnated, so to say, and the information stored travels through a *samskara* chain or stream. Thus the subconscious vehicles of remembering are used by the Buddhist in pretty much the same way as they are by the Nyaya philosopher and, by the way, practically all disputants on the classical scene.

But Udayana's counterargument is that the Buddhist's problem is that *samskara* are subconscious, not cognitive. They are not conscious moments within the stream that comprises a person. If they were, then, like all cognition on the Buddhist view, they would themselves be immediately grasped, not needing to be inferred to be known. Cognition is, Buddhists say (in agreement with Advaita Vedanta), self-luminous, self-manifesting. All knowledge is itself known. If instead the Buddhist views *samskara* as objects belonging to another stream and not part of that which comprises a person's identity, then remembering itself, as well as the psychological events that depend on remembering, would not belong to the consciousness stream. For how would they enter? Remembering is not perceiving. But something has to carry the information about the object, besides the object itself, in the period from yesterday's experience and today's remembering. This is not another psychological stream, since one person does not have another's memories. We remember only what we have experienced ourselves. Therefore, the resource of the psychologically dispositional property, the *samskara,* is unavailable to the Buddhist theorist.[17]

Whatever the Buddhist philosopher might say in reply, Udayana has homed in on a key feature of the Buddhist view, namely, that it is self-consciousness that matters most.[18] Karma and dispositional properties may shape a future personality, but the consciousness stream is taken to be what really matters. At each moment there is self-consciousness in that consciousness is aware of itself as consciousness. This *dharma* is privileged in the psychological continuum that not only is the person in this lifetime but also goes on past death (see below, figure 4B).

Thus in the end—and in wide overview, with an eye toward reincarnation—there seems little difference here from Nyaya, little difference between these staunchest of classical opponents, since consciousness, according to the Buddhist, survives death, as do many lines of karma.

Nyaya's idea of a self who is not necessarily but can be self-aware, whose presence underlying a stream of psychological properties secures identity, does not seem all that different, in cross-life perspective, from a consciousness stream around which accrues karmic dispositions and memories. Both are supposed capable of translife memories, as Ducasse would require (though only the Buddhists, and not the Nyaya philosophers, ever talk about this). Indeed, on the Buddhist theory, which is the one interpreted as reductionist, self-consciousness is more important than it is with Nyaya. The consciousness stream secures personal identity for the Buddhist in the current lifetime and beyond, whereas the Nyaya philosopher says we are often distracted and not conscious of ourselves, not only now but also after death. Perhaps we should say that it is on the Nyaya view that the "I" is elusive! The tantric Abhinava sides with the Buddhist about self-consciousness, and the individual he posits is not an eternal and independent entity, though it remains the same through multiple earthly incarnations. The Mahayana Buddhist, for her part, finds the bodhisattva to develop perfections over lifetimes, perfections understood as *dharma* streams accruing to a particular *santana* or psychological continuum of (self-)consciousness. And there is the Upanishadic conception of a spark soul or Hamsa, the great bird who flies over the highest mountains of life and death—ideas to which we shall return in chapter 5.

Translife Consciousness

We as "persons" do not survive death.[19] Personal identity is constituted in part by the physical body as well as by psychological continuity. Philosophers have shown that we use mixed criteria, physical and psychological, to make judgments about whether a person at time t_2 is the same as the person earlier at t_1.[20] Even the conservative Indian schools of Nyaya, Mimamsa, and others agree that what they call the self is not the person; the person is confined to the length of a particular life, whereas the self survives the death of the body.

Yoga philosophers disagree, however, about precisely what survives. Vedantins have somewhat different views from Nyaya (and Mimamsa, etc.) not only about translife continuity but also about the individual (*jivatman*) and the ontological underpinnings of self-consciousness, as do of course Buddhists: this is the "elusive I" one level up! So let us take a few steps down from the controversy about what's real to look at the psychological sides of the Yoga theories and what is said more concretely about processes and formations that form the bridgework between lifetimes.

We enter now the realm of the occult and nonmaterial and therefore of high speculation, where yogic and other mystical testimony is crucial as a launching pad. Nevertheless, we can also identify in ordinary experience the psychic sheaths, physical, pranic, and so on, central to one model of translife consciousness. Yogic testimony gets preeminent weight, but there are theoretical connections with everyday life on all the models, as we shall see.[21]

All Yoga psychology assumes a subtle body or nonmaterial psychological continua, whether simple or, more normally, complex consisting of multiple strands. Two models are dominant, a sheath conception, which corresponds to, roughly, a band or aggregate conception, and a chakric conception. Many tantrics use both the sheath/band model and the chakric, and some theorize on how the two relate. There are also complications about temporal limitations and the question of soul development mentioned at the beginning of the chapter. Let us try to disentangle Yogic thought about reincarnation by looking first at the psychological model of concentric or suffusing sheaths, *kosha* (figure 4A) along with its Buddhist stream or aggregate counterpart (figure 4B), then the chakric theory (figure 4C). Afterward, we shall return to the idea of soul development.

First, a little more about history. The Buddhist *skandha* model of our consciousness—*skandha*s are aggregates of currents of different phenenoma or entities, literally "parts" or "shoulders," of a translife complex or continuum (figure 4B)—is causal and antisubstantivalist, unlike the substantivalist *kosha* conception of the Upanishads, which is slightly earlier.[22] Nevertheless, there is at least a rough match with the sheath model, the *kosha* and the theory of the cosmic self, *atman*. The *rupa skandha*—anglicizing the Sanskrit, which in Pali is *khandha*—is sense data, form, matter corresponding to the food (*annamaya*) sheath; *vedana* is sensation, feeling corresponding to the pranic (*pranamaya*) sheath; *samjna* is cognition, thought corresponding to the lower-mind (*manomaya*) sheath; *samskara* (also *vasana*) is disposition corresponding to the higher-mind (*vijnanamaya*) sheath; and finally *vijnana* is consciousness corresponding to the bliss (*anandamaya*) sheath and the central self. Further convergence of traditions occurs in broad views of the relationship of karma and rebirth, as shown in both Buddhist and Hindu "mythological" stories of multiple worlds of after-death experience as well as in teachings of moral lessons to be learned from rebirth. But let us focus, if arbitrarily, on the substantivalist conception of the sheath, while keeping in mind that similar ideas are present in Buddhism. Shortly, we shall see that the sheath schema is consistent with the view of the afterlife in the *Tibetan Book of the Dead*, among other non-Vedantic ideas and texts.

According to the *kosha* or sheath model (figure 4A), consciousness has five spheres of embodiment: physical; vital—or "breath-made," pranic; lower-mind—the sensuous intelligence we share with animals; higher-mind—more profoundly connective intelligence; and blissful. The *Taittiriya Upanishad,* the earliest source, seems to have these bodies concentrically ordered, each interior (*antara*) to its predecessor, beginning with the most exterior, the physical body, the food (*annamaya*) sheath. However, the meaning of the word "interior" does not, in this context, concern relative location but rather relative essentiality and nearness to the immortal self. Some interpret "interior" as coincident. The ideas of essentiality and distance from the self are realized with respect to relative endurance, among other factors. The physical sheath perishes at the most rapid rate. Each sheath connects with a world or environment consonant with its constituents. The food sheath has as its external or universal counterpart the physical world, the pranic sheath has the life universe (or universes), the lower-mind and higher-mind sheaths connect with mental universes, and then bliss and spirit contain or suffuse all universes. The inner sheaths enliven the outer, and the outer can die or fall away while the inner continue on. The material world is suffused with *prana, prana* with mind energy, and so on. In other words, there is at least enough independence of the inner from the outer that the individual in her pranic body can and does survive the death and dissolution of the material sheath.

The individual self, *jiivatman*—or is it the universal self, *atman?*—chisels personality formations through its karma-making choices in the pranic and mental bodies as well as the physical. So not only do the nonphysical bodies—and the self's bliss (usually treated as intrinsic, if hidden from our waking consciousness)—survive, at least for a time, the dissolution of the physical sheath, but so do dispositions that mold the different substances into personality. Our strong talents and likes and dislikes and the whole range of emotional, mental, and intuitive resources that make up much of what we are right now will, so goes the core theory, continue on in a pranic or another world, enveloping this one, and shape our reincarnations.

Phenomenologically, our patterns of thought, our cast of mind, I should like to point out, do have unity comparable to that of the physical body. Each of us has a mental personality that is comparable to our physical "look," and our emotional or affective personality also has comparable unity. Thus it is not a stretch to imagine vital and mental bodies for an individual. The sheath model is of course metaphor, and beyond denial of causal closure, as discussed in chapter 2, the relationships among the parts of our being are not known. The tantric view of chakras has them connected by canals, *nadi,* which are sometimes viewed as strings of spiritual light also connecting the sheaths.[23]

In the tantric conception, nonmaterial substance or energy exists. The chakras are not material. From the epistemic point of view of our Yoga minimalism, this is the crucial part. Concerning details, my best guess is that like early physical theories, much of this occult physiology will be revised and changed, perhaps significantly. Nevertheless, the main point is that the emotional and thinking beings we are can and do survive death.

Now in due course there may well be, as some teach, dissolution of the pranic and mental bodies in turn. Not only do opinions diverge about the precise components of the "subtle body," *sukshma sharira,* that survives death and reincarnates, there is little consensus about the after-death adventure. Disputed in particular is what "exhausts itself" in experience in other worlds and what continues on to be reincarnated here, or whether, as in Tibetan Buddhism, by resisting the pull to reincarnation at various pivotal points one continues to progress toward enlightenment. Nevertheless, everyone agrees that formations in all four interior sheaths (or, in Buddhism, in all the *skandha*s, or at least bundled components from every *skandha*), are said to survive the dissolution of the physical.

The sheath model employs a substance metaphor that connects with the idea of worlds. Each sheath is made of a substance or energy that is a subkind of universal stuff, ordered asymmetrically in terms of successive containments such that the more interior formations are to endure the dissolution of the less. However, all are supposed to be interconnected, according to not only (rival) Buddhism as a fundamental principle of the universe but also Hinduism (for the most part), through the being of the Absolute Brahman (who is necessarily omnipresent).

In the mainstream Vedantic conception—which is absorbed into both Buddhist and Hindu tantra—the metaphysical correlate to the range of sheaths is the idea of the physical universe as one organized range of a continuum of manifested being, *sat.* The material universe is presumed to be a sector so distinctly organized that it appears to be separate from other universes, which are similarly distinctly organized and appear separate although none is in fact. All are sustained by the being of the Absolute, according to Vedanta, or are maintained by the cosmically constituent energy or shakti (or Shri), in tantric views. There are, strictly speaking, no "parallel universes" in Vedanta, tantra, etc., although we are encouraged to think like that by talk of various "worlds" in the Upanishads and elsewhere (*loka,* etymologically, field of vision), and indeed of separate sheaths.[24] But everything is interconnected; as pointed out, the "higher" are said to pervade and suffuse the "lower," for example, *prana*, enlivening the physical body and the mental suffusing *prana*.

According to Vedantic theism as well as the creationism of Abhinava and other tantrics, God is prolific. God self-determines its intrinsic aspect of energy/stuff to emanate a series of interconnected worlds or levels of being, ranging from the heavens of gods and goddesses through life worlds of typal beings down to our material level or, according to some, lower levels of hell.[25] The degree and type of power enjoyed by the individuals within a world as well as the character of the energy/stuff constituting a common nature and intersubjective objects distinguish heavens from hells and lower life worlds, as well as from our physical universe. Our physical world is apparently peculiar in manifesting properties typical of life and mind worlds, and as physical beings we live simultaneously in the physical extensions, so to say, of other universes.

At death, the subtle body (*sukshma sharira*) or astral body or, as is sometimes said, pranic body—which then would consist of not only the vital or pranic sheath but also the three sheaths interior along with the interiormost consciousness or self (variously interpreted, the metaelusive "I")—somehow "travels" to one or another life world, in the normal course of events. This would be, as explained, a universe largely separate from the physical world. However, there is much continuity, since, for example, the surviving being still thinks and has dreamlike experience continuous with her or his earthly embodiment. As suggested, opinions diverge about whether reincarnation is launched from this next world or whether there are a series of sheddings of bodies and travel through a series of worlds. Even Vedantins hardly speak in unison. The *Tibetan Book of the Dead* presents a complex series of realms into which the consciousness of the deceased can enter. Possibly there is no general rule.

Metaphysically, however, the ideas are clearer. The world of the physical sheath is at the boundaries of creation, viewed from the perspective of the essential consciousness. The soul sojourns here to practice yoga for spiritual development, say some tantrics. Mahayanins say that we should want to return to help others, progressively developing the necessary abilities. Embodied physically, we are also embodied pranically and mentally, living simultaneously in all the sheaths. The mental and vital sheaths help to determine what happens physically during a lifetime. Conversely, earthly choices and events and reactions shape the subtle body that survives.

Mental dispositions, including dispositions to desire and emotion, need not rest in the self, as says Nyaya, but in the pranic and mental bodies, as say Vedantins (of all stripes). Surely this is right. Some *samskara*

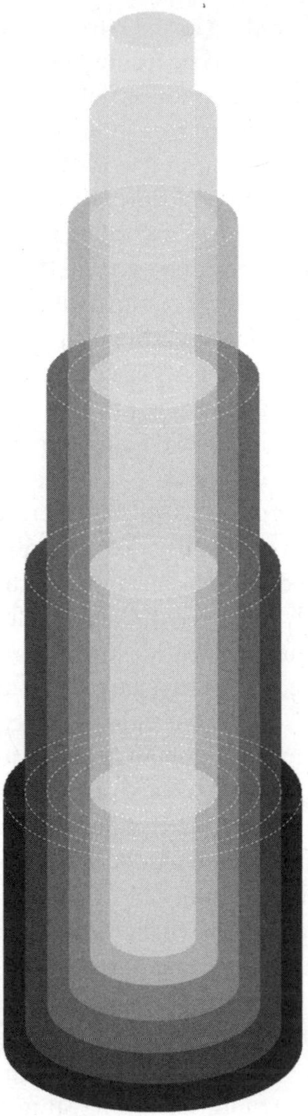
atman
self, that which is ensheathed but also all-suffusing
anandamaya-kosha
body made of bliss, *ananda*
vijnanamaya-kosha
body made of higher intelligence, *vijnana*
manomaya-kosha
body made of lower intelligence, *manas*
pranamaya-kosha
body made of life energy, *prana*
annamaya-kosha
body made of matter, "food", *anna*

FIGURE 4A. Koshas

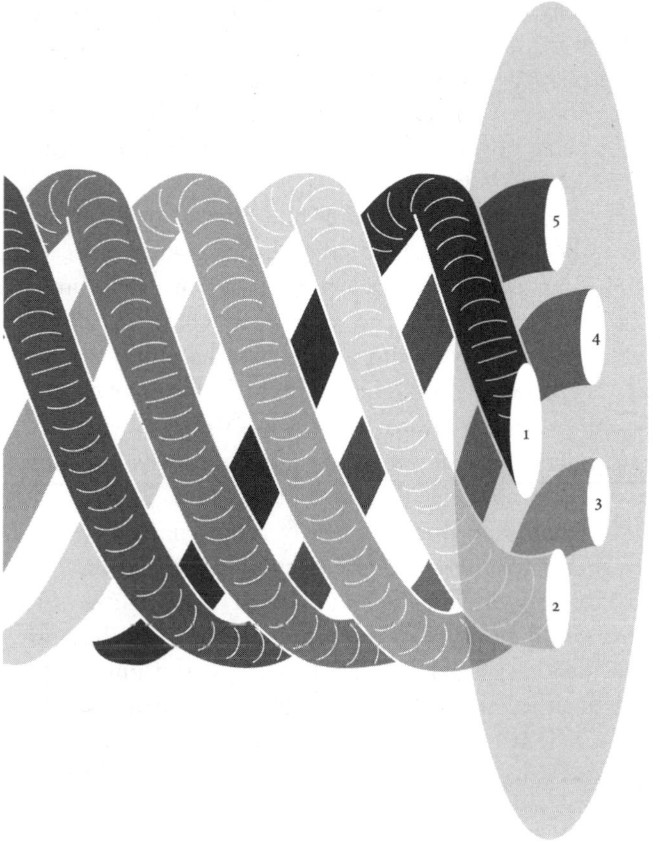

1. *Vijnana*, consciousness, self-consciousness
2. *Vedana*, sensation, feeling
3. *Samjna*, cognition, representational thought
4. *Samskara*, or *vasana*, disposition, connective thought
5. *Rupa*, sense-data, form, matter

FIGURE 4B. Skandhas

(mental dispositions) obviously rest in the brain. Formation of *samskara* percolate in, so to say, resonating through multiple levels, our actions etching patterns in nonmaterial energy/stuff as well as in the brain and physical body. Thus there would be, continuous with our earthly persons, aspects of ourselves that survive and act as individuals on other stages, like dream personas.

After appropriate adventures and rest in whatever worlds, the subtle body embodying the individual that died reincarnates along with the essential individual. Our Yoga minimalism prevents much further specification of the nature of the individual who dies and takes rebirth, but I shall close chapter 5 with a few remarks that are directed to practice. There is too much disagreement about the reality or unreality of the individual (*jivatman*) in broadest perspective, though there are convergences in practice. Advaitins would join Buddhists in saying that any individuality is ultimately illusory. For Advaita, Brahman is in the end the "I," and Brahman does not really reincarnate. Theistic Vedantins disagree sharply, Ramanuja, for instance, seeing the reincarnating *jivatman* as an eternal individual, as in Nyaya. There are other metaphysical variations, and the nature of the worlds we enter—there are so many possibilities to keep track of—is not clearly and uniformly conceptualized in classical literature or even in (Hindu) tantric texts specifically (I say this aware that I may be speaking in haste—this is a vast ocean of texts). Much seems to be left purposely vague, as though itself in honor of the minimalist attitude!

The *Tibetan Book of the Dead,* or *Bardol Thotrol,* is, in contrast, rich in details about an afterlife drama and opportunities for enlightenment.[26] Buddhist and antisubstantivalist, the text sets the adventure in phases or *bardo*s (transitions) where a common pattern of events occur, not as travel to other worlds. But the other-worlds schema of Vedanta and Hindu tantra translates pretty easily into the event-organized picture, although the conceptions of the three bodies of the Buddha and the five *skandha* or strands within the personality stream are, to be sure, peculiarly Buddhist. The overall plot structure as well as the forces and personalities encountered (hungry gods, bodhisattvas, wrathful deities, etc.) could be reconceived in substantivalist terms. Conversely, the other worlds of Hinduism and the Vedantic conception of sheaths could be accommodated to the Buddhist fantasia. The Tibetan tradition understands afterlife events as typal and invariable for everyone, although there are options (divergent routes) depending on choice or recognition and the karma of the deceased. New Yoga can accept this common denominator, the lines of emotional and intellectual continuity sketched, whatever the metaphysical truth about an underlying Self or self.

The *Bardol Thotrol* is most of all about enlightenment, about opportunities afforded the consciousness surviving a human death to become something other than someone destined for rebirth, realizing her true nature and merging with the *dharma kaya,* the "Dharma body," of the Buddha. Although treated as an individual unit in the directions given, i.e., as the addressee, the deceased is, in Buddhist conception, not really differentiated as an individual. Opportunities for enlightenment are sometimes talked about as though one's wave of light rejoined a larger and surer luminosity. The compassion of a bodhisattva is figured as a "light-ray hook." But note also the usage of the term *kaya,* body, in the compound *dharma kaya,* which in several places designates the supreme opportunity.[27] Furthermore, the deceased's "thought body" is mentioned expressly, and certain experiences and opportunities presuppose it.[28]

No chakric system of either a Buddhist or a Hindu variety is used very much in the *Bardol Thotrol.* Pranic energy is said to flow through a central channel (*avadhuti* = *sushumna*), but there is no express mention of energy centers. However, in other Buddhist texts—including, to be sure, Tibetan Buddhist—a chakric system is used to flesh out, so to say, a subtle body that survives and reincarnates.[29] We come now to our second prominent model of occult physiology, the chakric (figure 4C), which is also utilized to specify the continuity presupposed in the idea of reincarnation. As explained, I shall use Yogic and Vedantic terminology, not Buddhist, though the latter could serve as well. I shall also use what has become now in the twenty-first century a rather mainstream conception of global sway. But we should keep in mind that there is quite a diversity in details in the early texts, so scholars tell us.[30]

A series of chakras or occult centers of consciousness is depicted as joined, for an individual, by a central channel called *sushumna.* Pranic or life energy can be redirected from its regular channels throughout the pranic body, which suffuses and enlivens the physical frame, i.e., in the *nadi*s or ducts that constitute the main lines of flow of pranic energy. Thus it can be made to flow and "cleanse" the central channel, which joins the lowest realms of being with the spiritual. In the *Hatha Yoga Pradipika,* the central channel is talked about as itself divine, e.g., as Shambhavi (the "Kind Mother") (see appendix E, verse 3.4).

Other than the *sushumna,* the two most important *nadi*s are the *ida* and the *pingala,* which interweave from the nasal apertures through (or near) the chakric centers like the intertwining snakes around the caduceus of Greek mythology. Pranic energy can be redirected from these (by breath control as well as *bandha* engagement; see the discussion in the introduction as well as appendix E) to flow into the central channel, the divine axis said to correspond to the spinal column. This directly connects the principal chakras, which are seven (sometimes four, six, eight, nine, or ten). The chakras, like the sheaths, are thought to have cosmological dimensions, each connecting with a specific range of energies or substance or vibrational frequencies, depending on the otherworlds conception.

The seven principal chakras are, beginning with the lowest or "root" chakra (see figure 4C):

1) *muladhara,* the "root-support," which is said to feel as though located at the base of the spine and to connect the pranic with the physical, as well as to be the locus of the sleeping serpent energy, *kundalini* (more about which just below—some put *kundalini* in the second or third chakras instead);
2) *svadhishthana,* the "self-established," connecting with sexual energies (and so located);
3) *manipura,* the navel center, the "city of jewels," another life-world center and the beginning of the central channel in some Buddhist systems;
4) *anahata,* the heart center where the "unstruck" sound is heard, where *bhakti* is felt;
5) *vishuddhi,* the throat center, the "pure," connecting with voice and artistic expression;
6) the third eye, *ajna,* corresponding to the middle of the forehead, the "command center," the center of highest mind; and
7) *sahasrara,* the "thousand-spoked [wheel]," also *sahasra-dala,* the "thousand-petaled [lotus]," the divine center, the center of enlightenment, which is said to be located just above the crown of the head and connected occultly with the *brahma randhra,* the cranial cleft through which runs the central channel, *sushumna.*

A second kind of current or energy is said to flow in the central channel, shakti, also *kundalini,* the serpent power, a divine or more divine energy in contrast with *prana,* the energy of life and breath. Some tantric texts say summarily that the point of yoga is to replace *prana* with shakti in the central channel. "Kundalini yoga" is now an English expression referring to yoga practices focused on awakening *kundalini* so that we become aware of our diviner selves, considered to be more essentially embodied in our system of chakric centers, through which the divine energy flows unchecked by the ordinary limitations of being human.

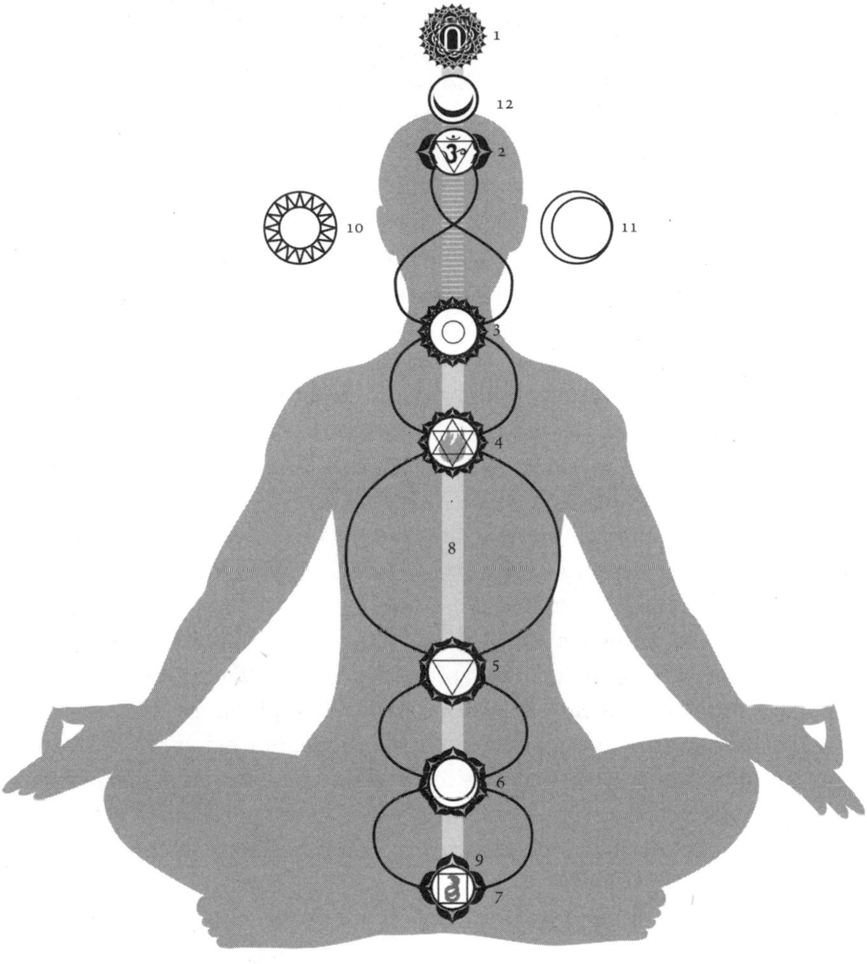

1. *Sahasrara,* "thousand-spoked wheel" of enlightenment
2. *Ajna,* "command" center, third eye
3. *Vishuddhi,* the "pure", center of inspiration
4. *Anahata,* life and heart center, center of the "unstruck" sound
5. *Manipura,* city of "jewels", life center
6. *Svadhishthana,* the "self-willed", life center
7. *Muladhara,* "root" center, where Kundalini sleeps
8. *Sushumna,* divine road
9. *Kundalini,* serpent energy
10. *Pingala,* pranic channel, "Sun"
11. *Ida,* pranic channel, "Earth"
12. *Brahma-randhra,* cleft of Brahman

FIGURE 4C. Chakras

There are also top-down Yoga teachings, *shakti pata,* descent of shakti (see the quote from the *Kularnava Tantra* in note 19 to appendix D). Divine energy is supposed to flow down from the thousand-petaled lotus above the body enlivening the central channel and the lower centers of consciousness, in the end awakening the *kundalini* energy—a reunion of lover and beloved throughout the manifestation of Brahman as the perfect individual (the bodhisattva).[31]

In the tantric Shaivism of Abhinava Gupta (see appendix D), the chakric model is employed in a top-down conception of creation including, in another Samkhya theme, very real individual conscious beings, a plurality of distinct *purusha*s. Abhinava posits a status for the individual beyond embodiment and embodiments, as in large part a manifestation, not just a development along lines continuous with previous births. Although Abhinava is a tantric monist, he finds a real, translife-constant, progressively manifesting individual. It's as though there are bare spiritual particulars, all exemplars of the chakric form, which is like a mold into which Shiva breathes—blows into full actuality like a glassmaker—life, the personalities assumed. The main thesis of the *Spanda-karika,* which is one of Abhinava's sources, is that the world is a tremor, vibration, *spanda* of the divine, an out-breath followed by an in-breath of enlightenment. The in-breath does not destroy but enlightens. The world is progressive manifestation, arranged from above, not below. In this complex of ideas, there is a clear step toward the antisubstantivalism of the Buddhist, since it is vertical integration in a moment of time that is important, not so much soul development, each instant a moment of unique beauty in a cosmic dance.

Inspiring visions employ the chakric system. But there is, in addition to the occult literature on chakras as matters of advanced yogic experience, rather mundane theorizing, some very crude, about chakric and occult determinations of events in everyday life. Please, yoga enthusiasts, don't expect me to champion everything. In order to be open to yogic teachings about chakras as they relate to our practices, we need not have too concrete a notion, I think, of occult flows of *prana* and shakti nor, especially, about the ties to everyday experience. Direct chakric openings in the course of asana work are not uncommon (especially in Corpse Pose, *shavasana*).[32] We don't have to have brittle beliefs in order to be ready for chakric experience.

Similarly, we have every right to be confident that at least something of our emotional and thinking beings survives—along with our best parts, our self-consciousness (in the Buddhist view) or our spiritual being. We shall look further at the concept of the spiritual individual in chapter 5.

The case for reincarnation is cumulative. No premise is the one and only hinge upon which all depends. Nevertheless, the reports of yogins and other mystics get special weight, and I shall devote the greater part of this section to the epistemology of yogic perception and mystic testimony. Then, in addition to several nonyogic considerations and evidence that provide further support for the reincarnation thesis, there are metaphysical considerations that help—for example, an argument put forth by Aurobindo that ties rebirth to the overall meaning of life. I shall look at all of these as well as, at the end, attacks by a famous atheist and psychic debunker, Paul Edwards. Thus, we shall take up yogic arguments, claims deriving from the results of yoga practice transmitted by testimony; nonyogic empirical considerations, such as xenoglossy, a child's ability to speak a language she has not learned; one metaphysical argument, which, though containing empirical premises, hinges on a nonempirical reason, namely, life having meaning; and arguments to the contrary.

Superstition finds fecund soil in the idea of rebirth. I have proposed that Yoga requires only a minimalist view of afterlife possibilities. But a kind of maximalist commitment, or dedication, to practices is required to make the discoveries the experts say connect best with survival. Such commitment, however, is not the same as belief. Indeed, mere belief is too bare-bones to inspire practice. It has to be surrounded by emotional attitudes as well as, when called for, assessment of degree of trust. I recommend as the Yogic attitude toward rebirth something like quiet interest and confidence in an adventure whose details are unknown but for which there is no better preparation than yoga practice. The epistemic or justificational component of such confidence is the subject of this section.

Yogic arguments trade on a parallelism thesis, an epistemic parallelism between yogic and sense experience implicit in the notion, common to all Yoga schools (with qualifications), of yogic perception, *yaugika pratyaksha*.[33] The move presupposes that ordinary sense perception has epistemic value (for the uncorrupted nonphilosopher, hardly a stretch), i.e., that in its normal operations it reveals facts and features of things around us; in other words, that it is a knowledge source, *pramana*—as say almost all the classical Yoga theorists. Yogic perception is a knowledge source for spiritual discoveries just as vision informs us of the lay of the land with respect to our physical environment.

The classical picture of the causal working of knowledge sources—perception, inference, testimony, a few other candidates—was sketched in chapter 3 in connection with the idea of *samskara*. Here we take a more purely epistemological or evaluative perspective. Yogic arguments have premises that are derived from yogic experience, such that at least one such premise—let us call it a yogic proposition, which is a lot like a claim made on the basis of sense perception—will figure crucially. Yogic propositions are warranted or justified by yogic perception, and the warrant carries over to conceptions and arguments developed from yogic propositions. The simple story ends here.

In both East and West, there have been many much more complicated stories just about the epistemic worth of sense perception, which is the launching pad for our parallelism thesis. The question of which sorts of claim sense perception makes certain has been a bugbear to theorists practically everywhere. To move quickly, I say, in line with Nyaya in classical India and successful criticism of Cartesian foundationalism in the West, that we should take for granted a certain fallibilism:[34] any claim made on the basis of sense perception is defeasible, that is to say, is possibly wrong, is correctable. So too, then I say, with yogic perception as a knowledge source. In both cases, we need a theory with a defeasibility condition. Normally our senses do generate knowledge, but sometimes appearances are misleading (astigmatic, I see two moons). Similarly, yogic experience of consciousness independent of the body (and death) is trustworthy by default, but this yogic proposition could be defeated by other evidence or arguments.

So far our discussion has proceeded from what is called an externalist point of view in epistemology, which has as byword, "innocent until proven guilty." As with sense perception in ordinary circumstances—and testimony based on firsthand experience—we do not question yogic perception's veridicality, or the truth of what we are told by the testifier (*guru*) who knows, unless specific reasons arise. Conscious certification is called for only when there are grounds for reasonable doubt. This externalist attitude is best defended in Yoga classically by the school of Nyaya.

But let us also put our parallelism thesis to the test of a different approach to knowledge, the internalist, which finds self-conscious justification to be required for a belief to count as knowledge. Yogic epistemic parallelism holds here too.

Following Roderick Chisholm and William Alston, I find a "Theory of Appearance" to capture the defeasibility of sense perception without denying its epistemic value from an internalist perspective.[35] This is an internalist view in that the subject knows that she is confronted with indications that might be misleading but is nevertheless sure about what she takes to be revealed. But note that the overall parallelism thesis does not hinge on Chisholm's or Alston's (or my or anyone's) version of perceptual warrant. Nevertheless, Alston's theory in particular does capture at least my intuitions about the role of sense perception in generating knowledge from an internalist point of view.

> A subject S who takes herself to be appeared to by object *a* F-ly (that is to say, who takes herself to perceive *a* as F) is *prima facie* justified in believing that *a* is F.

For example, S, looking at a banyan tree, takes herself to be appeared to banyanly (that is to say, takes herself to perceive the tree as a banyan), and is thereby *prima facie* justified in believing that the tree is a banyan. It may turn out to be a Hollywood movie prop or the like; the belief is justified *prima facie* only. Thus according to the yogic parallelism thesis, the belief "*a* is F" would be a yogic proposition, a basic yogic claim, insofar as a yogin or yogini self-consciously takes herself in her inner yogic experience to be appeared to appropriately. I daresay that the great teachers of yoga have been quite self-conscious about what they take themselves to perceive or experience. They articulate it in yogic propositions. Yogic arguments for rebirth have as a premise at least one yogic proposition, whose warrant derives from yogic perception.

For the externalist, the burden of proof is on the side of opponents of the parallelism thesis, since knowledge does not have to be justified. But this is also true for the internalist. For clearly yogins and yoginis self-consciously take their yogic experiences to be informative, as much as does anyone her sense experience. Thus, without countervailing evidence, they have a right to believe that F*a* (that, e.g., their consciousness is independent of the body), a right that passes on to us, their students, by their testimony. Furthermore, one level up, they themselves—or at least almost all the classical Yoga philosophies that defend and encourage yoga—assert the parallelism. Let me repeat that this is implicit in the very concept of *yaugika pratyaksha,* yogic perception, which in effect all the schools accept: yogic perception is a knowledge source, *pramana,* like sense perception.

Of course, for certain topics only a few people count as having the authority to make a yogic claim. Nonyogins and all levels of student depend on the testimony of those in the know. As argued in chapter 1, our guiding principle should be to give the benefit of the doubt. This is in fact the attitude we take in action in everyday life. Otherwise, we could not get along in the world. For example, by and large we have not personally experienced being named the names we carry. Even if as babies we were present, we cannot remember the ceremony. I take it on the testimony of (especially) my parents that the name I have is indeed mine. How crazy would it be to doubt such testimony, although we can easily imagine its falsity! The epistemic default is trust.

Let me once more emphasize that the parallelism thesis and what we may call the charity view of testimony do not entail the truth of yogic claims. All claims are corrigible. The faith to sustain practice does not depend on absolutely precise content of beliefs or on certainty. There may well emerge considerations that override the guru's teaching, as with an apparent perception of two moons. Nevertheless, we are to assume that meditation and other yogic experience has a noetic or cognitive quality, being both taken as informative about some pretty important matters, such as the death-spanning nature of our consciousness, and informative in fact. There is no general reason we should not trust our teachers' testimony. Of course, if materialism were true, testimony about the non-material nature of the subtle or pranic body that survives would be mistaken. But here (in chapter 2) we have successfully resisted the offending thesis of materialism, to wit, causal closure, and there is no other general consideration I am aware of that would undercut the healthy and open-minded attitude of accepting (provisionally, as with any testimony) what our teachers say. The Nyaya definition of testimony as a knowledge source (going all the way back to the *Nyaya Sutra,* sutra 1.1.7) is that it is the conveyance of information by an expert, i.e., by one knowing the truth, who wants to communicate with no intention to lie or deceive.

Opponents of the parallelism thesis purport to find a problem in the partial intersubjectivity of the (yogic, mystical) experience deemed to be, like sense perception, informative. Buddhists make different yogic propositions than do Hindus, objectors would allege using our terminology. The hasty (and illogical) conclusion is that disagreement cancels all views out, since the truth should be universally accessible and known. Religious pluralism is best explained as varieties of error, in this view. Yogic claims are undermined by the circumstances of their origin, peculiar histories leading to peculiar and diverse claims. I called this the historicist worry in chapter 1.

There are four main lines of response to the challenge, which through Yoga eyes looks like the problem of diverse lineages—the pluralism of views and traditions, some in sharp disagreement on certain issues—all of which promote yoga. So, in brief, the first line of answer is that, like Jaina positive perspectivalism and *syad-vada,* our Yoga minimalism includes the policy of relative and provisional acceptance, which does not mean that some claims might not on scrutiny be thrown out.

The second line, complementing the first, is that we are interested in convergences and divergences. We want to know why there are divergences. The convergences, such as between Buddhists and Hindus on the chakra system or even the *kosha* and *skandha* schemas, when appreciated, give us a better grip on truths of our psychology.

The third line is that partial intersubjectivity is well known to be objective within special activities that take sense perception to be informative, e.g., wine tasting, reading (knowing how the letters are sounded), jewel assessment, and so on (only the experts have the right to pronounce on the wine, the letters, the jewel, and so on). Yoga practice has physical, vital/emotional, intellectual, and spiritual dimensions, and there are high bars to cross in each sphere. Anyone in principle has the right to make a statement about, let us say, rebirth, that would count as initially acceptable, but only if he or she has passed all the disciplinary prerequisites should that person's testimony be accorded the status of a yogic proposition based on yogic perception. Not everyone counts as an expert.

Fourth and finally, with such overwhelming testimony as we have about survival, contrary testimony, for example, that water is fiery, appears to be defeated in advance, *badhita,* blocked, as a Nyaya philosopher would say. No belief is immune from revision and falsification, but some beliefs are well entrenched and unlikely to be dislodged.

A second group of arguments develop from nonyogic phenomena that indicate reincarnation in the absence of better explanations. Dean of rebirth research over the past fifty years, Ian Stevenson has published books and papers devoted to children's rememberings along with other abilities and bodily features that cannot be accounted for by genetics, experience, or the environment in the current lifetime.[36] The data range from the highly generic down to specifics, i.e., privileged knowledge to which it seems that only a very few particular people could have access.

Xenoglossy constitutes especially impressive evidence. But it is only one arrow in Stevenson's quiver. His research ranges wide, including birthmarks corresponding to wounds that the child's predecessor sustained along with birth defects, postures and gestures, and general countenance as helping to confirm a child's memories. Children, Stevenson explains, tend to be the only people who remember previous lives because they are not, like adults, so preoccupied with the affairs of this one. His cases are taken mainly from cultures where rebirth is a common belief. He argues that in the United States and other Western cultures there is built in discouragement of any talk that could lead to identification of the child's predecessor. "Don't say things like that, Martha. You're just daydreaming." Or it may be that simply a lack of encouragement results in such memories fading like dreams upon the child's immersion into worldly activity.

Overall, Stevenson makes an impressive showing. Surely he deserves a wider hearing among philosophers.[37] For Yoga philosophy, it is obvious that his evidence is not just compatible with our (minimalist) conceptions but also provides support.[38] However, the material is massive, and there is no point in reviewing cases. The main debunker I know of is Paul Edwards, and his mockery and ridicule and no-holds-barred assaults on the character of the testifiers means that details would have to be patiently reexamined to answer, for example, charges of lying. Suffice it to say that New Yoga has an ally in Professor Stevenson and other rebirth researchers.[39]

The standard argument in classical Indian philosophy focuses on voluntary action directed to a goal that has not been previously cognized by an infant or child in the current lifetime.[40] Goal-directed activity requires mental dispositions (*samskara*) formed by previous experience, and a child's first-time reaching for the mother's breast, or whatever the first action, is goal-directed, pushed by desire and informed by awareness of the breast as satisfying desire. *Ex hypothesi,* no such desire fulfillment has been had in the current life, and therefore must have occurred in a previous lifetime.

This proves rebirth, however, only of a generic consciousness, a generic human or animal soul that wants food and knows where to look. It does not prove that the hungry infant reincarnates particular lines of psychological continuity embodied previously in Mr. Smith.

Xenoglossy is similarly restricted as evidence; it holds that the child has inherited dispositions from prior generations of the speakers of the particular language. These *samskara* could be without content that is restricted to a particular life and person. Still, here we have strong evidence for some kind of reincarnation. Perhaps part of xenoglossy could be accounted for by the thesis of a universal grammar. Vocabulary, however, is entirely learned and conventional. Its proper use implies training. It is not inherited genetically. Nevertheless, being able to speak a particular language belongs to large communities (usually) and is a characteristic that does not differentiate individuals within large groups. At the other extreme, there are cases of rather privileged knowledge or recognitive abilities that indicates a specific line of continuity to one very particular person, Mr. Jones, from another, Mr. Smith.

Genetics is commonly cited as accounting for traits of personality, emotions, and even consciousness. But genetics provides only necessary, never sufficient conditions for psychological properties or states.

Furthermore, acquired characteristics are not, according to current theory, inherited. Thus Mr. Jones's memories formed by Mr. Smith provide evidence for reincarnation.

Personally, I think the memory cases recorded by Stevenson and others should not be accorded too much weight in shaping our overall theory since the rule is that we do not remember past lives. Past-life memories are the exception. Nevertheless, memory, as mentioned to open the chapter following Ducasse, is crucial in the soul space between incarnations, since without it the view would fall to the "Liebniz objection" that one person, Mr. Smith, died, and another, Mr. Jones, was born.

Finally, at the risk of running together arguments from categories one and two, the yogic proposition that there is available through yoga practice the power, *siddhi,* to remember past lives is common lore. The *siddhi* is expressly mentioned in the *Yoga Sutra,* among other places.[41]

A third group of arguments finds the rebirth idea intrinsic to a whole world vision. Here we may place a bit of abstract reasoning by the modern guru and philosopher Aurobindo.[42] He argues that since individuality is central to our lives as human beings, to our cultures, and indeed to our yoga practice—practice that can lead to spiritual enlightenment—it cannot be entirely illusory or so transitory as to end with death. Egoism is illusory and worse, but individuality itself is not all false. Now this is, to be sure, taking for granted a certain background metaphysics, namely, a variety of Vedantic and tantric monistic theism. Brahman, or God, working through divine shakti, suffuses the universe as "Sachchidananda," Being-Consciousness=Force-Bliss. Brahman "self-manifests" this nature for the purpose of delight and self-discovery. Life would not have meaning if the individual did not in some way survive, and such meaninglessness in the self-manifestation of Brahman would be metaphysically discordant. Rebirth is the necessary "machinery" for the persistence.[43]

The argument can be reconstructed as follows.

A) If God is X (Sachchidananda, loving, omnibenevolent), then life has to be meaningful.
B) Life would not be meaningful without persistent individuality.
C) Persistent individuality in our world demands rebirth as machinery.
D) God is indeed X (Sachchidananda, etc.).

Therefore,

E) Rebirth is real.

 Let me say a few words first about the third premise (C) and then address the argument as a whole.

Aurobindo shares with Vedantins and tantrics in particular a vision of worlds other than the physical universe where there are, to be sure, persistent individuals who are not reborn, not being subject to birth and death in the first place. Our world is a field of death and birth, and all individuals here have mortal bodies. If persistance as an individual is to include a material dimension—which means participation in ongoing life on Earth—then rebirth is called for.

This presupposes that a string of earthly identities is somehow more valuable or significant than a string of cross-world identities. The idea of Western religion that a life here is followed by life in heaven or hell or purgatory without a return is precluded, Aurobindo argues, by the value of human and cultural solidarities and other lines of continuity unavailable to a merely heaven-bound individual.[44] In sum, premise C could be replaced with C′: The best sort of persistent individuality for us demands rebirth as machinery.

This is in accord with Aurobindo's supposition that lines of earthly persistence are intrinsically valuable. As mentioned, it is also presupposed that there are individuals in other worlds who persist without rebirth. The idea is that we perfect specifically human virtues and contribute again and again to a communal life and history.

The most controversial premise may seem to be hidden in D, the reality of God or Brahman. But here the support is yogic perception and yogic propositions, as discussed above. Yogic testimony on this score is overwhelming, although there are differences about God's nature. It is crucial to Aurobindo's argument that God be Sachchidananda,[45] so D is controversial within Yoga.

However, a less elaborate description may be all that is required—for example, to borrow a favorite from Western theology, God's lovingness: (A′) If God is loving, then life has to be meaningful. Then the argument looks good, clear and cogent, given D. From another perspective, we might say that premise A is Aurobindo's development of classical Indian theodicy, using rebirth to defend God's goodness (see the end of chapter 3).

Finally, insuperable difficulties are alleged to face the rebirth conception, some of which have been collected recently in a book by philosopher Paul Edwards.[46] The book is badly organized, and employs rhetoric unbecoming of a philosophy professional ("On examination the theory turns out to be just as hopelessly absurd as it seems at first sight to all sane people" is typical). Nevertheless, a few comments suit our purposes.

Edwards's contentions may be grouped into three categories. First, there is his presupposition of the truth of materialism, of mind-body identity. "The weightiest argument against reincarnation . . . is based on the dependence of consciousness on the body and more particularly on the brain."[47] This, of course, has already been answered by us, in chapter 2. Please, Mr. Edwards, how can you prove causal closure? Unfortunately, this his main argument begs the question, but is employed time and again, particularly just when it looks, even in Edwards's hands, as though the evidence is favorable. Second, there is disparagement and ridicule of various translife conceptions, all of which, from our Yoga perspective, look like the fallacy "straw man." This is the (unfair!) presenting of a caricature or diminished version of a position to be attacked—in Edwards's case, infantile versions of the "astral body" and other theories, in a word, a straw opponent whom it is easy to beat up and bully. Not so, however, our small but muscular minimalist theories, which are unharmed by the alleged difficulties. Third, there are long-winded character assassinations of testifiers and tarring with a broad brush. I cannot find any other argument.

Just a word more about the straw men that Edwards advances. An alleged difficulty of population increase for rebirth theory is a good example. Where do the extra souls come from? Our answer is that the other world or worlds or, as in Vedanta, planes of being, in which we live, have the resources, and we do not presume to know the details. All Yoga theories of reincarnation assert an other-worlds hypothesis, and we have no extraterrestrial population counts. Edwards has an entire chapter on this pseudo-problem, presenting the theories of pseudo-science as though they were the final and best word on the subject. With the sensibilities of neither a researcher nor an interpreter, he consistently fails to look for the "grain of truth" in rebirth testimony and theories—unlike Jainas, we may emphasize, who try as hard as possible never to commit the straw man fallacy, seeing others as like themselves, fallible but trying to say what is warranted and true.

5
Powers

Holistic Health

This chapter addresses the goal, or goals, of yoga, particularly the tantric turn to harmony, integration, and transformation as yogic goal. The tantric ideal contrasts with but also is supposed to include spiritual transcendence. My aim is to connect Yogic ideas about this and other results of yoga practice—especially psychic powers, *siddhi*s—with contemporary ideas about health and well-being. Yoga need not be one-sided, should not be one-sided, I shall argue while exploring first *siddhi* teachings in connection with the idea of enlightenment (*samadhi*), then views about emotional well-being through *bhakti* and the yoga of art, and finally the holistic ideal of psychic transformation.

This last idea is tantric. It is symbolized in Buddhism by the bodhisattva, the perfect individual. In the Upanishads as well as tantric psychology, it is the ideal of living in the the soul, a translife consciousness "thumb size, forever dwelling in the heart of creatures" (*Katha* 6.17). A divine flame is depicted at the core of the individual, "behind" or otherwise related to the heart chakra (see figure 4C). The ideal of psychic transformation includes ethical and social well-being as well as mental, emotional, and physical well-being. And it connects with the *siddhi* theme of the *Yoga Sutra* (*YS*).

The *YS*'s fourth and final chapter is devoted to metaphysical conceptions. There is little instruction about practice. Despite the dualistic metaphysics that has already been drawn, there are arguments for a peculiar nature of *chitta*—thought and emotion or mind—distinguishing it from all other forms taken by *prakriti,* nature. The *YS*'s metaphysics may for this reason be described as a triple-ism, not a dualism. But be that as it may, the *chitta*'s being won over to the side of consciousness, away from the side of mechanical nature, is in general the way *siddhi*s, the powers of consciousness, are acquired.

Traditionally taken to be results of yoga, if not invariably a laudable goal, *siddhi*s are integrated into the larger theory in *YS* chapter 4 differently than is usually thought. The standard interpretation focuses on *YS* 3.37, which says that *siddhi*s are obstacles to the ultimate goal of *samadhi,* enlightenment or yogic trance ("These powers or wonders according to the ordinary human consciousness are obstacles to *samadhi*"). Against that single sutra we have in chapter 4, however, the claim that *siddhi*s follow upon thought and emotion coming under the control of the conscious being, the *purusha.* This is voluntarism *par excellence.* The admonishment of *YS* 3.37 is the sore thumb. In chapter 4, acquisition of powers turns out to be something that cannot be renounced. Let me explain.

The entire third chapter of the *YS*—except 3.37 and a few sutras at the beginning—lists *siddhi*s along with practices that bring them about. Then at the beginning of the fourth chapter is a wonderful overview of that whole long stretch of text, along with explanation of the possibility of *siddhi*s. This puts them—strangely, given the *YS*'s dualism as well as 3.37—as native capacities of consciousness.

Sutra 4.1 summarizes the practice themes introduced in chapter 3: "Powers (*siddhi*) come by birth, from herbs, mantras, asceticism, and *samadhi.*" Note that even this last item, *samadhi,* is given a voluntarist spin: *samadhi* is here not just goal but also instrument. In my reading, "yogic trance" or "enstacy" is itself a power of consciousness.[1] It is a part of *samyama,* we learn at *YS* 3.3–4, the pair of sutras that introduces the long list of powers. Most of these are said to come about through *samyama,* a conscious identification and control, and thus *samadhi* would be part of the *means* to powers, not blocked by them.[2] It would also not be the final goal, since it leads to something else. Let us dig a little deeper into the *samadhi* concept.

At *YS* 1.17–18, *samadhi* is said to have two forms, the second of which "is preceded by effort to hold steady ideas intent on contentment." As remarked in chapter 2, these create or reinforce *samadhi*-prone dispositions such that some people, on the basis of effort in previous lifetimes, are compelled into the yogic experience without much effort on their part in the current life. Sutra 4.1 repeats the idea with respect to *siddhis*, among which it seems we should count the ability to enter *samadhi*.

Powers come from accomplishments in previous lifetimes, "by birth." People born with metanormal abilities presumably have practiced yoga in a former life and *vasana* (translife *samskara*) are continuous from death to birth. They come "from herbs," as is taught in Ayurveda, traditional medical science. They come from "mantras," the practice of *japa*, which is the repetition of sacred syllables such as *om*. And they come from yogic austerities such as fasting (asceticism, *tapas*), and from *samadhi*. Note that, as I argued above (in the second section of chapter 2), if powers flow from *samadhi*, then *samadhi* cannot involve an entire separation of consciousness from its embodiments. And, as pointed out, *samadhi* is said to form part of *samyama*, the general power of conscious identification and control.

Sutra 4.2: "Transformation into a different type of being (or, into another birth) comes about from a superabundance of natural potentiality." The classical commentators emphasize that especially at death one has the opportunity to change into another type of being, not only through the loss of a particular persona but also by a core individuality becoming manifest in ways that were hitherto hidden. Vyasa insinuates that humans sometimes become gods.

More abstractly, the sutra itself suggests that practicing yoga does not change one's core nature but rather triggers wonders latent and intrinsic to consciousness. This reading is borne out by sutra 2.43 as well as the next sutra, 4.3. Sutra 2.43: "Powers of the organs of action (speech, hands, feet, evacuation, and sex) result from asceticism (*tapas*), which destroys imperfections." And sutra 4.3: "Practicing yoga does not impel transformations of nature. Rather, like a farmer (irrigating, weeding, etc., to help plants grow), yogic practices break up coverings or obstacles (so that one's true nature can become manifest)."

One's nature is not transformed from the outside, like a potter shaping a vessel of clay, but rather from the inside, like a caterpillar into a butterfly. Yoga practice removes obstacles to a self-manifestation that, once set off, unfolds on its own. That is, once obstacles are destroyed, the wonders of *samadhi*, etc., occur naturally.[3] The tantric ideal of perfect balance of body, life, mind, and self—psychic transformation—is thus precursed, and the Upanishadic idea of yoga as self-purification, which is reaffirmed in the *Gita* (e.g., in 6.12), is echoed. Self-perfection may have to be protected and tweaked, but in its essentials it is not created; it is rather the natural state or the natural state in expansion as the soul integrates its instruments into itself. (Compare, in appendix A, *Shvetashvatara Upanishad* 2.14: "With a knife smear a mirror with clay and just as when cleansed it shines again brilliantly, / So the embodied who knows the reality of the self (*atman*) becomes integrated, purposes fulfilled, parted from grief.") However, without prerequisites passed—including, most importantly, the *YS*'s "mental stillness" (*chitta-vritti-nirodha*), the cleansing of the mirror in the image of the Upanishad—the goal would remain elusive. This seems to be the idea. (Compare, in appendix D, *Kularnava Tantra* 2.33ff.)

This reading of the *YS* would show that the idea of the purpose of yoga as the particular power of *samadhi* is not all that the text holds forth. By putting aside only a few of the more metaphysical statements, we can see throughout the text the larger goal of powers taken more broadly and integrally, including balance and harmony among all the parts of our being. Let us look at one more sutra from chapter 4, in fact the very next, to seal this interpretation.

YS 4.4: "Thought and emotion (*chitta*) are shaped solely from egoity." By "egoity," *asmita,* the Samkhya principle of individuation might be meant, one of the twenty-four primary divisions or *tattva* of nature. According to the *Samkhya-karika,* the principle is responsible, in the unrolling of primordial stuff, for differentiations of individuals within a type, that is, on the side of nature, *prakriti.*[4] The *purusha,* the yogin himself, the one capable of shaping *chitta,* is intrinsically an individual.

However, assimilation to Samkhya is not even the route taken by the classical commentators here. The accomplished yogin capable of mental silence has the ability to individuate, i.e., create, new mind, *chitta,* new mental patterns, for himself *by* himself, or herself, as opposed to having one created for her by universal nature (to include karma from previous lives). In other words, normally a self or person is not very responsible, it is implied, for the cast of his or her mind. The current persona, the self in its current embodiment, would have *chitta,* mental and emotional patterns, determined by a combination of karma and the body and the environment. But the yogin has the ability to create new patterns.[5]

The interpretation of the classical commentators supports the power theme of Yoga philosophy: the yogin has metanormal capabilities, whereas ordinarily the mind is determined mainly by impersonal forces. Self-determination is at the core of all Yoga teaching, philosophic or practical, Patanjali's or another's, ancient or modern, defined by a commitment to yoga practices. A practice-oriented reading is put forth here by Vyasa and company: given that our minds are shaped to a large degree by our culture and social relationships, this sutra asks us to view the yogin as the artist and critic, the innovator capable of new *chitta*. At a minimum, he or she would not be as bound to convention as the non-yogin. In this way, the sutra seals the *siddhi* theme of chapter 3. Insofar as yoga is focused on transformation or creation of *chitta,* there need be no world denial. Aloneness, *kaivalya,* is not the only goal.

We have already dismissed the reading that would cram the meaning of all the sutras into the box of a dualistic metaphysics. But let me beat the dead horse (an exception to the rule of *ahimsa*). How could a disconnected individual shape *chitta?* Would the shaping of a mind be from the outside or from within? We are supposed to believe that in reality there is no relation between *purusha* and *prakriti,* but let us imagine, in line with the immediately preceding sutra, *YS* 4.3, that the the shaping is to be from within. Then we would have a nugget soul or *purusha* enveloped by nature, *prakriti,* somehow shaping and controlling her. The *purusha* would have no way out, though *prakriti* would be, thankfully, malleable and responsive. However, she would also be not conscious. The untenability of this picture is an argument for holism, for the deep unity, at some level, of matter and consciousness, as discussed at the end of chapter 2. It is not hard to discern holistic principles implicit in the sutras.

The *YS* in fact assumes about as much intrinsic power for consciousness as Vedantic theism assumes for God in its maximal version of self-determination. Sutra 4.23 asserts a kind of maximal capacity for knowledge: "The mind (*chitta*) that is conditioned both by awareness of the seer [i.e., the *purusha*] and that to be seen [i.e., *prakriti*] can cognize anything." Other kinds of mastery include the ethical (others' friendliness is said to flow from perfection of *ahimsa* at *YS* 2.35), as well as occult abilities and metanormal bodily capacities that have been better popularized (*YS* 3.46: "Perfection of the body means beauty, grace, strength, and adamantine hardness"—echoing an idea found in the *Shvetashvatara Upanishad* [2.11; see appendix A] of a body "made of the fire of yoga").

To be sure, the *YS* contains themes of world negation, joining with other early Indic mystical movements. In early Buddhist metaphysics and cosmology as well as in the early Jaina and several Upanishads, the reigning assumption seems to be that all embodiment is by nature suffering: *sarvam duhkham,* "All is suffering," is Buddhism's First Noble Truth. Pain and suffering arrive in practically infinite forms and degrees. The best one can do is to be calm and inactive, not creating disturbances in the cosmic web. This is the view prior to—or, less controversially, simply opposed to—tantrism and the tantric turn.

In a different interpretation of the truth of suffering, our experience is viewed as unfortunate in comparison with the Buddha's. "All is suffering" is matched by the third of the Four Noble Truths, the Truth of Nirvana. This is something positive, a void or emptiness (*shunyata*) vibrant with compassion and bliss that are the true self, or nonself, *anatman,* of everyone—much like the *atman* of the Upanishads. Thus regard for one's own self and consciousness, or future self, requires one to try to see life's pleasures as well as its pains as all in fact suffering, that is, in the light of the bliss that would be ours were we to awaken. In this Mahayana and tantric version of Buddhism, the void spills over into life in the perfection of the individual, the bodhisattva.[6]

Patanjali seems to side with the quietists at *YS* 2.15: "And because of conflicting fluctuations of qualities, there is suffering in change, in anxious, feverish states of mind, and in mental dispositions (*samskara*). Thus the person of discriminating judgment sees *all as suffering*" (my emphasis). This of course echoes Buddhism's First Noble Truth. But given the surrounding text (see appendix C), the judgment expressed seems based not on everyday experience alone—where of course we take ourselves to experience pleasure sometimes—but on a comparison with true self-experience. Furthermore, the tantric could agree with the sutra that there is suffering in *conflicting* fluctuations (*virodha*), while holding that there is the possibility of harmony and divine life. Abhinava Gupta holds that self-realization manifests in life as a spiritual tranquility (*shanti*) compatible with artistic expression, life as Shiva's dance.

But however we read the *YS,* a turn to world affirmation occurs in the philosophy and practices of tantra. North, south, east, and west in yogic traditions in India, in Vedanta, Shaivism, Vaishnavism, Buddhism, Jainism, and in new traditions too, there is the tantric turn. The old concern with discovery of a hidden or deeper self or consciousness remains, but is incorporated into a wider vision upholding enjoyment (*bhoga*) of all the flavors (*rasa*) of divine manifestation.[7] Celebration of the divine in life comes to be integrated into a world-oriented view of the person and self and the goals of life. Some early tantric texts (such as the *Kularnava Tantra;* see sppendix D) do keep to the idea that the highest good entails liberation from rebirth. But the ideal is shifting, coming to encompass development (through rebirth, partly) of a spiritual individual—the accomplished (*siddha*) yogin or in Buddhism, the bodhisattva. Swami Vivekananda (1863–1902), famous for bringing Vedanta to the West, proclaims that he no longer wishes to be free from rebirth, to renounce the world for the self, *atman,* but rather to be reborn again and again to worship God indwelling diversely in the material universe.[8] Self is not conceived as only the impersonal and cosmic *atman* but as the individual *jiva*, the living being, who is destined to become perfect in the terms of this mystically material universe.

The origins of tantra are obscure, but there are precursors in the Upanishads and especially in the *Gita*'s notion of karma yoga. Ethnographers have also pointed to "autochthonous" practices of people speaking Dravidian and other non-Indo-European languages. The worship of female "Earth" divinities seems especially important, permitting "homologies" and acculturation, to use the terms of academic specialists. Of course, much could be said about the material dimensions of tantric culture, but here we shall keep our eyes on the Yoga in tantra, i.e., Yoga philosophy.

The guiding idea of tantric outlooks is spiritual transformation. Everything may be one, or interdependent, but the processes of self- and world-development are real and meaningful. Yoga is the secret of self and nature, as the lower self and the body are transformed. On analogy to the transformation of desire into the higher emotions or aesthetic delight, spiritual transformation is said to occur in the purified "vessel" by the action of spiritual energy, or shakti. The flows of breath, *prana,* the vital energies of the body, are transmuted. The yogin or yogini is the remade person, a mage, with occult powers, *siddhi*s.

More broadly, pleasure and sexual fulfillment are viewed as intrinsically valuable throughout the highbrow literature of later classical Indian culture. The *Kama Sutra,* a textbook on lovemaking and sexual fulfillment that may be as early as the fourth century C.E., presupposes a theory of erotic dispositions as inherently good. Sexual desire is worthy of fulfillment so long as other values and duties are not neglected. "Let life be prosperous and full" is the attitude, not "Let us away from these things that are transitory."[9] A literature of philosophic aesthetics comes to accompany an increasingly refined poetry and drama, and the idea of the connoisseur, literally the "like-hearted" (*sahridaya*), who is capable of both universal empathy and uniquely aesthetic emotions prompted by art, is championed. The tantric philosopher Abhinava Gupta (see appendix D) draws on aesthetics to articulate a yoga of beauty and art—the topic of the next section.

To close this one, let us look at the unificational themes of tantra, the idea of unity in the notion of harmony, asanas requiring right alignment, and the holism of holistic health. Those who practice asanas know that some of the most difficult poses challenge balance. One cannot simply will balance, although one-pointed concentration helps. One has to be particularly responsive to feedback, as one limb or another normally in play is taken out of play. Balance poses reveal dependencies that are not absolute—they are really imbalance poses, teaching balance by imbalances that require compensation in effort or, more profoundly, alignment with other limbs.

All this is a metaphor or model for what yoga has to contribute to holistic health, as we get a better sense for the parts of our psychological makeup. If there is a teleology implicit in the practices of yoga prominent today, it is holistic health. This is wellness that is dynamic and expansive, including strength and flexibility for the body but also delight in the emotions, insight in the mind, and spiritual growth. There is movement toward integration of all the parts of the being (compare *Shvetashvatara Upanishad* 2.14, appendix A).

Better to grasp the concept of holistic health and tantric perfectionism, let us look back at the Platonic theory of a tripartite self.[10] Tantra would add a spiritual element to Plato's mix of, one, the appetitive, two, the enthusiastic or emotional, and, three, the rational. Thus, counting the body, four, we would have with the spiritual, five, a conception of the main parts of personality that is not too far from the *kosha* theory of the Upanishads (see figure 4A). However, there is unfortunately in the Western theory nothing spiritual. In Plato's view, the rational is to control and harmonize the activities of the appetitive and emotional parts. The vision of a society governed by a philosopher-king who alone comprehends the idea or form of the good corresponds with the psychological picture. The inadequacy of the political ideal thus helps to show the inadequacy of the tripartite view of the self. In Plato's closed society, poetry is banned as obscuring the rational message, and harmony is secured only at the expense of sensual gratification. Plato's would be a totalitarian state, where police keep us from unruliness. The problem lies in what does the harmonizing, the rational mind, which is clearly not up to the task—both socially and psychologically. Yoga proposes a role for the mind limited to its proper province, along with life-encouraging alliances and mergers with our other parts, all under the management of a psychic or spiritual element.

In the *Symposium,* which is perhaps Plato's greatest *literary* creation as opposed to work of philosophy, a view of harmony is presented that is much closer to the tantric conception. Here the form of the good is identical with ideal beauty. Through contemplation of the worthiness of the object of desire, a philosopher climbs the ladder of love, reaching the supreme (beauty = truth = goodness). In the process, feeling is transformed from desire into something very lofty, in what is more a mystical than a rational contemplation. And the result is not in the *Symposium* a set of rules for society but something rather more subtle, a bringing of beauty into life, something like Abhinava's yoga of art. The philosopher who has beheld the form of the beautiful turns back to the world to create works of delight—as does God in the harmony manifest in the great moments and rhythms of the natural universe. According to Plato, the philosopher also brings about harmony in the social universe, but here psychologically the integration does not, as in the *Republic,* have the rational part as the ruler, it seems to me. Clearly, it is not in tantra, although like other instruments the mind is a valuable tool and, indeed, according to Abhinava, its best and correct use the most important limb (*anga*) of yoga.

Holistic health in tantric yoga implies not just absence of illness and injury—which is a negative concept of wellness with perhaps too much play in contemporary medicine—but fulfillment of our capacities. Even disease and injury are afforded instrumental value in helping us achieve a complex balance and integration of all the parts of our being, including the highest but not restricted to it. As the *Kularnava Tantra* says (2.25; see appendix D), "Enjoyment becomes yoga practice; misbehavior becomes art (and the good deed); transmigratory existence (*samsara*) becomes liberation (spiritual transcendence)." This idea reverberates throughout tantra and yoga literature. Even the *Hatha Yoga Pradipika,* which is quite ascetic overall, advocates sexual practices bringing enjoyment (*bhoga*) as well as spiritual enlightenment (*HYP* 3.103), though its ideas of yogic perfection are much narrower than in more mainstream tantra. The broad ideal may be articulated best in Mahayana Buddhism's notion of the bodhisattva, which we shall continue to explore in the next section, along with Aurobindo's notion of psychic transformation, the topic with which we close.

Extraordinary Emotion: *Bhakti* (Devotional Love), *Rasa* (Relish), and *Ananda* (Bliss)

The discipline of devotional yoga, *bhakti yoga*, the "yoga of love" has been most famously articulated in the *Bhagavad Gita*, but also permeates tantra and almost all late Hindu religion. (The *bhakti* teaching of the *Gita* is expressed in its later chapters in particular; see appendix B.) To be sure, there are late-classical handbooks of yoga, such as the *Hatha Yoga Pradipika* (see appendix E), where *bhakti* is not in focus. But even there the "grace of the guru" figures prominently. Clearly, *bhakti* is predominant in, for example, the Kashmiri Shaivism of Abhinava Gupta (appendix D) as well as movements all over the subcontinent. It's not at all a stretch to say that in Vedanta and Vaishnavism more generally as well, *bhakti* reigns as the most important form of yoga in contemporary India. A more qualified statement would be needed to take in tantric Buddhism, but there too *bhakti* is conspicuous.

In the idea of God or the Divine or the Buddha that is crucial, there is both a general and a personal element. The general element connects with Western philosophy's "teleological argument," that is to say, with the kinds of consideration that Western philosophers have taken up—the beauty and order of the workings of nature and the miracle of our own being and faculties—to prove the existence of God on the basis of analogy to human arts and crafts (design requiring a designer). The practitioner of *bhakti* goes beyond the inference to perceive the beautiful body of the Beloved everywhere, in the great sights and sounds of Earth, the Mother, but also in every contact, in every sensation, both externally and internally in thought and emotion. The things and events of nature demand not only belief—the *bhakti* yogini would insist, implicitly granting the argument (of which there is an Eastern version much debated in Nyaya[11])—but principally delight in the whomever or whatever is their origin.[12]

The particular element in *bhakti* is a matter of personal relationship that extends, however indirectly or in however long a line, to this origin. That is, to use the first-person language of yoga, that whoever or whatever is the stuff of the stars and the Earth and the waters of life is somehow responsible for them too, through self-transformation. The idea that that divine X could be aware of and indeed somehow care for, if not me, at least something that does relate directly to me is the crucial propositional content of *bhakti,* in my opinion. There is my personal divinity, the spark soul in my heart, my higher self, my guru, who is intimate and responsive and moves my feelings by my sense of his or her connectedness, which makes me connected too. *Bhakti yoga* is all about training the emotions, and the emotions relate to the concrete, the divine or the divine representative in the here and now. The feeling is extended, as best one can, to transform all our everyday attitudes. In this way, *bhakti* would come to infuse all that we become and do. Our lives would be different.

Thus the sense of connectedness goes all the way back, grounded in the origin, the *ishvara* or *devi* or equivalent—about which it is necessary, then, to have some conception. I repeat, the particular element is more important in practicing *bhakti,* the devotional feeling rhapsodized in songs and literature. At the far end of the *bhakti* attitude is simply something or someone who need be conceived only vaguely. Nevertheless, the idea of total connection has to be there. Intimacy at the near end is divinely grounded. Thus the general is definitely intended.

Note that with the general and the particular put together, the whole universe stands as intermediary. For the Creator (mother, sustainer, etc., even emptiness) is the Creator (mother, sustainer, emptiness) of everything, the same with respect to the entire universe. Our existences conform to universal laws, exceptionless processes. The Creator has the whole to worry about, the workings of everything, and cannot be faulted for not weighting my preferences the way I do. Indeed, yogic preliminaries, such as nonharmfulness (*ahimsa*) and the other *yama*s and *niyama*s of the *YS*, are rules to which I have to conform to enter into the right relations that are the very essence of yoga. Thus a Yoga philosophy of *bhakti* turns to the intermediaries, the connectives joining the high and the low, which become manifest in practice.

Yoga is a matter of right relation, right alignment and connection among all the parts of ourselves. For whatever higher or deeper part there is—by definition, something of which I am currently unaware or aware only imperfectly—I need most of all a teacher, someone who knows the principles of yoga. I need a spiritual intermediary, a divine or human guru, who can show me right alignment. However found, the teacher naturally provokes a form of *bhakti,* gratitude mixed with devotion and happiness entailing confidence about our own destiny.[13] The universe, i.e., the sequence of events in a lifetime and its collective lessons or its sheer beauty, along with the conspiracies necessary to make us see it, can play the guru's role. So too can a tradition. The position is not filled only by a human representative or a god or goddess anthropomorphically conceived. But a book from a guru of the past as well as personal divinities and *avatara*s can serve, as can a living guru. Some teachers are charismatic, some not so charismatic. The essential prerequisite is having at least better connection with the divine than we have, and knowing how to bring us to know or realize it.

Classical Yoga philosophy in the *Gita* and elsewhere provides rich resources for theory of the teacher. At the high end is the notion of the *avatara,* the special divine "descent," put forth in the *Gita*'s fourth chapter. There is a special "divine descent" into finite form to uphold a moral order and direct the world in the right ways. *Gita* 4.6–8, Krishna speaking:

> Although I exist as the unborn, the imperishable self and am the Lord of beings, by resorting to and controlling my own nature I come into phenomenal being through my own magical power of delimitation (*maya*).[14] / Whenever there is a crisis concerning the right way (*dharma*), Arjuna, and a rising up of evil, then I loose myself forth (taking birth). For protection of good people and for destruction of evildoers, for establishment of the right way, I take birth age after age.[15]

Krishna as *avatara* is a person who is aware of himself as a manifestation of God, a person who shares somehow in God's awareness, power, and native delight.[16] In the *Mahabharata* as a whole, I admit, Krishna does more than teach yoga (see the introduction to appendix B). The "establishment of the right way" mentioned in verse 4.8, quoted here, is not to be understood as only a matter of yogic guidance. But in accordance with the openness and inclusivism of our Yoga, let us explore further the concept of divine descent and the guru. The *Gita* as a yoga manual is in rather surprising agreement here with the *Yoga Sutra,* as I intend to show.[17]

The *Yoga Sutra* has a conception of the Lord, *ishvara,* and a version of devotional yoga. In chapter 1, a handful of distinct methods to reach mental silence are laid out (mental silence being the goal of yoga according to *YS* 1.2, *chitta-vritti-nirodha,* stilling of fluctuations of thought and emotion, also called calming illumination of the mind at *YS* 1.33). One of these methods is *bhakti.*[18] *YS* 1.23 sums it up: Mental silence can result "from opening to (*pranidhana,* meditation on, surrender to) the Lord (*ishvara*)." Vyasa, the first commentator, glosses *pranidhana* as *bhakti,* which he says is an intense desire to be like the Lord in certain yogic characteristics and abilities.

The idea of such *pranidhana* is not as controversial in the Sanskrit commentaries as one might expect, knowing the diversity of renderings among modern translators. Still, on the idea of the Lord (*ishvara*) there is plenty of controversy among the classical authors.[19] The two-word expression recurs at *YS* 2.45, which connects the practice with *samadhi.* Interestingly, the immediately preceding sutra, *YS* 2.44, says that the practice of self-study (with respect to a yogic text), *sva-adhyaya,* brings the power, *siddhi,* of achieving contact with one's preferred divinity, *ishta devata.*[20] A person worships the form of the One that it is easiest to worship, the form to which she or he is personally drawn, who is their teacher or the teacher of their teacher, the founder of the lineage that extends to you. (See in appendix D, in the *Kularnava Tantra,* verse 1.2: Devi tells her guru Shiva that he is "easy to love" as she requests yoga teachings from him.) Others worship the forms and divinities they are drawn to. Behind them all stands the One.[21] In the tantric understanding of all this, the form of worship is *puja*, the ceremony of celebration of the divinity. The connection is occult but nonetheless real, a particular *puja* connecting with a particular divinity, the ceremony making, so to say, the right psychic space for that particlar divinity to manifest—this seems to be the tantric idea.

Skipping a couple of sutras that are systematic in character (in that they relate, or try to relate, the *ishvara* idea to the Samkhya system), we have at *YS* 1.26 what seems the essential conception: "The Lord is the guru even of the ancient teachers in not being limited by time." One of the arguments for the existence of God in classical Indian philosophy is what we may call the Criteriological Argument, which goes like this. Each craft, including speech, is by definition learned from a teacher who has learned from a previous teacher, e.g., grammar that, since the world has a beginning (a crucial premise that atheists such as Mimamsakas and Buddhists reject), has to have an originator, a first guru, traditionally, Shiva, the great god (*maha deva*), the founder of yoga. Shiva sets conventions, endowing words with meaning and patterns as grammatical rules, and fixing standards for excellence in all occupations. We learn these standards from our immediate teachers, who also learned them. Learning processes have to begin somewhere. Therefore, we must suppose an Original Teacher who knows the principles intrinsically without having been taught or who originally set them. Humans are rather obviously ruled out as incapable of these tasks (setting the conventions of language, etc.), so we must conceive of a Diving Being performing them, thus a "guru even of the ancient teachers in not being limited by time."[22]

That God is the original teacher of yoga converges with the *Gita*'s notion of Brahman as the foundation of *dharma* as well as the tantric idea of an individual's enlightenment as working for the benefit of everyone. It locks up with the Buddhist notion of the bodhisattva (as expressly pointed out by Abhinava—see appendix D: "Bodhisattvas, who are persons who know reality, appear again even after (their enlightenment) in a body that is perfectly appropriate for them in their intention, which is dharmic (righteous) and born out of concern for others' welfare, whose only consequence would be others actually being helped"). God is impartial. Similarly, the yogin "delights in the welfare of everyone," in the phrase of the *Gita* (*sarva-hite ratah*). Yoga brings us into right alignment, making us better sensitive to the general welfare. The principles of yoga have social ramifications.

It is not hard to see how the positive Buddhist tantric conception of the void's spilling over into life is connected to the idea of the perfect individual, the bodhisattva. Remarkably, there is a similar nexus of ideas in the "yoga of art" teaching of Abhinava Gupta (Abhinava's overall philosophy and *oeuvre* are introduced in appendix D). In brief, Abhinava uses the *rasa* theory of classical criticism, the *alamkara shastra,* to fill out the *Gita*'s teaching of karma yoga.[23] This genre of Sanskrit literature is rich and diverse, but throughout there is an amazingly durable theory of human nature. In the oldest version, the *Natya Shastra,* "The Science of Spectacle," by Bharata (c. 200 B.C.E.), eight dominant natural emotional states are matched to eight aesthetic flavors (*rasa*s) that a poet or dramatist should create his work to provoke in a (cultured) audience. Bharata lists eight types of *rasa,* which correspond to eight abiding natural emotions:

BHAVA (natural emotion)	*RASA* (relishing)
rati (sexual feeling)	*sringara* (the erotic)
hasa (laughter)	*hasya* (the comic)
shoka (grief)	*karuna* (the compassionate)
krodha (anger)	*raudra* (the furious)
utsaha (energy, vitality)	*vira* (the heroic)
bhaya (fear)	*bhayanika* (the frightening)
jugupsa (repulsion)	*bibatsa* (the disgusting)
vismaya (wonder)	*adbhuta* (the astonishing)

According to Bharata, *rasa*s arise out of "abiding emotional states," *sthayi bhava,* listed in the left column. Everyone is subject to these basic feelings, and the dramatist capturing an audience's interest and writing a good play evokes them in aesthetic versions, listed in the right column. This means that, unlike with ordinary fear, for instance, the spectator need not herself be afraid while savoring the *bhayanika,* the "frightening" (the "delightfully frightening," as is implied by its falling into the aesthetic category). She knows what it is like to be afraid (she has the appropriate mental dispositions, *samskara*s), and enjoys the representation, knowing it is only a play. The *rasa* is universal, however, and her individuality merges (ideally) with that of every member of the audience (all of whom meet the prerequisites for this type of experience) in relishing the presentation.[24] Thus the poet and dramatist work from knowledge of human nature, and the feelings are evoked by crafting situations in which the "abiding emotional states" occur.

Appendix D contains a bit of Abhinava's commentary on Bharata's *Natya Shastra,* where the theory of the eight flavors is in the immediate background (the argument is that there is a ninth *rasa* of spiritual peace, *shanta rasa*). More broadly, this tenth-century tantric critic and philosopher turns the older theory of *rasa* on its head by taking a more essentialist view of aesthetic response, a more internalist perspective. According to him, the *rasa*s are grounded not only in the corresponding *bhava*s but also in the *atman,* the impersonal and universal self. The delight intrinsic to all relishing derives from the *atman,* who is universal. The specialness of the ninth *rasa* (the reason, Abhinava says, Bharata did not himself mention it) is that it is doubly grounded in the self.

Bharata has what we might call a foundationalist view, that there are natural emotions that serve as material to be aesthetically transformed. Abhinava, in contrast, sees aesthetic experience as native to an interior realm closer to the self's own experience of bliss (*ananda*) than any natural feeling we are born with. Aesthetic experience draws on the *ananda* (delight) that is intrinsic to self-awareness. Relishing is not only impersonal and independent of petty circumstances of life experience but also preexistent. It is an inner sense or feeling that is not caused by the body or by mental dispositions (*samskaras*) created by experience storing memories. The circumstances portrayed by art may be physical, but the *rasa*s, like the universal self, are not physically caused. They are drawn out. In themselves, they belong to a separate domain of self-experience.

In line with this internalist, noncausal position, *rasa*s are viewed as self-authenticating, *sva-prakasha,* like the self. In this way, the perspective of the connoisseur is insider and privileged, the trained sensibility of the *sahridaya,* in Abhinava's view, the person of "like heart and mind," who is fit for aesthetic experience. Similarly, the self-disciplined yogin is fit to experience Shiva, the supreme self and reality. The analogy is explicit and total. The training that makes possible (but does not cause) our relishings undercuts their intersubjectivity no less than the training necessary to taste the supreme delight undercuts the reality of the One. Indeed, aesthetic training is a kind of yoga. Each world (*bhuvana*) or domain of the self's manifestation has objects that are proper to it and to a corresponding consciousness. The same is true of the aesthetic experience (*rasa*) of the *sahridaya.*

At risk of digression, it seems to me interesting that there is only one aesthetic state for which a radically different word and concept is used than that for the corresponding natural state: suffering or grief, *shoka,* which as a naturally occurring feeling is said to be matched in the audience not with a form of *shoka* but with something radically different, namely, *karuna,* compassion. The thesis that links the two is that when we contemplate suffering in the aesthetically interested but personally disinterested fashion of a connoisseur (*sahridaya,* "like-hearted" member of the audience), we taste the *rasa* of compassion—which, we may add, in the spirit of Abhinava's aesthetic Yoga, is right and proper because that's the true response of the *atman,* our deep self or, as in Buddhism, "nonself" essential consciousness.

Perhaps one side of the First Noble Truth—interpreting the "All" to refer to things that concern others as well as ourselves—is to acknowledge the selfness of others and to practice *ahimsa.* Abhinava would say that in a yoga of art, by empathizing with even an imaginary suffering we grow in our dispositions to compassion. Indeed, in all aesthetic experience we begin to enjoy the bliss of the true self, *ananda,* since *rasa*s as hedonic states are apparently closer to the self than are natural states, our everyday pleasures and pains. Thus aesthetic experience secures for us progress yogically toward the supreme good, now conceived as a kind of individual perfection. The supreme good includes developing an aesthetic and moral self. It is not just self-realization in the narrow sense in operation before or apart from the tantric turn.

In Buddhism, the change begins with the story of the bodhisattva's turning back from the personal annihilation of a solitary nirvana to help the world out of suffering. No end of embodiment for the buddha of unbounded compassion, not until every sentient being is enlightened. The bodhisattva is in every way beautiful and worthy of worship, worthy of *bhakti,* which is incorporated into the Mahayana path.

The history of the idea goes way back. Sermons and stories of the Pali canon, which are much earlier than the Mahayana literature to which the bodhisattva idea is proper, extol a triad of character traits as conducive to the *sumum bonum:* uprightness (*shila* in Sanskrit, *sila* in Pali), yogic trance or concentration (*samadhi, sammadhi*), and wisdom (*prajna, panna*). Practices consonant with their development are laid out in the early literature. In the hands of Mahayanins, the three are split to become the six marks, the six perfections, *paramita,* of a bodhisattva, and practice teachings are reorganized around the sextad of charity, uprightness, energy, patience, concentration (*samadhi*), and wisdom.[25] These qualities, whether as perfected through yoga practice over lifetimes or as natural traits of the awakened (unobstructed now for the master yogin or yogini), make a person efficient in helping others achieve enlightenment.[26] Thus like the supreme guru, Shiva, in Kashmiri Shaivism and the Lord of the *Yoga Sutra*'s conception, the bodhisattva is the ultimate teacher who inspires *bhakti*. The beautiful body of the bodhisattva also inspires love and delight.

In Buddhist tantra, yoga is auxiliary to the way of the bodhisattva. But assimilation is a two-way street. The Buddhist ideal converges strikingly with the karma yogin idea of the *Gita* we reviewed in chapter 3, although the intellectual foundations are different.[27] The Kaula goal and path as depicted in the *Kularnava Tantra* and elsewhere are also similar. In Vaishnavism we find just about everything we find elsewhere, and perhaps the best examples. Krishna, whom we are to make every effort to imitate and remake ourselves to be like, has certain qualities or characteristics. Rupa Gosvamin's sixteenth-century list of sixty-four qualities of Krishna includes: "Strong," "Truthful," "Eloquent," "Learned," "Witty," "Artistic," "Adroit," "Self-Controlled," "Generous," "Compassionate," "Happy," "Captivated by Love," "Beneficent to Everyone," "Partial to the Good," "Ever Fresh and New," and "Endowed with Spiritual Powers," among many more traits that are both yogic and world-directed.[28] One might add to this growing collection of paths the practice (the "yoke") of the imitation of Christ, in Christianity, which whether historically connected or not surely seems to have a *bhakti* element. Sufism is drenched in *bhakti*. These may appear remote disciplines, the trails of spiritual mountain-climbers. But *bhakti* is available in the yoga studio and anywhere else, to anyone, according to those who teach it. Music is also a particularly efficacious conduit, it is no hazard to say.

Finally, the concept of *shri*, divine beauty. This word, *shri*, is used in the Vaishnavism of South India in roughly the same ways as *shakti* in the Shaivism of Abhinava and company. The world is a manifestion of Shree (to use the phonetic spelling), of beauty, the Great Goddess. She is evident in nature. She gives meaning to life, both externally and internally. We are all her vehicles, but yoga is particularly efficacious in attuning us to her expressive energies.

Psychic Transformation

At the very end of the *Katha* or Story Upanishad (see appendix A, *Katha* 6.17), is an image that recurs throughout subsequent literature as a symbol of the individual soul: "thumb-size," seated in a "secret cave" (another Upanishadic symbol) located in or behind the heart (chakra), there is a conscious being (*purusha*) who survives death. "The inner self (*atman*) is a conscious being (*purusha*), thumb-size, forever dwelling in the heart of creatures. / It is to be extracted from the body patiently, with diligence, like the cane shaft from the *munja* reed. / The bright, the immortal, it should be known. The bright, the immortal, it should be known."[29]

From the spiritual autobiography of the Siddha yogin, Swami Muktananda (1908–82): "I would have a new movement in the heart, in which an egg-shaped ball of radiance would come into view. This is the vision of the radiant, thumb-sized being, who is described as follows in the *Shvetasvatara Upanishad* . . . 'The inner soul always dwells in the heart of all men as a thumb-sized being.'"[30]

There are other images, most notably the Hamsa (e.g., *Katha* 2.2.2), the symbol of the Sri Ramakrishna Math, the Bihar School of Yoga, and other modern institutions, which, despite being sometimes depicted as a swan, is the Siberian crane—I hazard, following Kalidasa and other classical authors—a bird that flies over the Himalayas each spring from India, where it winters, to summer in Siberia.[31] There is also the image of the spark soul, the same in divine substance as the spark in everyone else, transmigrating from death to birth.

All this has become part of the mainstream Tantric psychological picture, in accordance with the *Shat-chakra-nirupana* (Description of the Six Chakras) of Purananda (sixteenth century).[32] In *Kundalini Yoga*, Swami Satyananda writes about the heart chakra (*anahata*), "In the center of the pericarp of the lotus is an inverted triangle, within which burns the *akhanda jyotir*, unflickering eternal flame, representing the *jivatman* or individual soul."[33] As we saw in chapter 4, there is wide diversity of opinion about the *jivatman*, the individual consciousness, especially in its relationship to Brahman or God. But there is interesting commonality too. All Yoga traditions teach that the intention to practice yoga is a wedge of light coming up from our truest self or consciousness, turning us toward other right attitudes in life as well as to our longer-term self-interest, that is to say, our self-interest considering survival and reincarnation.

Thus amid great diversity of opinion about an individual soul, I wish to strike the common theme of yoga as tool of—let us say, following the coinage of Aurobindo—psychic transformation.[34] Our minimalist commitment is only to the value of yoga for this life and an indefinite future. But just to consider asanas, there are some it would take, for most of us, at least another lifetime to master! There is also the ability to turn one's thought and emotion to the sattvic, that is, to the healthy and good and beautiful. One way to think about all this is that we are being influenced by the *purusha* or soul, the psychic spark in the heart that survives death, the *jivatman*, a part of ourselves deeper than thought that has leverage over it, capable of changing it and all our instruments for the better. In the terms of the *kosha* system (figure 4A), it's as though the innermost sheath of bliss (the *anandamaya kosha*) expands to suffuse the other sheaths, the mental, pranic, and physical, so that—to use the aesthetic terminology of Abhinava—everywhere there is *rasa*. To paraphrase the line from the *Kularnava Tantra,* all life becomes yoga and even our flaws and failures the stuff of art.

Aurobindo weaves a theory of psychic transformation into an overall Vedantic philosophy, and has much to say about an occult individual in the heart, which he calls the psychic entity.[35] The psychic entity develops psychic personality, which he calls the psychic being and the true person, over the course of lifetimes of embodiment, incorporating transformed mental and pranic energies and dispositions into an enduring individual complex that survives the death of the body.

> The true secret soul in us—subliminal, we have said, but this word is misleading, for this presence is not situated below the threshold of waking mind, but rather burns in the temple of the inmost heart behind the thick screen of an ignorant mind, life and body, not subliminal but behind the veil—this veiled psychic entity is the flame of the Godhead always alight within us, inextinguishable even by that dense unconsciousness of any spiritual self within which obscures our physical nature. It is a flame born out of the Divine and . . . the inner light or inner voice of the mystic. It is that which endures and is imperishable in us from birth to birth, untouched by death, decay, or corruption, an indestructible spark of the Divine.[36]

In a poem by Abhinava translated in appendix E, the divinities of the directions offer all our efforts to the divine core represented by Bhairava/Bhairavi and the central channel descending from the thousand-petaled lotus above the head down into the heart chakra. Here Aurobindo's conception is a little different. The soul in a secret temple behind (but immediately connected to) the heart center—our spark soul—is constantly doing *puja,* offering everything to the divine in joy and adoration, all the while luring, not coercing, our parts—body, life, and mind—to the side of its quiet spirituality. This is the interpretation Aurobindo gives to the "Nachiketas fire" of the *Katha Upanishad* (see appendix A, the introduction to the *Katha*), "the immortal in the world of mortals."

Our minimalist attitude responds, like the Jaina logic, with a *syat,* "maybe," maybe this is true. There surely are other views about a *jivatman*. Personally, my response is that it would be wonderful if such a theory were even roughly right. Here is not only survival but also meaning and purpose to an individual life; life has meaning as, we might say, psychic expansion, involving increased psychic incorporation of mind, life, and body. The tantric turn is from an idea of withdrawal from the outer to the inner and a turn to an idea of transformation of the outer by the inner. Such a reversal is expressly championed by Aurobindo. It's the *kosha* theory inside out, or the flowering of the inner in the outer, to change metaphors. Translife continuity is crucial, partly because our lives are short. It takes more than a single lifetime for a soul to perfect its instruments.

Like other tantric endeavors, Aurobindo's is a rather maximalist spiritual philosophy that departs from the traditional Vedantic emphasis on transcendence to include affirmation of spirit in life. It is a world-affirming theism in which psychic transformation is key. The soul or psychic entity emerges from behind its veil into what Aurobindo calls the surface consciousness, urging us to practice yoga with all our instruments, body, life, and mind, and inspiring works—of wisdom or saintliness or beauty or at least comparatively greater wisdom, et cetera. The soul oversees and, in this view, progressively becomes the perfection of the body, life, and mind. Thus, as in the tantric turn more generally, the supreme good is not simply discovery of Brahman, as classical Vedantins claim, but just as importantly a kind of occult self-making, the making of a spiritual but also world-oriented individual.[37]

This is a process for which the divine and the embodied psychic being are said to share responsibility. As we saw in connection with Aurobindo's reincarnation argument, psychic development—alternatively, manifestation—through a series of lives is the linchpin of his, and in general the tantric, view of self and indeed the world and God. In particular, Aurobindo's stress on individuality echoes Abhinava's concept of *svatantrya,* the freedom of self-determination that belongs to Shiva, who is ourselves. Actually, here Aurobindo's theory diverges a little from the Kaula philosophy of Abhinava, since Aurobindo puts much more emphasis on the theory of soul development (deriving from the *Gita*) than does Abhinava, who views the individual as manifesting from the top down (an idea inherited from Samkhya), although of course he accepts karmic continuities. But both tantric theists have a common denominator with modern existentialism, since God is not external to us but rather the source of our spontaneous acts. With both Aurobindo and Abhinava, reality is enriched by our personal delimitations of the universal creativity. The point of life is not just to recover or recognize the self as source but also, according to our own appropriations, individual natures, and styles, to manifest the divine energy and to relish beauty.

Rupa Gosvami (c. 1525), in a shocking use of a worldly metaphor, says that the prerequisite (*adhikara*) for the most advanced type of *bhakti* is simply longing (*lobha*), intense longing, veritable greed for amorous contact with Krishna. This contrasts with scriptural injunctions that he specifies must be followed as a prerequisite for less perfect forms of *bhakti*. But here, in what seems like Aurobindo's "soul emergence," both logic and scripture are swept aside as the desire for the divine takes over, assuredly bringing the *rasa* and delight of divine contact and love play in all the events of life.[38] The seeker's *prana* and thought are transformed as a spiritual identity is forged in erotic rendezvous of the divine with the individual soul.[39] This is the tantric turn with a vengeance, spirit coming into life and psychic transformation.

To round off this book, I want to bring out a virtue of Yoga in the context of political philosophy, that is, to draw out the most important political ramifications of rebirth and the yogic goals we have surveyed. What sorts of institutions would we want, were we confident of rebirth along the lines of individual and karmic continuity and justice, unseen force (*adrishta;* see the final section of chapter 3; alternatively, God's grace), affirmed throughout Yoga philosophies? The question presupposes continuity of some mental dispositions (*samskara*) as well as individual translife identity. It also presupposes some sense of the workings of unseen force.

The answer to the question is, fortunately, pretty clear, at least in broad outline. We would want the world into which we will be born to be one where our talents can flourish.[40] The political philosopher John Rawls famously imagines an "original position" where all parties to a fundamental social contract—namely everyone—would choose the first principles of government without knowledge of their particular place in society, parents, sexual identity, likes and dislikes, and so forth.[41] All one would know is that one is a human being in a society governed by law, along with, to be sure, science, including principles of bureaucracy and administration. Such a perspective is strikingly similar to that which we take when we contemplate our next birth according to Yoga, albeit one may be aware of a certain karmic carryover in translife consciousness.

According to the most prominent rebirth theory, which we are calling soul making, each of us will be reborn as a human being, in all likelihood. Otherwise, there could be little karmic continuity. Musical talent and a person's developing it, or not, throughout a lifetime seems a good example. Surely Paul McCartney, who cannot read music, has been a musician previously. And, like a musical ear, so on through a range of inherited and acquired characteristics that help to secure continuity from one life to the next. According to this Yoga theory, each of us is or is making a translife personality through making karma and individualized realizations of human capacities.

Thus as beings with multiple human futures, we have tremendous interest in worldly institutions. When we die we are not going away; for us there is no final heaven or hell beyond the planet, and we are not just "food for worms."[42] Thinking, then, with Rawls, about the institutions that we would like to be in place for our future births, we have, I should like first to point out, tremendous incentive for those institutions to be fair.

Contemplating future births according to the principles of *samskara* continuity and karmic justice, we have added reason to want what Rawls calls the Liberty Principle ("maximal liberty compatible with a like liberty for another"). We would also accept something like his Equality Principle, which has two parts, Equal Opportunity and the Difference Principle. Yoga, as I will explain, might want to quarrel with the Difference Principle. Rawls thinks that the two principles would be unanimously adopted in the original position. Yoga's theory of rebirth and karmic justice would mainly reinforce his conclusions. Yet there is one departure that stands out.

Distribution of wealth looks a little different to Yoga than it does to Rawls. The philosopher abstracts from positions of people in society, considering a unit to be a single life. If a person knows, however, that her current birth is only the most immediate of a long series, then it seems she would be a little more willing to gamble with unequal distributions than is Rawls, who argues that institutionalized inequalities should work out to the advantage of the least well-off. Karmically, a super-rich birth is not necessarily desirable, since with great wealth comes great responsibility for beneficence. The danger of forming negative unseen force is particularly great, and a modest patrimony may be a godsend.

Furthermore, what we really want are institutions that allow us to develop our talents, no matter to what class or caste we are born.[43] So long as we have schools aplenty for everyone and yoga studios, we would not mind that a few have especially great wealth. We ourselves may have such a birth in the future, or had one in the past, and we have a healthy respect for the addictive qualities of the pleasures that wealth makes possible. In any case, we should like to be secure in having yoga instruction available, and if this requires wealthy patronage other than the State's, then we might differ from Rawls. In contrast, a case can be made for yoga instruction in State-sponsored schools, an easy case, since yogic skills are transferable to all occupations, mental and physical. Furthermore, yogic instruction need not be sectarian, although it cannot help but make a person more self-conscious in the good sense. The poor should not have to depend on charity to get yoga instruction. Furthermore, as parties to an original contract, à la Rawls (and earlier social contract theorists), we might be especially mindful of the least fortunate out of a sense, like Rawls's, of longer-term self-interest.[44] May everyone be prosperous and find the opportunity to practice.

Finally, let me share some mantras and further ideas about setting an intention (*samkalpa;* see the introduction), especially as such a practice is relevant to a yoga class. First, a Vedic mantra (taught to me by Shri Jagannatha Vedalankara, whose interpretation I follow) that seems appropriate for the beginning of a yoga class. In English it goes as follows: "I call the fire, ancient priest of the sacrifice, the divine who summons (the divinities), bringing here jewels."[45] The mantra is particularly significant because it is the first verse of the Veda, of the *Rig Veda,* to be precise, verse 1.1.1, part of a short hymn to fire (*agni*). I interpret this fire (following Jagannatha) not as earthly or heavenly but rather as psychic fire, the Hamsa, the spark soul.[46] In the verse, such fire bridges the worlds—it is able to bring here the sacred and its enrichment. The fire is the ancient priest of the inner or yogic sacrifice, and appropriately invoked at the beginning of a class of asanas. The idea is that we enliven the soul's intention when we call the psychic flame. In other words, we call the fire, the Hamsa, the "thumb-size" consciousness in or behind the heart, dwelling in a cave or inner sanctum of the body as temple.[47]

APPENDIX A
Select Yogic Passages in the Upanishads

The historical setting of the Upanishads is outlined at the beginning of the third section of chapter 1. There are two translations that I recommend: Roebuck (2000), which is the more accurate, and Easwaran (1987), which is the more poetic. Here I translate and discuss only those passages in the very earliest Upanishads where the word *yoga* is used in the sense of self-discipline[1] (see the list of early Upanishads in figure 1A in chapter 1). My style is occasionally to include a short explanation in parentheses within the translation. In other words, expressions in parentheses are not on the surface of the Sanskrit text. But as glosses they are practically synonyms with the words glossed, and so are visible just below it. It is also my practice throughout these five appendices to restore ellipsis and sometimes to substitute for pronouns their referents.

Every Upanishad is a text that, like the *Yoga Sutra,* relates to yoga practices philosophically. So practically any selection is arbitrary, from the perspective of Yoga. No thematic criterion is available for homing in on the most important passages. Even only the Upanishads that the earliest commentators knew—which indologists consider the oldest, numbering 13 or 14 out of 108 counted traditionally, or more than 200 by the largest count[2]—present more than one theory about a spiritual reality. Classical Vedanta assumes, erroneously, that there is a single metaphysical view. Unfortunately, this assumption defines the school, which from the *Brahma Sutra* (c. 200 B.C.E.) on takes its task to be extraction of the single philosophy of the Upanishads. However, Upanishadic unity lies elsewhere than in a Vedantic system spun around the conception of Brahman or God. In fact, some Upanishads are theistic; some are not. Some have one view of the relation of Brahman to the individual; some another. Upanishadic unity comes from other quarters—from yoga advocacy and occult discoveries through yoga.

Not all Upanishadic passages are explicitly Yogic or yogic, however, in that there are puns, jokes, and stories with morals for everyone, not only for yogins and yoginis, at least now that the Upanishads have been brought out from their secret lineages. Nevertheless, Upanishadic psychological claims and doctrines of self and self-consciousness, as well as the metaphysics of Brahman, all presuppose yoga practice. This is not just an epistemological point (the third section of chapter 4 addresses the epistemology of yogic experience) but also pedagogical, according to Vedantic as well as Yogic traditions: only by yoga practice does one become capable of understanding the Upanishads, the "secret doctrines."[3]

The twelve or thirteen or fourteen earliest and principal Upanishads are old texts, some very old, whose abstract metaphysical claims are susceptible to multiple interpretations, as is shown by the very existence of Vedanta subschools. There is less possibility of controversy with passages about methods of yoga, so less commentary is required, although all Upanishadic readings need a little contextualization and commentary. The passages rendered here pertain to yoga practice and psychology in the first place and speculative philosophy in the second place.[4]

The translations here are not of the very most famous Upanishadic passages. Through the eyes of Yoga philosophy, they (or any other passage from the early Upanishads, for that matter) carry significance other than what classical Vedantic commentators find. Views about Brahman, the Absolute, and the relationship to the self or Self, *atman,* and our psychology as individuals are the Vedantic stock-in-trade. From a Yoga perspective, these doctrines are interesting. Vedanta is a philosophy encouraging yoga practice. However, it is also exciting to find *practice* teachings in the Upanishads typically ignored by Vedantins.[5]

To begin, there is a story about how different yogas are appropriate for different psychologies that shows especially well several concerns of ours, including the background of all Upanishadic teaching, though it is only a minor part of the overall case for highlighting yoga.[6] The passage occurs in what scholars consider the oldest or one of the two or three oldest Upanishads, the *Brihadaranyaka* (c. 800 B.C.E.), 5.2.1–3. Made famous in the West by T. S. Eliot's 1922 poem, *The Waste Land,* it shows yoga eligibility conditions while setting out different "disciplines" for different personality types or distinct parts of ourselves. It is also a forerunner of the *Gita*'s teaching of karma yoga.

Prajapati, father of creatures, becomes the guru for three groups of children: gods, humans, and demons. At the end of a period of service and self-discipline—a first stage of a two-stage yoga—all three receive a special mystic teaching and prescription called an *upanishad*—in each case the single syllable *da*, but each group understands it differently. The gods take *da* to mean that they should restrain themselves (*damyata*), and Prajapati says, "Yes (*om*), you have understood." The humans are then also confirmed by him in their hearing that they should give (*datta*). And the demons say it means they should be compassionate (*dayadhvam*), with Prajapati again concurring. The thunder repeats the message endlessly, *da, da, da,* and the passage closes with the refrain, "Peace, peace, peace" (*shantih shantih shantih*). Shankara and other classical commentators differentiate types of person and dispositions as targets of Prajapati's injunction: gods have desires, men are afflicted by greed, and demons are prone to anger. But the unity of *da*'s message is also emphasized: *yoga,* yoking or self-discipline, as appropriate according to your nature, is a prerequisite for mystical knowledge of your highest self, the Brahman.

Despite all the disagreements among Vedantins of the various subschools, the message that through yoga we can have mystical knowledge of the Absolute, the Brahman, can hardly be missed, in this or in any other early Upanishad. Knowledge of Brahman, which is a single self of everyone, *atman,* brings freedom from fear (see the beginning of section 3.2). Cosmologically opinions differ, but insofar as any individual consciousness remains, it is no longer subject to an otherwise inevitable reincarnation or any other natural force or law. There is liberation, *moksha.* Yoga makes this possible if it does not directly bring it about. *Katha* 2.23 is interpreted by some to mean that the grace of the higher self is the trigger, making itself known to the lower self, which has been made ready by yoga. But yoga would still be necessary prep.

As mentioned in chapter 1, the word *yoga* derives from the verbal root *yuj,* which comes to be used in the Upanishads in the sense of restraining or yoking the mind (*manas*).[7] The sense of *yoga* as union, as in union with God or union with the higher self, which is a later usage, seems to be introduced in the *Maitri Upanishad,* though the passage may be an interpolation and, in any case, it is difficult to date that Upanishad or know the linguistic history with much confidence.[8] Despite that and other stray occurrences of the meaning of (spiritual) union, self-discipline is the sense common among Upanishads, the *Bhagavad Gita,* the *Yoga Sutra,* and other classic texts.

Now the word itself in this precise sense is used in the early Upanishads relatively rarely, compared with more than one hundred occurrences in the *Bhagavad Gita* alone and hundreds more in later sections of the *Mahabharata.* But yoga practices go by many names; *tapas,* heat, the spiritual heat generated by asanas, etc., is a general word that is practically a synonym as employed in many Upanishads (cf. the later usage of *tapasya,* asceticism).[9] Furthermore, often the focus is on yogic experiences and realities revealed, not on the practices which are presupposed.

One final remark before we turn to the texts. The Vedantin Shankara identifies eighteen "great statements" (*mahavakya*) throughout ten or eleven Upanishads, among which is a line from *Brihadaranyaka* 4.5.6 that has wide resonance within all the classical schools: "Verily the self is to be learned about (from scripture), thought about, and made immediate in meditation."[10] *Practices of yoga are implied in the final prescription.* This is not, let me emphasize, an uncommon reading. Almost all of the philosophers of the classical schools on record, including, notably, Nyaya philosophers as well as Vedantins, read it this way.[11] It's as though the three (only marginally) separate classical *darshana* (ways of viewing the world)—Vedanta, Nyaya, and Yoga—are each sanctioned: Vedanta with its emphasis on learning from scripture, Nyaya with its emphasis on intellectual reflection, and Yoga with its emphasis on practice and immediate meditational experience.[12]

From the *Taittiriya Upanishad* (2.4–5)[13]

In what may be its first recorded occurrence in the sense of self-discipline, the word *yoga* is used in the midst of explanation of the *kosha* (sheath) theory that we reviewed in chapter 4 (see figure 4A). This is the teaching of five sheaths or bodies dwelt in simultaneously by the self or soul: the physical or made-of-food sheath, the breath or pranic sheath, the lower mind, the higher mind, and the bliss-made *kosha*. Specifically, the word *yoga* is used in connection with description of the fourth sheath, the higher mind, *vijnanamaya*, understood by Shankara as the understanding, *buddhi,* as opposed to the synthesizing sense mentality, *manas* (the stuff of the third sheath). The word for that of which the fourth sheath is made, *vijnana,* is commonly translated "understanding." Shankara says that through it we understand truths. He also says that such understanding guides action. The overall message of the Upanishad is that by *tapas*—as noted, usually translated "austerity" but definitely including practices we know as yogic, such as meditation—one discovers that each of the sheaths is the Brahman, the Absolute, progressively, beginning with the food sheath. But first we have to be able to identity the sheath itself, and in the following passage we are told about that which is made of knowledge or the higher mind.

The *Taittiriya* is an early prose Upanishad (see figure 1A) that has come down to us through the Taittiriya lineage of the *Yajur Veda*. In fact, all the passages that follow, except for those from the *Mundaka,* come from that lineage, from that school of keepers, to be precise, of the "Black," *Krishna Yajur Veda* as opposed to the "White." (The former has explanatory prose intermixed with its poems, while the latter does not.) There is much overlap in Vedic literature among lineages and repetitions of the *Rig Veda* in particular, including other forms and derivations from the root *yuj* occurring in the *Brihadaranyaka* and Upanishads from other lineages. Thus nothing much should be made of the fact that all the early and principal Upanishads (except the *Mundaka*; see below) in which the word *yoga* is used in the sense of self-discipline belong to this Taittiriya line. As mentioned, yoga practices are referred to as *tapas* and named in a variety of manners. Perhaps with the noun *yoga,* however, it was in this *shakha,* this branch or Vedic school, that the linguistic convention originated.

> There is, interior to and other than the body made of mind (*manas*), a body made of knowledge (*vijnana*). By that this is filled. This too has just the form of a person. According to that one's personal form, this one has personal

form. Just trust (*shraddha*, faith) is its head. The right way (*rita* = *dharma*) is its right side. Its left side is truth. Its body (trunk) is *yoga*. The great unmanifest is its lower part, its base.

The point here concerning the assimilation of yoga to the fourth sheath seems to be that yoga requires mental direction, a plan intellectually understood. Cognition directs action. Yoga (*tapas*) is to be carried out in the terms of the other sheaths too, the body, the breath, and so on. But in all cases there are mentally discernible rules. Furthermore, our knowing faculty, despite its confusions and the difficulties it makes for other parts of our being, is also the Brahman—so the Upanishad goes on to conclude.

From the *Katha Upanishad* (2.12, 2.23–24, and 6.7–18)

The *Katha* or Story Upanishad, unlike the *Taittiriya,* is written in verse. Its poetry is nevertheless antique, complex, and ideatively dense and imagistic in comparison with, for example, the *Bhagavad Gita,* which often echoes it. The teacher or guru is Yama, God of Death, the Controller. His pupil is Nachiketas, a young man in ancient India whose father, in accordance with prevailing religious practice is, as the Upanishad opens, sacrificing his possessions, offering all to the gods in the hope of attaining heaven.

As the grand procession is led past, Nachiketas argues that his father's efforts are useless. "Giving away everything will get you nowhere," he tells him. When the father ignores the impertinence, the son asks, "Then to whom will you give me?" The father doesn't respond. Nachiketas taunts him with the question a second and a third time. In exasperation, the father shouts ("Go to hell") "To Death, I give you to Death."

Nachiketas, being a serious and dutiful son, follows his father's orders and travels to the gates of the afterworld through a yogic trance. (The notion of yogic prerequisites is thus built into the plot.) There he waits for three days on the doorstep of Yama himself, Lord of Death. Now Nachiketas is not only a guest but a Brahmin, of the priestly caste. Yama violates a higher law, it seems, by ignoring him, particularly for so long a time. To make amends, he grants Nachiketas three wishes or boons, one for each day he had to wait. The boy's first wish is that his father no longer be angry with him. Yama readily grants the request. For the second, Nachiketas asks about the meaning of the sacrificial ritual. Death gives him an explanation in which fire is symbolic of a divine being concealed in matter. Nachiketas's inner fire of discontent or aspiration is "the immortal in the world of mortals." Whoever lights this sacrificial flame, Yama says, crosses to the farther shore. When the boy seems to grasp what his teacher is talking about, Death, pleased at finding so receptive a pupil, names it the Nachiketas fire.

For his final boon, Nachiketas asks: "When a person dies, is he there or not?" Death complains that not even the gods or the *rishi*s can answer the question.

 He begs him to choose some other boon: elephants and gold, beautiful wives, sons and grandsons, a kingdom, long life. Nachiketas dismisses these as transitory. He insists that only Yama can reveal the mystery and that this is his single wish. Death, who cannot go back on his word, instructs Nachiketas in a yoga of immortality.

Verse 2.23 is extremely important to Yoga theism, including tantric readings of the Upanishads, for its apparent reference to God's choice and activity. If one takes the supreme self, *atman,* of the Upanishads to be Brahman in the theistic sense of a Supreme Lord and Inner Controller, *antaryamin,* who emanates all the worlds by voluntary choice, then yoga is not in itself sufficient to attain the supreme good. God's grace, the self's "choice," is also necessary. Indeed, it is the trigger of enlightenment. (The idea recurs in the *Mundaka;* see below.)

In all the following verses except the last, the speaker is Yama, Death. The last verse closes the Upanishad by telling us in effect that Nachiketas, by following the teaching, attained the supreme state of consciousness called the Brahman, the Absolute. The first verse rendered, 2.12, tells us that as a first step to this knowledge one knows by yoga the immortal, indwelling self or soul (as discussed in the last section of chapter 5).

> 2.12. That one that is difficult to know, hidden, immanent, set in the cavern (of the heart), resting in the depths, / A wise man realizing it through knowledge of yogic method with respect to the self leaves behind joy and grief. . . .

> 2.23. Not through words is this the self (*atman*) to be got. Not by being smart. Not from wide learning (in scripture). / Just by whom the self chooses is the self obtainable. Only the one the self chooses gets the self's own form.

> 2.24. (Not by everyone) not by one who still behaves badly, not by one who is not calm and peaceful (*ashanta*), not by one incapable of *samadhi* (yogic concentration and trance), / Nor even by someone wise and insightful if the mind is not calm and peaceful, would this one (the self) be got.

> 6.7. Higher than the sense faculties is the *manas*, the mind (the organ of inner sense). Essence (the *sattva* mode or *guna* embodied in intelligence) is superior to the *manas*. / The great self is above essence. Beyond the great (self) is the unmanifest.

> 6.8. But the (supreme) person is superior to the unmanifest, pervasive and without distinguishing mark— / By knowing whom a creature is liberated and goes not again to the estate of death.

> 6.9. The form of that one (the supreme person) lies not within the expanse of vision. No one sees that one with the eye. / Through the heart and mind and

intelligence is that one apprehended by them who by knowing that one have become immortal.

6.10. When the five (sense) cognitions are stilled along with the sensual intelligence, / And the (higher) mind does not wander (in thought), the highest state that is called.

6.11. This they consider (true) yoga, the firm control in concentration of the organs and faculties. / Then one becomes vigilant; for yoga is the origin and ending.

6.12. Never by speech, not by the sensual intelligence, not by vision is that one got. / How is it to be known except by one proclaiming, "It is (real)" (as a matter of immediate experience)?

6.13. "It is (real)" is just the way that it is to be known, and it is to be known in its essential principles—both. / For the person who knows indeed "It is (real)," the essential principles become clear.

6.14. When all the desires that dwell in the heart have been let go, / Then the mortal becomes immortal. He enjoys here (in this life) the Brahman (the Absolute).

6.15. When all the knots of the heart have been cut through here (in this life), / Then the mortal becomes immortal—this is the teaching.

6.16. A hundred and one are the channels (*nadi*) of the heart. One of them issues at the crown of the head. / Through it departing, one goes to immortality. The others lead out in all directions.

6.17. The inner self (*atman*) is a conscious being (*purusha*), thumb-size, forever dwelling in the heart of creatures. / It is to be extracted from the body patiently, with diligence, like the cane shaft from the *munja* reed. / The bright, the immortal, it should be known. The bright, the immortal, it should be known.

6.18. Nachiketas, having obtained this knowledge proclaimed by Death (Yama) and all the principles of yoga (*yoga-vidhim . . . kritsnam,* the entire method of yoga), / Attained the Brahman. He became free from passion, free from death. Any other would do so too, who likewise knows about the self.

The edition glossed by Shankara has one more line, a ritual closing. The fact that verse 6.18, which is the last with real content, mentions yoga, using our word, indicates that we are to understand the entire teaching to be about that which is attainable through yoga. Rather arbitrarily, we have begun at 6.7 the stretch that culminates in 6.18. But in these dozen verses there are in summary form several key theses: the Samkhya disidentification theme (also called the "elusive I") in verses 6.7 and 6.8 (ideas that also occur at *Katha* 3.10–14); the practice of *pratyahara,* sense withdrawal, which is the fifth limb of the *Yoga Sutra*'s eight-limbed yoga, *ashtanga,* in verse 6.11; the mental silence idea in 6.10 and other verses; suggestions of the tantric occult psychological system in verses 6.14–16; and the doctrine of the psychic individual in verse 6.17.

From the *Mundaka Upanishad* (3.1.1–10 and 3.2.3–6)

The *Mundaka*—which has three main sections or chapters, each with two subsections—is composed in elegant verses. It belongs to the *Atharva Veda,* the "fourth" Veda, which is not mentioned in some Upanishadic passages that mention the other three. *Atharva* hymns have impressed scholars as distinctive, and are usually dated a few centuries later (c. 1000–800 B.C.E.) than other Vedic hymns. But there are repetitions and echoes that unify Vedic literature—including the presence of the subgenre of Upanishads.

Stylistically, the *Mundaka* seems separate from the oldest group of Upanishads. Its concept of Brahman borders on paradox: see below, 3.1.7, which directly echoes the koanlike *Isha*. The Advaitin Shankara lucidly glosses each verse, commenting on practically every word, occasionally polemically (but only occasionally), seemingly letting his Advaita commitment distort his reading (e.g., of 3.2.3, below).

The yoga or self-discipline recommended in this Upanishad seems severe, extreme heat, *tapas,* built up through renunciation (*samnyasa,* 3.2.6) presumably of hunger, thirst, and desire for sex. But 3.1.8 seems to recommend balance along with meditation, and 3.1.5 says that the *rishi*s, the mystic knowers of self, would be "ones whose desires have been obtained" (*apta-kamah*). Also in 3.1.8, as in the *Katha* (above, 2.23), what Vedantic theists call Grace seems to be thought the trigger for self-discovery, yogic prerequisites being in place.

At the beginning of this stretch of text, an image of two birds occurs, one absorbed in eating, the other watching, and it recurs at *Shvetashvatara* 4.6–7 and reverberates throughout Yoga and Vedantic literature. Here we have an icon of self-monitoring consciousness. Shankara glosses the word *sayuja* as *sarvada yuktau,* joined, or united (*yukta*), all the time, a word thus fraught with overtones (our two selves forever yoked in yoga). The yogin transcends both good and bad karma, according to *Mundaka* 3.1.3, but nevertheless has flawlessly moral character. The distinction between yogic immediate knowledge and intellectual understanding seems implied in 3.1.4. The word *yati,* striver, in 3.1.5 and 3.2.6, refers to the yoga practitioner. It derives from the root *yat,* to strive after, to devote oneself to, and in the *Gita* is used synonymously with *yogin* (e.g., *Gita* 5.26). Verse 3.1.10 anticipates the *siddhi* theme of the *Yoga Sutra.*

The word *yoga* occurs in our sense in 3.2.6, within a context, it seems, of a world-denying mysticism in that the yogin would enter "Brahman worlds." But the word in Sanskrit translated "world" is *loka,* sometimes used in the sense of field of vision.[14] The verse may be interpreted as saying that whatever world the yogin finds himself in will be a "Brahman world" in the sense that he or she sees everything as the Brahman.

3.1.1. There are two birds (with beautiful wings) who are constant companions (as though always together yoked), clutching the same branch of a tree. / One of them eats the sweet berry; the other, not eating, watches.

3.1.2. On a common branch, a person (a conscious being, *purusha*) sits sunken in sorrow at his helplessness, deluded. / The other sits contented. When the first person sees him to be (self-)lord, magnificent, his grief departs.

3.1.3. When he becomes a seer, seeing the golden-hued doer, the lord, the conscious being (*purusha,* person) born in the womb of Brahman, / Then as the Knower shaking off good deeds and bad, of flawless character, he attains the supreme equality (*samya,* equanimity; unity [with Brahman]).

3.1.4. This is the life energy (*prana*) that radiates out from every being. Knowing this, the Knower tends not to excessive disputation. / Playing and relishing the self (*atman*), with self as his delight, doing works this one becomes the best of Brahman knowers.

3.1.5. This is the self (*atman*) obtainable by truthfulness (*satya*), by *tapas* (heat of yogic austerities), by right cognition, by the constant practice of the student's life of chastity (*brahmacharya*). / For there is within the body something made of light, beautifully radiant. They perceive this one, the strivers (*yati*) do, whose faults have been diminished (by these means).

3.1.6. Only truthfulness wins, not falsehood. By truthfulness was the divine path laid out. / By following it, *rishi*s, having obtained their desires, come to that which is for truthfulness the highest home.

3.1.7. And that is the vast. Its form inconceivable, divine, subtly that radiates, so subtly. / Farther away than that which is far and at the same time right near at hand, it is here and now for those who see (it), set in a secret place.

3.1.8. It is not grasped by the eye, nor through speech. Not by other faculties, nor by *tapas,* nor action. / With (inner) being (*sattva*) purified through knowledge and serenity, then in meditation one perceives that one, the partless (the imperceivable).

3.1.9. This minute self is to be known by a consciousness into which *prana* (breath, life energy) has in five ways entered (and become controlled). / The intelligence (*chitta*) of creatures is altogether shot through with *prana* (that is out of control). Once purified, in it this self appears.

3.1.10. Whatever world the person of purified (inner) being turns to, illuminating mentally, and what desires he makes his own, / He wins just that world and those desires. Therefore, if you want (true) prosperity, you should hold the self-knower as the ideal.

3.2.3. Not through words is this the self (*atman*) to be got. Not by being smart. Not from wide learning (in scripture). / Just by whom the self chooses is the self obtainable. Only the one the self chooses gets the self's own form.

3.2.4. This the self is not to be realized if you are not strong, and not if there is distraction or carelessness, nor if the discipline (*tapas*) is off the mark, flawed. / But if by these methods and means you strive, a knower you become. For you, the self has its home in Brahman.

3.2.5. *Rishi*s having realized that one, satisfied in their knowledges, perfected in the self, free of passion, calm and serene, / These wise ones find the Omnipresent everywhere. Disciplined in yoga (*yuktatman*), they enter the All.

3.2.6. Ascetics, strivers (*yati*), who know well the meaning of the Upanishads (*vedanta*) through their own experience, purified in their (inner) being through renunciation and yoga practice— / All of them become at the end absolutely liberated into the worlds of Brahman, having passed beyond death (possessing the supreme nectar of immortality, *amrita*).

Five varieties of breath are introduced in the *Brihadaranyaka* (3.9.26) and other Upanishads: *prana* proper as well as inhalation, *apana,* down-breath, *vyana*, wide-breath, *udana,* up-breath, and *samana*, equalizing breath. The translations are problematic in that for yoga practice these are terms of art and perhaps best left untranslated or anglicized.[15] Probably these are the five breaths that are referred to in *Mundaka* 3.1.9. However, the word *prana* is also used in the sense of life energy in general (see, e.g., 3.1.4), energy that in tantric teaching can be redirected up the central channel of the occult body, *sushumna* (see appendix E, *Hatha Yoga Pradipika* 2.41–42).

As noted, verse 3.2.3 repeats the theistic idea of grace that we encountered in the *Katha* (2.23)—at least in the theistic interpretation of Ramanuja and company. Shankara takes the verse to express the idea of the self's power of self-illumination in such "choosing." Verse 3.2.4 goes on to spell out yogic prerequisites in general terms. The last two verses give us a conception of the goal of yoga.

From the *Shvetashvatara Upanishad* (1.1–3 and 2.8–17)

The *Shvetashvatara* is referred to generously by Ramanuja and other classical Vedantins, including Advaita Vedantins, although, like the *Katha*'s, its philosophy is theistic. The oldest commentary is by Shankara, as for almost all the early and principal Upanishads. According to expert indological opinion, the *Shvetashvatara* is in style like the *Kena,* the *Mundaka,* and the *Katha,* and thus probably belongs to a second period of Upanishadic composition, around 400 B.C.E., although some would assign it a still later date. In any case, it is older than the *Gita,* which borrows lines from it and dates from 300 or 200 B.C.E. at best estimate. All four Upanishads appear to be prior to the advent of Buddhism and the *Gita* afterward.

The *Shvetashvatara* repeats ideas and phrases from other Upanishads, the long prose *Brihadaranyaka* and the cryptic and short *Isha* as well as several others. In it philosophy and yoga coalesce in a theistic vision that is world-affirmative, precursing tantra (though this is not true according to Shankara's reading). The directness of the metaphysical questioning at the beginning is striking. The passage constitutes part of the evidence that there were public debates about the Brahman in kingly courts and elsewhere in Upanishadic times.

In verse 1.3, there is mention of yoga and meditation together in a compound (*dhyana-yoga*), and it is impossible to say whether the Sanskrit is to be rendered "the yoga *of* meditation" or "yoga *and* meditation." I think the ambiguity does not matter much, for everything is spelled out in verses 2.8–15. Clearly, the method prescribed includes meditation. Note, however, that it is with *bhakti yoga* that the passage ends, verses 16–17, which are the last lines of section 2 (the Upanishad is divided into six sections or chapters).

1.1. They say who debate about Brahman: "What is the cause (of the phenomenal display)? Is it Brahman? From what are we born? By what do we live? And on what are we based? / We live experiencing pleasures and their opposites—governed by what or whom? (Tell us) you Brahman-knowers.

1.2. "Should we think time is the answer? Each thing's own nature? Necessity? Chance? The elements? A (cosmic) womb? A (cosmic) person? / No, not these nor a combination of them, since there is the (individual) self (which is something other than these and their combinations). The self too is not the answer, since it cannot determine its own pleasures and pains."

1.3. Those who follow the yoga of meditation have perceived the hidden energy (*shakti*) of the divine self (*devatman*), hidden its own workings and strands. / Who governs all those causes including time on through the (individual) self, it is this one.

2.8. Holding the body balanced and steady (*sama*), the three upper parts (torso, neck, and head) erect, pulling the senses with the mind into the heart, / The knower would cross all fear-carrying currents by the boat of Brahman.

2.9. Squeezing the *prana*s (the five breaths) here (in the heart), let the yogin of disciplined movement, the knower, breathing through the nose with constricted breath, undistractedly control the mind like a vehicle yoked (*yukta*) to wild horses.

2.10. In a clean level spot, free from pebbles, fire, and sand, which is pleasing to the sensuous intelligence (*manas*), not paining the eye, by such qualities as sounds of water, let yoga be practiced by one who lives in a secluded and sheltered place.[16]

2.11. Mist, smoke, rays, (vital) air (*anila*), (interior) fire (*anala*), fireflies, lightning, crystal, the moon— / These forms are precursors of Brahman awareness in yoga, manifesting (by its imminence).

2.12. (The elements) earth, water, the fiery element (*tejas*), air, and ether (*kha,* sky) are presented (subtly) when yoga practice is under way in its fivefold character. / For the accomplished whose body is made of the fire of yoga, there is no disease nor old age nor death.

2.13. Lightness (or clarity of mind), health, steadiness, clarity of complexion, and excellence of voice, / A beautiful smell, slight urine and stool—they say these come first in the processes of yoga.

2.14. With a knife smear a mirror with clay, and just as when cleansed it shines again brilliantly, / So the embodied who knows the reality of the self (*atman*) becomes integrated, purposes fulfilled, parted from grief.

2.15. One disciplined in yoga would perceive here in this life the reality of Brahman by the reality of the self that is like a lamp. / Then knowing the unborn, the constant, that which is untouched by all (other) realities, the God, he becomes liberated from all bondages.

2.16. For this God extends in all directions. Everything follows in accord with him. For he was born before. In the womb in the end it is just he. / It is he who has been born and who will be born. In front of all creatures, he faces in all directions.

2.17. Who is in fire, who is in the waters, the God who is everything has entered the world. / Who is in plants, who is in the forests, to this God salutations, let there be salutations (*namo namah*).

The yogic progression seems to be from asanas and the body through meditation and control of the mind to discovery of an indwelling self. That discovery then becomes the means, the lamp (2.15), whereby the God is discovered.

The *bhakti* sentiments at the end are not spelled out as a method of yoga. They belong rather to the substance of the discipline.

Along the way, *siddhi*s come as signs of progress, indicators of imminent yogic experience and spiritual transformation. Apparently in this way a practitioner would receive feedback from the higher self and keep confidence in the end to be achieved, not let up or fall away from the path. The precise nature of the conveyance seems less important than the fact simply that there would be such encouragement. The mist, fireflies, and so on mentioned in 2.11 comprise nonetheless a (fascinating!) sequence of events in meditation, according to the common interpretation.[17]

APPENDIX B
Yogic Passages in the *Bhagavad Gita*

The *Gita* is a small section of an epic poem, the *Mahabharata* (c. 400 B.C.E.–200 C.E.). The epic is enormous, with more than 100,000 verses; the *Gita* has about 900 verses, arranged into 18 chapters. The main story line is about princely succession. The *Mahabharata* describes city-states of urban and agricultural centers amid dense forests along the Ganga and other rivers of north India. The warrior Krishna rules a neighboring state, and though able, just, and politically astute, is not the divine guru (*bhagavad*) in the main part of the poem that he is in the *Gita* (see the discussion in chapter 5 on Krishna as *avatara*). The political issues are complex, but one side of a quarreling family, and not the other, has the just claim. The rightful heir with his four brothers and their allies and troops and elephants are arrayed on this, the side of justice; Arjuna is the third of the five brothers. The usurpers along with, unfortunately (from Arjuna's perspective), many venerable sages and heroes are lined up on the other side. Arjuna's own archery teacher, who has guided him to incredible proficiency, "best in the three worlds," is in the enemy camp. At the opening of the *Gita,* Krishna joins the battle line as Arjuna's charioteer. Then ensues a dialogue between the two just before the fighting begins. In the poem, this is reported by a blind holy man who has the *siddhi* of being able to hear at a distance, guaranteeing that the words have been recorded accurately.

Arjuna insists that it cannot be right to kill his kinsmen, teachers, and friends who face him on the far side of the battlefield. Verses 1.31b–35:

> No good do I see in killing my own family in battle. I desire not victory, nor rule, nor pleasures, Krishna. What is power to us, enjoyments, or life, Govinda? Those who make rulership desirable for us, and enjoyments and

> pleasures, it is they that are arrayed in battle (against us), abandoning life and wealth. Teachers, fathers, sons, grandfathers, uncles, in-laws—these I do not wish to kill even if it means that I must die, Krishna—not even to rule the three worlds, why then for the earth?[1]

Despite the sincerity of moral feeling, Krishna says the right thing to do is to fight, to kill the opposing warriors, and to win the battle—all the while taking a yogic attitude, which, in apparent paradox, involves *ahimsa,* nonharmfulness (*Gita* 10.5, 13.8, 16.2, and 17.14), as discussed in chapter 3.

Traditionally the *Gita* is not identified as an Upanishad; it does not form part of Vedic literature. Furthermore, its language is more direct and less symbolic and playful than that of the early and principal Upanishads. But in many Vedantic circles as well as by generations of yogins and yoginis, it is treated as an Upanishad, a "mystic doctrine" meant to guide practice and to encapsulate results. The selections below tend to avoid controversial metaphysical statements in favor of direct instructions in yoga. Sometimes, however, the line is hard to draw, particularly with *buddhi yoga,* the discipline for the higher intelligence (*buddhi*) that is laid out in chapters 2, 8, and 13, in particular, but also here and there throughout.

Krishna's teaching of karma yoga is meant to overcome the tension between the ethical value of nonharmfulness, *ahimsa,* and the duty of a soldier to fight. More broadly, it is a yoga for anyone who has to act in the world (see the third section of chapter 3 in this book). Apparently any action can be done with the yogic attitude specified, including killing. However, in my reading karma yoga demands giving to a recipient whom one loves and adores, and this factor surely shrinks the range of permissible acts. It seems to me crucial that the cause for which Arjuna is fighting is just, although some commentators say that any action may be the stuff of karma yoga.[2]

Krishna also embeds his karma yoga teaching in a metaphysics that has God's creative act, or continuing acts, as the cosmic foundations of human action, using a ritual image of sacrifice. Brahman creates the world as a gift (see above, the last section of chapter 3), maintaining it in "Brahman action" (*Gita* 4.24).

We should keep in mind too that in the *Gita* Krishna reveals himself to Arjuna as God incarnate, an *avatara,* literally a divine descent or manifestation (see again the second section of chapter 5). In chapter 11 (little of which is included here since it depicts Krishna, not his teaching), Krishna shows Arjuna his divinity after first giving him the "divine eye" necessary to see it—below, 11.8, a verse that includes an interesting mention of the word *yoga.* Krishna reveals his own yoga, which would be presumably the laws of the universe, like principles of alignment in asana.[3] Thus Krishna's yoga instruction is not to be understood as simply a friend's encouragement or the teaching of just any guru. His words are the voice of God speaking to a human being in personal crisis—so the *Gita* is and has been understood by theists who would emphasize its teaching of *bhakti yoga,* the yoga of love and devotion. In my reading, this yoga is to be seen as completing or complementing the karma yoga teaching.

Also laid out are practices of meditation, breath control, and other forms of what is called *jnana yoga*, the yoga of meditation, as well as a yoga for the higher rationality, the *buddhi* or intelligence. Indeed, the sixth chapter has rather detailed instructions for meditation, and the metaphysical themes of the entire text may be taken to inform *buddhi yoga*. This latter, by the way, is mentioned explicitly at *Gita* 2.49, 10.10, and 18.57, but is not always recognized as on a par with the karma yoga, the *jnana yoga*, and the *bhakti yoga* often together taken to be the threefold path of the *Gita*.

It is through such discipline in general that one comes to live a transformed life. One would come to be in the end a person, like Krishna, aware of one's immortal soul or self, transcending the universe and its karmic laws, and directly aware of God, the Brahman, the personal/impersonal Absolute.

Textually, the *Gita* often echoes Upanishadic passages, and there are several outright repetitions of lines. For example, *Gita* 8.6 (see below) echoes *Mundaka* 3.1.10 (see above), though few of the words are identical. Of course, the epic's meter, which is rarely used in the Upanishads, would demand a change of wording even if a quotation were intended. In the Sanskrit edition I use, which contains the commentary of Shankara, a title for each chapter is given in a colophon at the end of the chapter.[4] These seem to me to be useful indicators of content, and are translated below though they are not to be thought of as part of the text. Except for the title of chapter 11, each includes the word *yoga*, which I omit: "(The Yoga of) X." Chapter 1 (not excerpted) is entitled "The Yoga of Arjuna's Despondency."

Chapter 2: Analysis (*Samkhya*)

(Krishna, Shri Bhagavan, the Blessed One, said:)

2.39. So much for the (metaphysical) truth, which is for the intellectual (the philosopher, *samkhya*), for you spoken thus. Hear it now for yoga (practice). Son of Pritha, if you practice yoga according to this teaching, the bondage of karma you will escape.

2.40. With this yoga (unlike with a ritual act), there is never loss of effort, never an obstacle that can prevail. Just a little bit of this *dharma* saves from the great fear. . . .

2.47. (In this yoga of inner sacrifice unlike with Vedic rituals) to the action alone is a person entitled, never to the results. Do not be moved by the fruits of action; do not be attached to inaction.

2.48. Given to yoga, perform acts, giving up attachment, Dhanamjaya. Becoming one for whom success and failure do not matter, equal-minded; yoga is called equanimity.

2.49. For the act (itself) is far less important than the attitude (*buddhi*) taken in practice, in yoga, Dhanamjaya. Put your trust in the attitude; pitiable are those moved by fruits.

2.50. Practicing yoga with this attitude, a person pushes away, right here and now, karma both good and bad. Therefore, direct yourself toward yoga; yoga is skill in works.

2.51. For sages practicing yoga with this attitude reject the fruit due to karma. Free from the bondage of birth, they go to the place beyond misery.

2.52. If your mind (*buddhi*) transcends the chatter of delusion, then you'll become indifferent to scriptural texts, both those known (to you) and those still to be learned.

2.53. Averse to scriptural lore, unshaken (by controversy), unmoving in yogic concentration (*samadhi*), if your mind were so, then you would have (true) yoga.

Arjuna said:

2.54. How to describe one of fixed intelligence, the person who has attained yogic concentration (*samadhi*), Keshava? How does the person of fixed thought talk, how sit, how walk?

The Blessed One said:

2.55. One is of fixed intelligence if all the desires that come into the heart, son of Pritha, have been rejected, (that is to say) if he is content living solely in the (universal) self (*atman*), content through the self.

2.56. A sage is of fixed intelligence if his heart is undisturbed in the midst of sorrow and unclinging in the midst of happiness, if he is one whom passion, fear, and anger do not touch.

2.57. Who in all circumstances is free of preference, whether this or that good or ill fortune comes about, who does not rejoice nor gripe (whatever happens), that person has a firm and stable intelligence.

2.58. If, like a turtle that draws in its limbs totally, he draws in his faculties and organs (of sense, digestion, etc.) from their objects, that person has a firm and stable intelligence.

2.59. Objects presented desist (in their attractiveness) for one who, (though) embodied, indulges (eats) them not—except for an impersonal relish, which also desists for him when he perceives the Supreme.

2.60. For even striving, Kaunteya, a person of discernment has organs and faculties that, churning and disturbing, carry away his heart (his attention, *manas*) violently.

2.61. Integrating and controlling (*samyamya*) them all, a person sits engaged in yoga, intent on me (the divine). For he whose organs and faculties are in control is a person of firm and stable intelligence.

2.62. A man thinking about objects becomes attached to them. From attachment is born desire, and from desire anger is engendered.

2.63. From anger bewilderment comes to be; from bewilderment loss of memory. From the breaking off of memory, his (yoga-directed) mental attitude (*buddhi*) perishes; from the perishing of his mental attitude, he comes to nought.

2.64. But ranging over objects presented with organs and faculties separated from passion and dislike, submissive to the self (*atman*), self-governing, he achieves tranquility.

2.65. Once there is tranquility, all suffering is for him banished. For he whose heart and mind are tranquil quickly achieves a mental attitude that is stable and firm.

2.66. There is no right mental attitude without practicing yoga, no self-enlivening (*bhavana*).[5] There is no (spiritual) peace (*shanti*) without self-enlivening. How, if one is without peace, can there be happiness?

2.67. For if the heart and mind follow the churning organs and faculties, they carry away one's intelligence, like the wind (does) a boat on the sea.

2.68. Therefore, strong-armed warrior, a person has a firm and stable intelligence if he has organs and faculties in every way pulled back from their objects.

2.69. What is night for all beings is a time of wakefulness for the person of (integral) control (*samyamin*).[6] That which is their waking is night for the sage who sees.

2.70. Waters enter the ocean forever being filled up (yet) unmoving fundamentally. For whom, like that, all desires enter (without disturbance), that person attains (spiritual) peace (*shanti*), not one who welcomes desires (the *kama-kami*).

2.71. The man who, rejecting all desires, acts without longing, without a sense of "my" and "mine," without egoism, he attains (spiritual) peace.

2.72. This is living in Brahman, the Absolute, O son of Pritha, attaining which a person is no longer deluded. Coming to live in it even at the last hour, to the nirvana that is Brahman he goes.

Chapter 3: Works (*Karma*)

Arjuna said:

3.1. Krishna, if you consider mental attitude (*buddhi*) superior to action, why then do you urge me on to an action so terrible?

3.2. It seems you would confuse my mind (*buddhi*) with contradictory words. So tell me definitely that whereby I can attain the supreme good.

The Blessed One said:

3.3. There are in this world two fundamental stances declared by me of old, Arjuna: the yoga of knowledge (insight) for intellectuals (philosophers, *samkhya*), and karma yoga, the yoga of action for yogins.

3.4. By abstaining from works, a person does not enjoy a mystical actionlessness; nor by renunciation alone is perfection attained.

3.5. For no one is able to remain even for a moment without acting; everyone willy-nilly is made to work by the impulsions (*gunas*, modes) of nature (*prakriti*).

3.6. Self-deluded is he who sits controlling the organs of action while at the same time remembering with heart and mind their objects. His is a false practice.

3.7. But one controlling organs and faculties with heart and mind and commencing disciplined practice (*karma yoga*) with the organs of action, unattached, he excels, Arjuna.

3.8. Do controlled work, for action is better than inaction. The very maintenance of your body would not be accomplished without work.

3.9. Without personal attachment undertake action, Arjuna, for just one purpose, for the purpose of sacrifice. From work undertaken for purposes other than sacrifice, this world is bound to the laws of karma.

3.10. Bringing forth creatures along with sacrifice, the Creator said of old, "With this may you bring forth fruit; let it be your horn of plenty (your wish-fulfilling cow).

3.11. "With this, may you make the gods flourish and may the gods make you flourish. Mutually fostering one another, you will attain the supreme good.

3.12. "For made to flourish by sacrifice, the gods will give you the enjoyments you desire. One who without giving to them enjoys their gifts is nothing but a thief."

3.13. Good people eating the remains from sacrifices are free from sin. But those sinners eat evil who cook for their own sake.

3.14. From food beings come to be; the origin of food is from rain. Rain comes to be from sacrifice. Sacrifice has its origin in works.

3.15. Know works to have their origin in Brahman, and Brahman its foundation in the Immutable. Therefore is the omnipresent Brahman established through all time in sacrifice.

3.16. The wheel is thus set in motion. One who does not follow its rounds, evil in intention, sensual in delights, he lives in vain, son of Pritha.

3.17. But the person delighting only in the higher self (*atman*) and satisfied living in it—for such a person, thoroughly contented in the self alone, there is nothing that must be done.

3.18. Nor is there for him any gain in what he has done or has not done. Nor do his interests depend in any way on anyone or anything else.

3.19. Therefore, ever unattached, do the work that has to be done. For the person who is unattached in performing action attains the supreme good.

3.20. For by work alone did Janaka and others attain perfection.[7] Considering also the holding together of the worlds (i.e., of society), you should be doing works.

3.21. Whatever the superior person does, that indeed is what others try to do. The standard he sets, the world follows.

3.22. For me, there is nothing whatsoever that has to be done, son of Pritha, in the three worlds; nor anything unattained that I need to attain. Still I continue in action.

3.23. For if I did not continue ever tirelessly in action, my example people would follow, son of Pritha, as they always do.

3.24. Societies would come apart if I were not to do works, and I would be the author of chaos in the world. I would destroy these creatures.

3.25. The unenlightened, who are attached to their actions, proceed in works, Arjuna; so should the enlightened, unattached, to hold together society.

3.26. One should not engender a division in the understanding of ignorant folk who are attached to their works; rather, knowing, one should inspire them, performing all actions, disciplined in yoga.

3.27. Works in every fashion are being done by the impulsions (modes, *guna*) of nature. The person deluded by egotism thinks, "I am the doer of this work."

3.28. But the one who knows what is real, strong-armed warrior, concerning those impulsions and the different types of action, realizing that the impulsions operate on themselves, he is not attached.

3.29. Deluded by the impulsions of nature, people are attached to its works. One whose knowledge is complete should not disturb the dull-witted whose knowledge is incomplete.

3.30. Concentrating on the higher self, entrust all your actions to me. Be free of expectation and possessiveness. Fight, with your fever departed.

3.31. People who always follow this teaching of mine, with faith and without griping, they too are freed from (the karmic consequences of) their actions.

3.32. But those who, finding fault with this teaching of mine, do not follow it, know them as confused by every bit of knowledge, lost and unaware.

3.33. Even a person with knowledge (insight) acts in accord with his own nature. Beings follow their nature. What would coercing avail?

3.34. Attraction and repulsion are set in the object of each sense. One should not allow oneself to come under their sway; for they are highwaymen endangering the path.

3.35. Better one's own right way (*dharma*), though flawed, than the way of another perfectly followed. Death following one's own way is better. The way of another is perilous. . . .

Chapter 4: Renunciation of Action in Knowledge

The Blessed One said:

4.1. This imperishable yoga I proclaimed to Vivasvan (the Sun God); Vivasvan declared it to Manu (the first human); Manu told it to Ikshavaku (a primeval king).

4.2. Thus passed from one to another, the royal sages and seers knew it. Then with a long lapse of time, Arjuna, the yoga was lost.

4.3. Today that very yoga, that ancient yoga, is by me explained to you. You are beloved to me, and a friend. So this is indeed the highest secret.

Arjuna said:

4.4. Later is your birth, sir; (much) earlier Vivasvan's. How am I to understand that you declared this yoga in the beginning?

The Blessed One said:

4.5. Many are my past births; yours also, Arjuna. I know them all; you do not.

4.6. Although I exist as the unborn, the imperishable self, and am the Lord of beings, by resorting to and controlling my own nature I come into phenomenal being through my own magical power of delimitation.

4.7. Whenever there is a crisis concerning the right way (*dharma*), Arjuna, and a rising up of evil, then I loose myself forth (taking birth).

4.8. For the protection of good people and for the destruction of evildoers, for the establishment of the right way, I take birth age after age.

4.9. Arjuna, he who in this way knows my divine birth and work comes to me upon abandoning the body, not to rebirth.

4.10. There are many who have come to my (divine) state, their passion, fear, and anger gone, who have been made pure by the ascetic heat (*tapas*) of knowledge.

4.11. In whatever way people approach me, just in that way I give them a share of myself. Humans in all their ways (and approaches) follow a path that is mine, son of Pritha.

4.12. People offer sacrifices to divinities (perform Vedic rituals) in this world when they want success in their activities. For (it is said) quickly in the human world comes success born of (sacrificial) action.

4.13. The social order has been created by me, fourfold, according to distinctions among modes of nature (*guna*) and karma (along with karmic law). Although I am its maker, know me as the nonmaker, the imperishable.

4.14. Actions do not stain me. Nor do I have desire for the fruits of works. The person who recognizes me as this way is himself not bound by his works.

4.15. So knowing, ancient seekers of liberation and enlightenment carried out works. Therefore, simply do actions as were done of old by them.

4.16. What action is, and what inaction, even *rishi*s (seer-sages) are confused on that score. To you I will explain that kind of action, which when (you have) understood, you will be free from all ill.

4.17. For action must be understood, and wrong action as well; inaction must be understood—deep, dark, and dense is the nature of action.

4.18. If one were to see inaction in action and action in inaction, that person among mortals would be wise; he would be spiritually disciplined, yoked in yoga, in all his works.

4.19. One whose instigations and undertakings are all free from the motive of personal desire, the wise see that person as the genuinely learned, the one whose karma has been burned up in the fire of knowledge.

4.20. Having abandoned attachment to the fruits of works, constantly satisfied, independent, one does nothing whatsoever even while thoroughly engaged in works.

4.21. Transcending hope and expectation, controlled in heart and mind, with all possessiveness renounced, one doing simply physical actions accrues no (karmic) adversity.

4.22. Satisfied with whatever gain comes, passed beyond oppositions and dualities, untouched by jealousy, equal-minded and balanced in the face of success and failure, such a person, though he acts, is not bound.

4.23. All karmic dispositions dissolve and wash away when a person is free from attachment, liberated, with a mind firmly fixed in knowledge, acting in a spirit of sacrifice.

4.24. Brahman is the giving, Brahman the oblation; by Brahman into the Brahman fire it is poured. It is just to Brahman where one goes, achieving the ecstatic trance of Brahman action.

4.25. Some yogins practice sacrifice directed to the gods. Others offer the sacrifice into the fire of Brahman.

4.26. Others offer the sense organs of hearing and so on into the fires of control. Still others offer the sense objects of sound and so on into the fires of the senses.

4.27. And others (offer) all the actions of the sense organs and the actions of the life breaths as well into the yogic fire of self-control kindled by knowledge.

4.28. Likewise, some perform material sacrifices, some sacrifices of austerity, and some sacrifices of yoga. There are seekers who with strict vows perform sacrifices both of religious study and of knowledge.

4.29. Similarly, some offer the incoming breath into the outgoing breath and the outgoing breath into the incoming. These restraining the courses of the breaths are devoted to the practice of breath control (*pranayama*).

4.30. Others controlled in diet offer the breaths into the breaths. All these understand sacrifice, and through sacrifice reduce the stains (of karma).

4.31. Those who eat the nectar of immortality left over from a sacrificial action, they go to the eternal Brahman. This world does not belong to one who fails to sacrifice, so how could the next, Arjuna?

4.32. In this way, numerous diverse sacrifices are spread wide in the mouth of Brahman. Know them all as born in action. Thus knowing, you will be liberated and enlightened.

4.33. A sacrifice in knowledge, Arjuna, is superior to a sacrifice with material things. All action in its entirety culminates and is fulfilled in knowledge.

4.34. Come to have this knowledge through submission to those who know, by questioning and service. They, the seers of what is real, will initiate and teach you.

4.35. Knowing that, you will not ever be confused again, Arjuna—that whereby you will see beings without exception in the self (*atman*) and then in me.

4.36. Even if of all sinners you are now the very worst evildoer, once in the boat of knowledge you will safely cross over the crookedness of evil.

4.37. As a fire kindled reduces its fuel to ashes, Arjuna, so the fire of knowledge makes ashes all karma.

4.38. For here in this world there is no purifier the equal of knowledge. A person perfected through yoga practice finds it himself in the self (*atman*) after a time.

4.39. A person of faith gets that knowledge, (having) concentrated on it, with senses controlled. Having the knowledge, he at once gets the supreme peace.

4.40. A person not only not knowing but having no faith, his mind full of doubts, is lost. Neither this world nor another, nor happiness, comes to the doubting mind.

4.41. Actions do not bind him who has transcended works through yoga and cut through doubt with knowledge; he is self-possessed, Arjuna.

4.42. Therefore, having cut through the doubt that is born of ignorance and set in the heart, having cut through it with the sword of self-knowledge, in yoga, Arjuna, take your stand. Stand up and fight.

Chapter 5: Renunciation

Arjuna said:

5.1. Renunciation of actions but also yoga (in action) you praise, Krishna. Which one is the better of the two? That tell me very definitely.

The Blessed One said:

5.2. Both renunciation and karma yoga (the yoga of action and sacrifice) bring about the supreme good. Of the two, however, great-armed warrior, karma yoga is better than the renunciation of action (altogether).

5.3. The person to be known as a renunciant, a constant renunciant, is neither happy nor griping (whatever happens). For, strong-armed warrior, transcending dualities, he easily is liberated from the bondage (of rebirth).

5.4. Metaphysical truth (*samkhya*) and yoga (practice) children speak of as separate, not the learned (or wise). Putting your heart in either perfectly, you find the fruit of both.

5.5. The state obtained by the intellectuals (and their method, their analysis, *samkhya*), that is also gained by yogins (and their method, *yoga*). Who sees *samkhya* and yoga as one, genuinely does that person see.

5.6. But renunciation, strong-armed warrior, is difficult to carry out without yoga. Not in a long time is it that the sage disciplined in yoga practice attains Brahman.

5.7. Disciplined in the practice of yoga, self-purified, self-controlled, with organs and faculties conquered, he whose self has become the self of all beings, however acting, is not stained.

5.8. The knower of the truth of things, disciplined in yoga practice, would think, "I do nothing whatsoever," while seeing, hearing, touching, smelling, eating, moving about, sleeping, breathing.

5.9. Conversing, eliminating, taking in, opening or closing the eyes, "The organs and faculties are working on their objects," contemplating (all the time).

5.10. Depositing actions in (the fire of) Brahman, giving up attachment, he who then acts is not stained by sin, like a lotus leaf by water (is not touched).

5.11. By the body, with the heart and mind, by the intelligence, even only with the organs and faculties, yogins perform actions, abandoning attachment, to purify themselves.

5.12. Disciplined through yoga practice, abandoning attachment, one finds the peace of the deepest foundation. A person who does no yoga practice, attached to the fruit of what he does because of desire, is bound (by his karma).

5.13. Renouncing in heart and mind all actions, a person sits easily (happily) in control. In the nine-gated city (the human body), the embodied never acts, never causes to act.

5.14. The Lord lets go (creates) neither agency nor actions for people, nor the connection between actions and their fruits. These operate according to the law of nature.

5.15. The Omnipresent accepts neither the sin nor the good deed of anyone. Knowledge is enveloped by ignorance; thus deluded are creatures.

5.16. But for whom this ignorance is destroyed by knowledge (insight), concerning the self (*atman*), for them, like the sun, knowledge reveals that supreme (Brahman).

5.17. With their mental attitude set on that, taking their selves as that, taking their stand on that (their consciousness set in that), on that intent, they go to freedom from birth, their stains cleansed by knowledge.

5.18. The learned (the wise) with respect to an educated and cultured Brahmin, a cow, an elephant, a dog, and an outcaste see the same.

5.19. Here and now, by them whose heart and mind are set in equality and equanimity, is birth conquered. For the faultless Brahman is (everywhere) the same. Therefore, they take their stand in Brahman.

5.20. One who would not get excited when something good occurs, nor depressed at something unfortunate, a person of fixed and stable mental attitude (*buddhi*), no longer deluded, is the Brahman knower, (his consciousness) set in Brahman.

5.21. One by nature unattached to outward contacts, finding what pleasure he finds in the self, one who is by nature disciplined by the yoga of (the yoke of, union with) Brahman, easily (sweetly, *sukham*) tastes the Imperishable.

5.22. For the enjoyments that are born from contacts with other things are only a source of suffering. They have beginnings and endings, Kaunteya. The wise person does not in them delight.

5.23. The man who just here, before leaving the body, is able to bear the impetus that builds from desire and anger, is the one disciplined in yoga, happy.

5.24. It is he whose happiness is within, whose enjoyment is inner, and whose light is only within, who is the yogin. Having become Brahman, he attains nirvana in Brahman.

5.25. Seer-sages (*rishis*) gain nirvana in Brahman with their sins effaced, cutting through dualities, working for the good of all beings, delighted in the good of all.

5.26. Separating themselves from desire and anger, the disciplined, with their thought streams under control, possess nirvana in Brahman here and now and all around, having knowledge of the self (*atman*).

5.27–28. Outside having put external contacts and directing the visual organ (to the inner center) between the eyebrows, making the upward and downward breaths (inhalations and exhalations, *prana* and *apana*) equal (in duration), moving through the nostrils (not the mouth), with organs and faculties, heart and mind, and (higher) intelligence (*buddhi*) all under control, the sage intent on liberation, with desire, fear, and anger gone, is (already) liberated forever indeed.

5.29. Such a person, knowing the sweet inner heart of all beings, comes to (spiritual) peace (*shanti*), comes to me, the enjoyer of sacrifice and asceticism, the lord of all the worlds.

Chapter 6: Meditation (*Dhyana*)

. . .

(Krishna, the Blessed One, said:)

6.10. Let the yogin ever practice on himself (or, ever unite with the self) in a retreat, becoming solitary, controlled in thought and emotion (*chitta*) and without expectations and (any sense of) possessiveness.

6.11–12. Setting himself in a clean place in a steady asana (posture, seat) that is neither too high nor too low (to be comfortable), on a cloth, animal skin, or *kusha* grass, there fixing heart and mind on a single point, working to bring his thought and emotion along with his organs and faculties under control, let him practice yoga for self-purification.

6.13–14. Holding the body, head, and neck motionless, drawing in the vision to fix it (on midline) at the tip of the nose and not looking in any direction, steady, consciously identifying with the thought and emotion and controlling it, let him sit practicing yoga with his thought and emotion directed to me, intent on me.

6.15. Practicing yoga on himself in this way constantly, the yogin with fixed heart and mind attains the peace supreme of nirvana, (that is to say) attains to the station of me (the station of my consciousness).

6.16. Yoga is not for one who eats too much, nor for one who does not eat at all. Arjuna, it is not for one who sleeps too much, nor for one who stays awake (constantly).

6.17. Yoga banishes suffering for one who practices asleep and awake, eating and playing, in working (always) acting like a yogin.

6.18. Insofar as a person's thought and emotions (*chitta*) are directed solely to himself (that is to say, to the universal self, *atman*), such a person is rightly called a yogin, free of wishing, practicing with respect to all desire.

6.19. As a lamp set down out of the wind does not flicker—this analogy is used for the yogin whose thought and emotion are restrained, practicing yoga for himself (or, for the universal self, *atman*).

6.20–21. Checked by yoga practice, the thought and emotion (*chitta*) having come to stillness, seeing (everywhere) the self by the self, being satisfied in the self (alone), a yogin knows a supreme and endless pleasure, which is graspable by the intelligence though it is not within the range of the senses, becomes in it fixed and stable, and never moves away from the reality.

6.22. It is that which, once (having) obtained (it), a person would not regard obtaining anything else as better. Fixed in it, a person is not disturbed by even (occasions for) the fiercest grief.

6.23. May this (state) be known—yoga is known as the disjunction from all contact with pain and grief. Such yoga should be practiced with determination (never despairing), with thought and mind engaged.

6.24–25. Rejecting desires born of intentions, all of them without exception, with the *manas* alone, the attention, completely checking the pack of sense organs, then gradually, step by step, one should become still, holding the attention (*manas*) in the self (*atman*) with the intelligence (*buddhi*), the intellegence itself held tight with fortitude, one should think of nothing at all; nothing whatsoever should come into consciousness.

6.26. Wherever the attention would roam, restless and not steady or firm, just there checking it, one should put it in the control of the self alone.

6.27. For a pacified mentality carries the yogin to the highest pleasure and happiness, his passion quietened, absorbed in Brahman, without flaw.

6.28. A yogin constantly practicing on himself in this way, flaws departed, effortlessly enjoys the supreme pleasure that is the touch of Brahman.

6.29. Seeing the same everywhere, disciplined through yoga practice, one perceives the self seated in all beings and all beings in the self.

6.30. A person who sees me everywhere and everything in me is never lost to me, and I am never lost to that person.

6.31. However he may live, the yogin lives in me who, stationed in oneness, is devoted to me who am set in (the heart of) all beings, sharing in me.

6.32. Who sees through the lens of likeness to self the same everywhere, Arjuna, whether pleasure and happiness or pain and suffering, that yogin is to be deemed the very best.

Arjuna said:

6.33. The yoga declared by you, Krishna, as practicing equality (and equanimity), well, I do not see it becoming firmly fixed because of the restless nature (of the mind).

6.34. For the sense mind (*manas*) is restless, Krishna, whirling, forceful, and tough. I think it is as hard to control as the wind.

The Blessed One said:

6.35. Doubtless, O strong-armed warrior, the sense mind is hard to control, (always) wandering about. But with practice (*abhyasa*), Arjuna, and dispassion (*vairagya*), it can be checked.[8]

6.36. My view is that this yoga would be difficult for someone who is not self-controlled. But for one who is self-controlled it can be done through the proper means with effort.

Arjuna said:

6.37. Someone of insufficient accomplishment but of good faith, whose heart and mind wander off from the practice, what becomes of such a person, Krishna, one who (tries but) does not attain success in yoga?

6.38. Is he not like a cloud split apart, dissolving bit by bit, separated from both (success in the world and success in yoga)? O great-armed warrior, would not the person who is not firmly set (in yoga or in making gains in life) be self-deluded on Brahman's path?

6.39. This is my doubt, Krishna. You are fit to make it disappear (if anyone is). For other than you, there is no one who could get rid of this worry.

 The Blessed One said:

6.40. Not at all in this world, son of Pritha, nor hereafter is there for him such loss. For, set on doing good, he does not, child, come to a bad end.

6.41. Winning the worlds of the doers of good deeds, living there immemorial years, someone (like you describe) fallen from yoga would be born in a household of people who are pure (of good habits) and beautiful.

6.42. Or he would be born just into a family of yogins and yoginis, people of wisdom. For such a birth is very difficult to obtain in this world.

6.43. There he would recover the purposefulness of his previous life, and would strive, O joy of the Kurus, from that point on toward perfection.

6.44. For even without trying he would be carried just by the practice in his former birth. Even one who merely wants to know about yoga transcends the revealed word (conventional religion).

6.45. The yogin is the person who willfully is making effort, his flaws being washed away. Through many births becoming accomplished, he attains then to the supreme condition.

6.46. The yogin is superior to those who practice austerities; he is (to be) deemed superior to intellectuals (theologians) too. The yogin is superior to ritualists. Therefore, be a yogin, Arjuna.

6.47. I deem the person the most accomplished of yogins who with inner self given to me with trust takes his share of me.

Chapter 7: Knowledge and Higher Insight (*Vijnana*)

The Blessed One said:

7.1. Listen, son of Pritha, to how, by practicing yoga with your mind attached to me, relying on and given over to me (*mad-ashraya*), you will come to know with certitude me in my entirety.

7.2. I shall tell you in full the knowledge that is accompanied by the higher insight, the knowing of which will leave it unnecessary to know here anything else.

7.3. Among thousands of human beings, occasionally there is one who strives (*yatati*) for perfection (*siddhi*). Among those strivers who are accomplished (*siddha*), occasionally there is one who knows me in my essential principles.

7.4–5. Earth, water, fire, air, ether (the medium of sound), the sense mind (*manas*), and the rational intelligence (*buddhi*) too, along with the ego sense (the principal of individuality, *ahamkara*), make up the divisions of my eightfold nature. This is the lower nature. Know my higher nature to be other than this, O great-armed warrior. It is by my higher nature having become the living individual (*jiva*) that this world is supported.

7.6. The womb of all creatures it is—realize this. I am the origin of the entire universe, its dissolution too.

7.7. There is nothing whatsover superior to me, Arjuna. On me all this is strung like gems on a necklace.

7.8. Kaunteya, for water (of all its qualities) I am taste, I am the light of the sun and the moon; *om* among everything Vedic, sound (words) in ether, among persons what makes them persons.

7.9. I am both the sweet smell of earth and the fiery light of fire. Life am I of living beings, and the *tapas* (ascetic heat) of those who practice austerities.

7.10. Know me, son of Pritha, to be the abiding seed of everything. I am the intelligence of the intelligent. I am the *tejas* (enthusiasm and energy) of the *tejas*-endowed.

7.11. The strength of the strong I am, strength devoid of ambition and liking. Desire in creatures I am, desire in accordance with *dharma*.

7.12. And those (further qualities found in things)—sattvic, rajasic, and tamasic (illuminative, passionate, energetic, and dull, inert)—know them to come from me alone. But I am not in them; they are in me.

7.13. This entire universe deluded by the emergent states (and combinations) of these three qualities (*guna*) does not know me beyond them, the Imperishable.

7.14. For this my divine *maya* is difficult to cross beyond. They cross over this Maya who come over (*prapatti*) to me. . . .

7.29. Those who strive (*yat*, i.e., practice yoga) for freedom from old age and death by taking their resort in me, Brahman is what they come to know, the whole, the spiritual, who is karma (action) in its entirety (or, the integral action).

7.30. Those who know me as I am in both material and spiritual being, and in my sacrifical nature too, at the end of life as well (as at any other time), with their consciousnesses disciplined in yoga (*yoga-yukta,* yoked by yoga practice, yoked by union [with Brahman]), they are knowers of me.

Chapter 8: Perseverance

. . .

(The Blessed One said:)

8.6. Whatever state (world or state of consciousness) remembering upon abandoning the body at death, to just that state one goes who has enlivenened (the idea of) it continuously (through meditation thereon).

8.7. Therefore, at all times remember me and fight. As a person whose mind and higher intelligence are on me, holding me as the ideal, you will come to me alone, no doubt about it.

8.8. With a consciousness disciplined by yoga (*yoga-yukta*) practiced diligently, not wandering off to some other thing, one goes—hereon keeping the attention—to the supreme Person, the Divine, O son of Pritha.

8.9–10. The ancient Poet-seer, the Preceptor, more minute than the minute, whoso should (thoroughly and intensely) meditate on this one that supports everything, of unthinkable form, the color of the sun, beyond darkness, / That person, disciplined in yoga with a motionless mind and *bhakti* made strong through practice, who at the time of death makes the breath enter (the center) between the eyebrows properly, attains the supreme Person, the Divine.

8.11. That Imperishable talked about by those who know the Vedas, entered into and realized by ascetics (*yati*) with preferences gone, desired by students practicing chastity, that station perspicaciously I shall explain to you.

8.12–13. Consciously controlling all the gates (of the body, the sense organs, etc.) and checking the sense mind in the (lotus of) the heart, collecting the self's breath into the head (center), engaged in holding on to the yoga (*dharana,* concentrated perseverance), chanting *om*—meaning the One, the Imperishable, the Absolute Brahman—thinking about me, whoso abandoning the body goes forth (at death), that person goes to the supreme goal (the supreme ongoing goal, *gati*).

8.14. Whoso constantly thinks about me, the consciousness continually on nothing else, for such a person, O son of Pritha, I am easy to find, for such a yogin ever disciplined in yoga.

8.15. Those the great-souled (*mahatman*) who have realized me do not obtain another birth, no rebirth that is a place of suffering, that is transitory. They go (rather) to supreme perfection (*samsiddhi*).

. . .

Chapter 9: The Royal Knowledge and the Royal Secret

. . .

(The Blessed One said:)

9.26. Whoso presents a leaf, a flower, fruit, water, to me with devotion (*bhakti*), I consume that offering of such an aspiring soul, that offering made with *bhakti*.

9.27. What you do, what you eat, what you offer, what you give, what *tapas* you perform, Arjuna, do it as a present to me.

9.28. In this way, you will become free from the good and bad consequences of your acts, the bindings of karma. Entirely liberated, disciplined by a yoga of renunciation, you shall come to me.

9.29. I am the same in all beings. To me, none is despicable, none dear. However, whoso worship me (taking their share of me) with *bhakti,* they are in me and I too in them (consciously).

9.30. Although the behavior has been very bad, if I am loved with unswerving devotion, the judgment should be that the person is indeed a good person. For now the intention would be correctly set.

9.31. Quickly the person comes to be *dharma*-minded, attaining everlasting peace. Understand, Arjuna, my *bhakta,* my devotee, does not perish.

. . .

Chapter 10: Special Divine Manifestations (*Vibhuti*)

. . .

(The Blessed One said:)

10.8. The wise (the awakened), adoring me (taking their share of me) in the knowledge that I am the origin of everything, that from me everything comes forth, come to be filled with emotion.

10.9. With thought and emotion (*chitta*) on me, with their lives (their life energies, *prana*) given over to me, enlightening one another, constantly telling stories about me, they are happy and delighted.

10.10. To them thus constantly disciplined in adoration, *bhakti,* that is accompanied by intense affection, I provide the discipline, the yoga, of the higher intelligence whereby they realize me.

10.11. Out of compassion for them, I destroy the darkness born of ignorance. Sitting in the seat of their emotions, I radiate with the light of knowledge.

. . .

Chapter 11: The Vision of (Krishna's) Totality

. . .

(The Blessed One said:)

11.8. With just your own organ of vision you are not able to see me (as I am in my totality). Divine vision I give to you. See my majestic discipline (*yoga*)![9]

. . .

11.54. But, Arjuna, I can be known as such (as you have beheld, not only by the grace of divine vision but) by undeviating love and devotion (*bhakti*). And I can be so seen and realized in essential principle, O scorcher of the foe.

11.55. Whoso acts for my sake, for whom I am the supreme ideal, devoted to me (*mad-bhakta*) without self-interest, whoso has no enmity toward any creature, that one comes to me, Arjuna.

Chapter 12: Love and Devotion (*Bhakti*)

. . .

(The Blessed One said:)

12.6–7. But those who giving all their actions up to me, focused on me, worship meditating on me through an absolutely undeviating yoga (of *bhakti*), I rescue them before long from the ocean of death and transmigration. Their consciousnesses are absorbed in me.

12.8. Put your mind on me alone (your sense mind, *manas*); occupy your higher intelligence (*buddhi*) with me. (Then) you shall live in me alone, transcending this (mortal existence), no doubt about it.

12.13–14. Not hating any creature, friendly and compassionate too, without possessiveness or egotism, facing pleasure and pain with equanimity, patient and enduring, contented always, the yogin whose (lower) self is under control, whose resolve is firm, whose *manas* and *buddhi* are given over to me, this my *bhakta* (*bhakti yogin*) is dear to me.

12.15. Who does not trouble people, and who is not troubled by people, who is free from excitement, impetuosity, fear, and vexation, he too is to me dear.

12.16. Independent, pure, capable, indifferent, having transcended perturbations, who has surrendered all (separate) initiatives to action, this my *bhakta* to me is dear.

12.17. Neither rejoicing nor cursing, neither mourning nor hankering after, having no concern whether what happens is fortunate or unfortunate, endowed with *bhakti,* he to me is dear.

12.18–19. Equipoised in the face of friend and foe, likewise in honor and dishonor, the same in cold or heat, pleaure or pain, free from attachment, balanced in the face of praise or blame, silent, contented no matter what comes about, beyond home, steady, having intense *bhakti,* the person is to me dear.

12.20. But those who put into practice this principled, immortal nectar of teaching, as it has been laid out, having faith, entirely focused on me, such devotees (*bhakta*s) are to me intensely dear.

Chapter 13: The Field and Knower of the Field

. . .

Chapter 14: The Triad of Qualities

. . .

Arjuna said:

14.21. By what marks, lord, is the person known who has transcended these three qualities, *gunas* (*sattva, rajas,* and *tamas,* the illuminating, the passionate, energetic, and the dull, inert, respectively, that make up all of our lower psychology)? How does he act? And how does he come to be beyond the three *gunas*?

The Blessed One said:

14.22. That person does not loathe (the workings or manifestation of any of the three) the illuminative, the active, or the dull and confused. He does not hanker after (the one or the other's) working in himself nor its ceasing to be.

14.23–25. The one seated as though high above, indifferent, who does not move with the movements of the qualities, who thinks just, "It is these *gunas* doing what they do," standing apart, unflappable, the same whether facing pleasure or pain, self-possessed, equal-minded toward clay, stone, and gold, balanced in the face of both the pleasant and the unpleasant, such a wise one who is balanced in the face of both praise and blame, balanced in honor and dishonor, balanced whether facing a faction of friends or enemies, who has surrendered all (separate) initiatives to action, that is the person to be known as transcending the *gunas*.

14.26. And whoso with an unswerving discipline (*yoga*) of *bhakti* performs service (*seva*) for me, does go beyond the *gunas* completely, becoming fit for Brahman experience.

14.27. For I am the basis of Brahman, the immortal and the imperishable, and of *dharma* (the right way) ever ongoing, and of the pleasure that is absolute and unsurpassed.

Chapter 15: The Supreme Person

. . .

Chapter 16: The Divine and Demonic in Us

. . .

Chapter 17: Three Types of Faith

. . .

(The Blessed One said:)

17.23. "*Om tat sat*" ("*om,* That, Being [Reality]") is known as the triple designation of Brahman. By it, priests, the Vedas, and sacrifices were consecrated of old.

17.24. Therefore, the Brahman-professing commence acts of sacrifice, giving, and *tapas* (asceticism) as laid down in rules only after uttering *om*.

17.25. Uttering "*tat*" ("That"), (to suggest) intending not to aim at the fruit, seekers of liberation perform acts of sacrifice and *tapas*, acts of giving too, as laid down in rules.

17.26. The utterance "*sat*" ("Being, Reality"), is used in the sense of being and in the sense of good. The word *sat* is thus used, Arjuna, for commendable work.

17.27. And "*sat*" is said when a person is steadfast and persevering in sacrificing, performing *tapas*, or giving. And any action whose purpose is sacrifice, etc., is to be designated just by uttering "*sat*."

17.28. An oblation poured without faith, without faith a gift given or *tapas* performed, or whatever is done without faith, that is to be called *asat* (nonbeing, unreal, bad), Arjuna. On dying, that is negative, as it is negative too here in this world.

Chapter 18: Renunciation and Liberation

. . .

(The Blessed One said:)

18.45. A person delighted in the work that is to him natural (that he seems cut out for) obtains complete perfection. Hear now how perfection is got by him who is intent upon the work that is to him natural.

18.46. A human being finds perfection by honoring through his own work (the work he finds natural) the one from whom all creatures come forth, by whom all this is pervaded.

18.47. One's own *dharma*, though imperfectly carried out, is better than the *dharma* of another performed to perfection. A human doing work determined by his own nature does not get stained.

18.48. Work that is natural, Arjuna, though flawed should not be rejected. For all undertakings are enveloped by flaws, like smoke around a fire.

18.49. With an intelligence (*buddhi*) not attached to anything, with (lower) self conquered, far gone his preferences, he attains the ultimate perfection of actionlessness by renunciation.

18.50. Hear and learn from me perspicaciously, Arjuna, how once attaining such perfection a person attains to the Brahman. What I shall tell is the deep basis of knowledge (here).

18.51–53. Disciplined in yoga by means of a purified higher intelligence (*buddhi*), firmly restraining the (lower) self, renouncing (the distractions of) sound and other objects, casting far away liking and disliking, living in a secluded place, eating lightly, with constrained speech, body, and (sense) mind (*manasa*), all the time intent on practicing the yoga of meditation, completely settled in dispassion (*vairagya*), distanced from egotism, violence, pride, sexual desire, anger, possessiveness, such a person, nonacquisitive and at peace (*shanta*), is fit for Brahman experience.

18.54. Living in Brahman, self-content, such a person, neither grieving about nor hankering for anything, and the same with respect to every creature, obtains (although taking the route of meditation) a state of supreme *bhakti* for me.

18.55. Such a person, coming through *bhakti* to recognize me as who I am in essential principle, thus knowing me in essential principle, enters me (my state) immediately thereupon.

18.56. Whatever action such a one may perform at any time—such a one who has me as wide basis—obtains by my grace the everlasting, the condition (of consciousness) that is imperishable.

18.57. In emotion and thought depositing all your action in me, focused on me, practicing the yoga of the higher intelligence (*buddhi yoga*), be one whose thought and emotion (*chitta*) are all the time given to me.

18.58. One whose thought and emotion are given to me will cross over all difficulties through my grace. But if from egotism you do not learn (how to live yogically), you will come to nought.

18.59. If, retreating into egotism, you should think, "I will not fight," false then would be this "resolve" of yours. Nature (*prakriti*) would be controlling you.

18.60. Arjuna, you are bound by the karma that is your own in virtue of your peculiar nature. What you do not, because of delusion, want to do, that you will do though (cluelessly and) willy-nilly.

18.61. In all creatures the Lord abides, Arjuna, in the place of the heart, controlling all creatures (by their desires) through (the magic of) *maya* (illusion, power to self-delimit) as though working a machine.

18.62. Make him alone your refuge, Bharata, in every condition and state of mind. Through his grace you will obtain the supreme peace (*shanti*), the condition, the abode that is imperishable.

18.63. This is the teaching that, (though) more secret than secret, has been by me now told to you. Considering it without leaving anything out, do what you want to do.

18.64. Listen again to the most secret secret, my final word. You are very dear to me. Thus for your sake I shall tell you.

18.65. Be one whose mind is on me, devoted to me (in *bhakti*). Sacrificing to me, honor me. You will come to me alone. This is the truth, I promise. You are dear to me.

18.66. Abandoning all *dharma*s, take refuge in me alone. I shall free you from every evil. Do not worry.

APPENDIX C
The *Yoga Sutra*

The *Yoga Sutra* (*YS*) defines a worldview and spells out exercises of yoga practice. That is, it spells out a system—really system*s*—of practices framed by a metaphysics. The Yoga philosophy of the *YS* is distinct from, for example, the theism of the *Bhagavad Gita,* though the *Gita* also advocates yoga practices. As we have discussed (in the first section of chapter 5 in particular), the supreme good according to the *YS* is a rupture separating an individual conscious being, *purusha,* from nature, *prakriti.* To explain this possibility, which it calls aloneness (*kaivalya*), it presents a metaphysical dualism of an infinite plurality of such individual conscious beings, on the one hand, and a single nature, on the other. That is to say, its dualism may be interpreted as an explanation of how liberation from nature (*prakriti*) is possible. It is so because in reality the individual conscious being (*purusha*) is already liberated.

Thus, in addition to its delineation of yoga practices in the style of a how-to book or meditation manual, the *YS* attends to questions about reality, especially about the relation of consciousness to nature. There is also an intermediate level of psychological theorizing, which models various cognitive and motor functions. The psychology constitutes a bridge between the practice teachings and the metaphysics of Yoga, and, as I have argued (chapter 2), is valuable despite the inadequacy of the *YS*'s brand of dualism.

The textual and commentarial tradition is discussed in the last section of chapter 1. Although the commentary by Vyasa (see figure 1A) fixes a classical reading, probably many of the sutras were formulated in distinct philosophical settings other than his and Patanjali's. Modern commentators sympathetic to traditions of Indian spirituality try to restore a sense of the sutras outside the systematic interpretations of classical commentators—with some success, in my opinion. Furthermore, some classical philosophers, such as the tantric Abhinava Gupta (c. 950), also read the aphorisms differently than Vyasa and his followers.

A telltale tension in the text concerns the theory about God, the Lord (*ishvara*), in connection with practice teachings of *bhakti* (love and devotion to God). As discussed in chapter 5, here theory seems to undermine practice, and many classical theists find value in the psychological and yogic teachings of the *YS* while rejecting its theology. God, according to the *YS* (or, more precisely, according to the classical Yoga interpretation of the text by commentators, beginning with Vyasa in the fifth century), is the archetypal liberated conscious being, never sullied by contact with the world (although somehow also the primeval teacher). This is a very different notion from that of the *Gita*, where the Supreme Being is conceived along lines a lot closer to the theology of Western religions.

Indologists have seen the *YS* as a compilation of distinct texts. Classical commentators, in sharp contrast, presuppose its unity. Modern yoga sympathizers, such as B.K.S. Iyengar (1993), Georg Feuerstein (1979), and Swami Satyananda Saraswati (1976), not only try to restore an original "experiential" or "phenomenological" sense but also, in the case of Iyengar in particular, import much traditional folklore in their commentaries. My method has been to try to learn from everyone.

The text is taken from the critical edition of the first chapter and Vyasa's commentary by P. Maas and, for the remainder of the text, from a critical edition of two important commentaries by V. Karnatak.[1] The transliteration of the *YS* text into roman characters follows the standard indological rules and not the phonetic schema (without diacritics) used here elsewhere than with full sentences. Sanskrit words used in the translation are, as always, defined in the glossary. See p. 163 in this book for an explanation of the translation style. In general, my reading expands on the ideas of a paper, "The Conflict of Voluntarism and Dualism in the *Yoga-sutra*,"[2] which is summarized in chapter 2, the third section.

The Yoga Sutras of Patanjali

Salutations to Patanjali!
oṃ namo namaḥ.

samādhi-pāda

1.1. atha yogânuśāsanam.
Now instruction in yoga.[3]

1.2. yogaś citta-vṛtti-nirodhaḥ.
Yoga is the stilling of fluctuations of thought and emotion (*chitta*).[4]

1.3. tadā draṣṭuḥ sva-rūpe 'vasthānam.
Then the seer (the conscious being, *purusha*) rests in its true form.

1.4. vṛtti-sārūpyam itaratra.
At other times, fluctuations are identified with.

1.5. vṛttayaḥ pañcatayyaḥ kliṣṭâkliṣṭāḥ.
Fluctuations are of five types, and are detrimental or nondetrimental (to the practices of yoga).[5]

1.6. pramāṇa-viparyaya-vikalpa-nidrā-smṛtayaḥ.
The five are knowledge sources (and knowledge), the opposite, thought and imagination, sleep (and dreaming), and memory.

1.7. tatra pratyakṣânumānâgamāḥ pramāṇāni.
Among these, the knowledge sources (along with the veridical awarenesses to which they give rise) are perception, inference, and testimony (including scriptural tradition).

1.8. viparyayo mithyā-jñānam atad-rūpa-pratiṣṭham.
The opposite to the knowledge sources amounts to misapprehension indicating that something is what it is not.[6]

1.9. śabda-jñānânupātī vastu-śūnyo vikalpaḥ.
Thought and imagination (*vikalpa*, the third item on the list of five), which are devoid of real objects, are dependent on words and concepts.

1.10. abhāva-pratyayâlambanā vṛttir nidrā.
Sleep (along with dreaming) comprises the mental fluctuation whose object is a stream of ideas about things not present.

1.11. anubhūta-viṣayâsampramoṣaḥ smṛtiḥ.
Memory is not letting experienced objects get away.

1.12. abhyāsa-vairāgyābhyāṃ tan-nirodhaḥ.
Restriction of them (all five types of fluctuation) is accomplished through practice and disinterestedness.

1.13. tatra sthitau yatno 'bhyāsaḥ.
Practice is effort to hold fast the restriction.

1.14. sa tu dīrgha-kāla-nairantarya-saṃskārâsevito dṛḍha-bhūmiḥ.
But that effort becomes firmly established when its mental (or memory) dispositions (*samskara*) become habitual through long and continuous practice.

1.15. dṛṣṭânuśravika-viṣaya-vitṛṣṇasya vaśīkāra-saṃjnā vairāgyam.
Disinterestedness is the consciousness of being in control (of appetites), on the part of someone who has no thirst for objects directly perceived or reported.[7]

1.16. tat-param puruṣa-khyāter guṇa-vaitṛṣṇyam.
Superior to that is (the absolute disinterestedness of) lack of desire for (manifest or unmanifest) phenomena (*guna*, qualities) because of perception of the *purusha* (true person).[8]

1.17. vitarka-vicārânandâsmitā-rūpânugamāt samprajñātaḥ.
Samadhi (yogic trance or enstacy) has two forms, one of which is supported by wisdom in accordance with reasoning, discrimination, bliss, and sense of identity ("I-amness").

1.18. virāma-pratyayâbhyāsa-pūrvakaḥ saṃskāra-śeṣo 'nyaḥ.
The other, in which only mental dispositions (*samskara*) remain, is preceded by effort to hold steady ideas intent on contentment.

1.19. bhava-pratyayo videha-prakṛti-layānām.
Disembodied yogins and those merged with nature attain *samadhi* through being intent on birth (i.e., just by being born).

1.20. śraddhā-vīrya-smṛti-samādhi-prajñā-pūrvaka itareṣām.
Others attain it through faith, energy, remembering (i.e., meditation), and wisdom deriving from *samadhi*.

1.21. tīvra-saṃvegānām āsannaḥ.
It settles in for those who are exceptionally intense.

1.22. mṛdu-madhyâdhimātratvāt tato 'pi viśeṣaḥ.
Even among those (who are exceptionally intense), there are differences: the barely so, the moderately so, and the extremely so.

1.23. īśvara-praṇidhānād vā.
Or, (restriction occurs) from opening to (devotion to, meditation on, *pranidhana*) the Lord.[9]

1.24. kleśa-karma-vipākâśayair aparāmṛṣṭaḥ puruṣa-viśeṣa īśvaraḥ.
By "Lord" is meant a particular conscious being (*purusha*) who (unlike us) is untouched by obstacles to enlightenment or by stores of ripening karma.

1.25. tatra niratiśayaṃ sarvajña-bījam.
The seed of omniscience (present in everyone) is unsurpassed in the Lord.

1.26. sa pūrveṣām api guruḥ kālena anavacchedāt.
He is the guru even of the ancient teachers in not being limited by time.

1.27. tasya vācakaḥ praṇavaḥ.
The Lord is indicated by the syllable *om*.

1.28. taj-japas tad-artha-bhāvanam.
(Devotional yoga consists in) repetition of *om* and enlivening its meaning.

1.29. tataḥ pratyak-cetanâdhigamo 'ntarāyâbhāvaś ca.
From that comes understanding of inward consciousness as well as negation of obstacles.

1.30. vyādhi-styāna-saṃśaya-pramādâlasyâvirati-bhrānti-darśanâlabdha-bhūmikatvânavasthitatvāni citta-vikṣepā antarāyāḥ.
Obstacles are illness, listlessness, doubt, heedlessness, laziness, nonabstention, wrong outlook, and failure to attain a certain level or to stay there. They make the *chitta* unsteady.

1.31. duḥkha-daurmanasyâṅga-mejayatva-śvāsa-praśvāsā vikṣepa-sahabhuvaḥ.
Symptoms of unsteadiness include pain, bad mood, shaky limbs, and uneven in- and out-breaths.

1.32. tat-pratiṣedhârtham eka-tattvâbhyāsaḥ.
For the purpose of checking them, practice should be maintained within a single system (or, by a single principle, *eka-tattva*).

1.33. maitrī-karuṇā-muditôpekṣāṇāṃ sukha-duḥkha-puṇyâpuṇya-viṣayāṇāṃ bhāvanātaś citta-prasādanam.
Calming illumination of the mind (*chitta*) is furthered through practicing (or, enlivening), toward objects pleasant, painful, virtuous, and full of vice, (respectively the balancing attitudes of) friendship, compassion, gladness, and indifference.[10]

1.34. pracchardana-vidhāraṇābhyāṃ vā prāṇasya.
Or, it (calming illumination, stilling of the *chitta*) can be brought about by controlled exhalation and holding of the breath (i.e., by *pranayama*).

1.35. viṣayavatī vā pravṛttir utpannā manasaḥ sthiti-nibandhanī.
Or, (it arises from) the advent of sense-object-centered activity binding the sensuous mentality.[11]

1.36. viśokā vā jyotiṣmatī.
Or, (it arises with) activity that is free from sorrow and luminous (such as concentration on the heart center or the center between the eyebrows).

1.37. vīta-rāga-viṣayaṃ vā cittam.
Or, when the mind (*chitta*) contemplates beings who have transcended passion.[12]

1.38. svapna-nidrā-jñānâlambanaṃ vā.
Or, (another means is) the mind brought to knowledge of sleep and dreams.

1.39. yathâbhimata-dhyānād vā.
Or, from meditation in accordance with (an individual's) proclivities.

1.40. paramâṇu-mahattvânto 'sya vaśīkāraḥ.
The (self-)control of the yogin extends from the smallest atom (of his body) to the largest magnitude (known in meditation).

1.41. kṣīṇa-vṛtter abhijātasya iva maṇer grahītṛ-grahaṇa-grāhyeṣu tat-stha-tad-añjanatā samāpattiḥ.
The person whose mental fluctuations have become attenuated achieves *samapatti,* yogic balance, with respect to things subjective, sensational, and objective, like a polished jewel that takes on the color of that on which it lies.[13]

1.42. tatra śabdârtha-jñāna-vikalpaiḥ saṃkīrṇā savitarkā samāpattiḥ.
The type of *samapatti,* yogic balance, called the higher rational, *savitarka samapatti,* has verbal and other cognitions blended in.

1.43. smṛti-pariśuddhau sva-rūpa-śūnyā iva artha-mātra-nirbhāsā nirvitarkā.
The type of *samapatti,* yogic balance, called beyond the rational, *nirvitarka samapatti,* occurs after the memory has been purified, (the *chitta*) shining in pure awareness of whatever object, devoid of self-consciousness, as it were.

1.44. etayā eva savicārā nirvicārā ca sūkṣma-viṣayā vyākhyātā.
This explains both types of mental balance no matter how subtle the content.

1.45. sūkṣma-viṣayatvaṃ ca ā-liṅga-paryavasānam.
Content can be subtler and subtler until it is the unmanifest (i.e., nature undifferentiated).

1.46. tā eva sabījaḥ samādhiḥ.
All these (stages and types of mental balance) are called *samadhi* with seed, *sabija.*

1.47. nirvicāra-vaiśāradye 'dhyātma-prasādaḥ.
After becoming expert in nondiscursive mental balance and *samadhi*, the spiritual opens its light.

1.48. ṛtam-bharā tatra prajñā.
"Truth-conscious," *ritam-bhara* (bearing the divine mind, in tune with the cosmic order), is the yogin's wisdom and awareness (*prajna*) there.[14]

1.49. śrutânumānābhyām anya-viṣayā viśeṣârthavattvāt.
Its object and scope is other than that of the wisdom of scripture and reasoning, since its purpose (or value, *artha*) is unique (or, since its objects are absolute particulars).

1.50. taj-jaḥ saṃskāro 'nya-saṃskāra-pratibandhī.
The mental disposition created by this state blocks the firings of other mental dispositions.

1.51. tasya api nirodhe sarva-nirodhān nirbījaḥ samādhiḥ.
When it too is checked, there is seedless *samadhi*, since all have been checked.[15]

sādhana-pāda

2.1 tapaḥ-svâdhyāyêśvara-praṇidhānāni kriyā yogaḥ.
(The second limb of *ashtanga yoga*—see below, 2.32—the *niyamas*, include what is called) Kriya yoga, which consists of asceticism (*tapas*), self-study (in the light of a yogic text), and opening to (or meditation on) the Lord.

2.2. samādhi-bhāvanârthaḥ kleśa-tanūkaraṇârthaś ca.
(It is practiced) to enliven *samadhi* as well as to attenuate afflictions (*klesha*).

2.3. avidyā-asmitā-rāga-dveṣâbhiniveśāḥ pañca kleśāḥ.
Spiritual ignorance, I-identification, liking, disliking, and the proclivity to remain in one's own form (or, clinging to life) are the five afflictions (*klesha*).

2.4. avidyā kṣetram uttareṣāṃ prasupta-tanu-vicchinnôdārāṇām.
Spiritual ignorance is the field for the others (to flourish) in degrees from dormancy and attenuatedness to suppression or expression outright.

2.5. anityâśuci-duḥkhânātmasu nitya-śuci-sukhâtma-khyātir avidyā.
To be spiritually ignorant is to mistake the noneternal, impure, painful, and nonself for the eternal, pure, delightful, and true self.[16]

2.6. dṛg-darśana-śaktyor ekâtmatā ivâ asmitā.
I-identification is the distinct powers of the seer (the conscious being, *purusha*) and the seeing (nature, *prakriti*) seeming one and the same.

2.7. sukhânuśayī rāgaḥ.
Liking follows pleasure.

2.8. duḥkhânuśayī dveṣaḥ.
Disliking follows pain.

2.9. sva-rasa-vāhī viduṣo 'pi tathā rūḍho 'bhiniveśaḥ.
Proclivity to remain in one's own form (clinging to life) is sustained by its own relishing, being self-perpetuating even for the learned.

2.10. te pratiprasava-heyāḥ sūkṣmāḥ.
Subtle (though they be in their disturbances), these afflictions can be banished by countermeasures.

2.11. dhyāna-heyās tad-vṛttayaḥ.
These detrimental fluctuations can be banished through meditation.

2.12. kleśa-mūlaḥ karmâśayo dṛṣṭâdṛṣṭa-vedanīyaḥ.
(Action-inducing) karmic latencies, which are to be experienced in the current or a future birth, are rooted in afflictions.

2.13. sati mūle tad-vipāko jāty-āyur-bhogāḥ.
So long as the root endures, its fruit will endure, the (triple) fruit, namely, of birth, life, and enjoyment.

2.14. te hlāda-paritāpa-phalāḥ puṇyâpuṇya-hetutvāt.
These three bring joy or suffering according to moral merit or lack thereof (in accumulated karmic latencies).[17]

2.15. pariṇāma-tāpa-saṃskāra-duḥkhair guṇa-vṛtti-virodhāc ca duḥkham eva sarvaṃ vivekinaḥ.
And because of conflicting fluctuations of qualities, there is suffering in change, in anxious, feverish states of mind, and in mental dispositions (*samskara*). Thus the person of discriminating judgment sees *all as suffering*.[18]

2.16. heyaṃ duḥkham anāgatam.
Future suffering is to be banished.

2.17. draṣṭṛ-dṛśyayor saṃyogo heya-hetuḥ.
That which is to be banished is caused by a conjunction of the seer (the conscious being) and that to be seen (nature).

2.18. prakāśa-kriyā-sthiti-śīlaṃ bhūtêndriyâtmakaṃ bhogâpavargârthaṃ dṛśyam.
What is to be seen (i.e., nature) is characterized by the (three qualities or strands) of intelligence, activity, and dullness or inertia (*sattva, rajas,* and *tamas*); it includes the gross elements and the sense organs, and has as its *raison d'être* enjoyment for, or liberation of, the conscious being.

2.19. viśeṣâviśeṣa-liṅga-mātrâliṅgāni guṇa-parvāṇi.
The (three) qualities (nature comprises) are expressed in distinct stages, that is to say, stages where predominate individuals, general forms, subtle forms, and the trans-subtle.

2.20. draṣṭā dṛśi-mātraḥ śuddho 'pi pratyayânupaśyaḥ.
The seer (the conscious being), although pure (i.e., although pure consciousness), appears to see through thoughts and ideas.

2.21. tad-artha eva dṛśyasya ātmā.
Only for the sake of the seer is the seen in its essence.[19]

2.22. kṛtârthaṃ prati naṣṭam apy anaṣṭaṃ tad anya sādhāraṇatvāt.
Although destroyed (for the liberated) yogin whose purpose is accomplished, nature is not destroyed for others (who are not liberated), because she is common to everyone.

2.23. sva-svāmi-śaktyoḥ sva-rūpôpalabdhi-hetuḥ saṃyogaḥ.
The conjunction (of the conscious being and nature) causes perception of the true nature of the powers of the owned (nature) and of the owner (the conscious being).[20]

2.24. tasya hetur avidyā.
Spiritual ignorance is its cause (i.e., the reason the conjunction endures).

2.25. tad-abhāvāt saṃyogâbhāvo hānaṃ tad-dṛśeḥ kaivalyam.
When spiritual ignorance is no longer, the conjunction is no longer. This is the relinquishment, the aloneness (*kaivalya,* i.e., the *summum bonum*) of the seer (the conscious being).

2.26. viveka-khyātir aviplavā hānôpāyaḥ.
Unbroken practice of discriminative discernment is the way to that relinquishment.

2.27. tasya saptadhā-prānta-bhūmiḥ prajñā.
For such a yogin, sevenfold wisdom and insight (*prajna*) are the boundary of his attainment.

2.28. yogâṅgânuṣṭhānād aśuddhi-kṣaye jñāna-dīptir ā-viveka-khyāteḥ.
By practice of the limbs of yoga (*ashtanga yoga*), impurity is attenuated. Cognition is illuminated up to discriminative discernment.

2.29. yama-niyamâsana-prāṇâyāma-pratyāhāra-dhāraṇā-dhyāna-samādhayo 'ṣṭāv aṅgāni.
Ethical restraints, personal constraints, asanas, breath control, withdrawal of the senses from their objects, (and three stages of meditation) *dharana* (concentration in movement), *dhyana* (meditation proper), and *samadhi* are the eight limbs of yoga.

2.30. ahiṃsā-satyâsteya-brahmacaryâparigrahā yamāḥ.
The restraints (*yama*) are nonharmfulness (noninjury, *ahimsa*), truthfulness, nonstealing, sexual restraint, and nonpossessiveness.

2.31. jāti-deśa-kāla-samayânavacchinnāḥ sārvabhaumā mahā-vratam.
These practiced universally, irrespective of station and circumstance of time and place, constitute the "great vow."

2.32. śauca-santoṣa-tapaḥ-svâdhyāyêśvara-praṇidhānāni niyamāḥ.
The personal constraints (*niyama*) are cleanliness, contentment, asceticism (*tapas*), self-study (in the light of a yogic text), and opening to the Lord (or, meditation on the Lord).

2.33. vitarka-bādhane pratipakṣa-bhāvanam.
In order to check disturbances one should enliven counterattitudes.[21]

2.34. vitarkā hiṃsâdayaḥ kṛta-kāritânumoditā lobha-krodha-moha-pūrvakā mṛdu-madhyâdhimātrā duḥkhâjñānânanta-phalā iti pratipakṣa-bhāvanam.
Disturbances are a feeling of injuriousness and so on, perhaps actually acted out, perhaps caused to be acted out, or perhaps simply approved of and acknowledged. Their symptoms or precursors are greed, anger, confusion, and they come in slight, middling, and extreme intensities. Their fruits are endless suffering and ignorance.—This thought itself is an enlivening of a counterattitude.

2.35. ahiṃsā-pratiṣṭhāyāṃ tat-sannidhau vaira-tyāgaḥ.
When nonharmfulness (*ahimsa*) is firmly established, then in the person's presence all animosity disappears.

2.36. satya-pratiṣṭhāyāṃ kriyā-phalâśrayatvam.
When truthfulness is firmly established, then what has been said becomes the basis for action and results (i.e., promised and foretold results come about).

2.37. asteya-pratiṣṭhāyāṃ sarva-ratnôpasthānam.
When refraining from stealing is firmly established, all jewels come near.[22]

2.38. brahmacarya-pratiṣṭhāyāṃ vīrya-lābhaḥ.
When sexual restraint is firmly established, (great) energy and vitality are gained.

2.39. aparigraha-sthairye janma-kathantā-sambodhaḥ.
Upon achieving steadiness in nonpossessiveness, the yogin or yogini comes to know the how and the why—the meaning—of his or her birth.[23]

2.40. śaucāt svâṅga-jugupsā parair asaṃsargaḥ.
From cleanliness comes aversion (or indifference) to one's own body and noncontact with others.

2.41 sattva-śuddhi-saumanasya-ekāgryêndriya-jayâtma-darśana-yogyatvāni ca.
(Other results are:) The yogin or yogini becomes fit for, and capable of, sattvafication (sattvic transformation), (unshakeable) cheerfulness, concentration (one-pointedness of mind), and sight of the self.

2.42. saṃtoṣād anuttamaḥ suḥkha-lābhaḥ.
From (firm establishment of) contentment, unparalleled pleasure is gained.

2.43. kāyêndriya-siddhir aśuddhi-kṣayāt tapasaḥ.
Powers (*siddhi*s) of the organs of action result from asceticism (*tapas*), which destroys imperfections.

2.44. svâdhyāyād iṣṭa-devatā-saṃprayogaḥ.
From self-study (in the light of a yogic text, *svadhyaya*) comes contact with one's preferred divinity, *ishta-devata*.

2.45. samādhi-siddhir īśvara-praṇidhānāt.
The *siddhi* of *samadhi* comes from opening to (or meditation on) the Lord.[24]

2.46. sthira-sukham āsanam.
Postures (*asana*) should be firm but easy (comfortable).[25]

2.47. prayatna-śaithilyânanta-samāpattibhyām.
(Postures become perfect) in relaxation of effort or by the mental balance, *samapatti,* called the infinite (or, the serpent Ananta, Without End).[26]

2.48. tato dvandvânabhighātaḥ.
From that (mastery of asanas), a person becomes impervious to dualities (of hot and cold, hunger and satiety, happiness and sorrow, etc.).

2.49. tasmin sati śvāsa-praśvāsayo gati-vicchedaḥ prāṇâyāmaḥ.
An asana practice in place, "breath control," *pranayama,* involves checking (holding voluntarily) the in-breath and the out-breath (for regular intervals).

2.50. bāhyâbhyantara-stambha-vṛttir deśa-kāla-saṃkhyābhiḥ paridṛṣṭo dīrgha-sūkṣmaḥ.
Three types of *pranayama* practice are the outer (e.g., using one's fingers to close and open nostrils and counting), the inner (e.g., without use of props), and the suppressed (an advanced practice). Modulated by location (within the body, from the abdominal muscles to the nose), time (i.e., duration of each of the three factors), and number (i.e., proportional time being spent on each breath as well as number of repetitions), the breath is to be both protracted (i.e., deepened, slowed) and made subtle (practically soundless).

2.51. bāhyâbhyantara-viṣayâkṣepī caturthaḥ.
A fourth type transcends both the external and internal focuses.

2.52. tataḥ kṣīyate prakāśâvaraṇam.
From that (mastery of *pranayama*), the lid covering the light (above the head) is diminished.[27]

2.53. dhāraṇāsu ca yogyatā manasaḥ.
And (then) the mind (*manas,* the internal organ of sense) becomes ready for *dharana,* concentration (in movement) (limb number six).

2.54. sva-viṣayâsaṃprayoge cittasya sva-rūpânukāra iva indriyāṇāṃ pratyā-hāraḥ.
(Limb number five) "pulling back," *pratyahara,* is the disconnection of the sense organs from their objects as if in imitation of the talent of the *chitta,* "feeling and thought" (to be still).

2.55. tataḥ paramā vaśyatā indriyāṇām.
From that comes utter control of the sense organs.

vibhūti-pāda

3.1. deśa-bandhaś cittasya dhāraṇā.
Concentration (in movement, *dharana*) is binding the *chitta* down to the spot (of movement).

3.2. tatra pratyaya-eka-tānatā dhyānam.
Of the three (stages of meditation), meditation (*dhyana*) is a single ideational focus.

3.3. tad eva artha-mātra-nirbhāsaṃ sva-rūpa-śūnyam iva samādhiḥ.
Samadhi is illumination of an object as object only, bereft, as it were, of its being anything other than an object of consciousness.[28]

3.4. trayam ekatra saṃyamaḥ.
The three together are called conscious identification (*samyama*).

3.5. taj-jayāt prajñā-ālokaḥ.
Through its mastery comes the light of wisdom and insight (*prajna*).

3.6. tasya bhūmiṣu viniyogaḥ.
It is to be applied to different spheres (subtle objects as well as gross ones).[29]

3.7. trayam antar-aṅgam pūrvebhyaḥ.
The three together are internal to the first five limbs.[30]

3.8. tad api bahir-aṅgam nirbījasya.
But, just as with the first five, these three are external to seedless *samadhi*.

3.9. vyutthāna-nirodha-saṃskārayor abhibhava-prādurbhāvau nirodha-kṣaṇa-cittânvayo nirodha-pariṇāmaḥ.
The restriction transformation correlates with *chitta* in a moment of conquest of stimulating mental dispositions (*samskara*) and the arising of mental dispositions of restriction.

3.10. tasya praśānta-vāhitā saṃskārāt.
That transformation is borne along tranquilly because of mental dispositions (restriction) (becoming dominant).

3.11. sarvârthatā-ekâgratayor kṣaya-udayau cittasya samādhi-pariṇāmaḥ.
The transformation of *chitta* called the *samadhi* transformation occurs when distraction has become attenuated and one-pointedness (*ekagrata*) has become natural for the *chitta* (the natural state of the mind).

3.12. tataḥ punaḥ śāntôditau tulya-pratyayau cittasya ekâgratā-pariṇāmaḥ.
After that, there is the transformation of *chitta* called the one-pointedness transformation. It occurs when the ideative contents disappearing and appearing are identical.[31]

3.13. etena bhūtêndriyeṣu dharma-lakṣaṇâvasthā-pariṇāmā vyākhyātāḥ.
By what has already been said, three further transformations are explained with respect to both the material elements and the sense organs: the *chitta*'s becoming transformed in its properties, the *dharma* transformation, its becoming transformed in its (temporal) character, the *lakshana* transformation, and its becoming transformed in its state or condition, the *avastha* transformation.

3.14. śāntôditâvyapadeśya-dharmânupātī dharmī.
The property bearer (i.e., the *chitta* as a substance) takes shape according to its properties: quiescent, active, and unmanifest.

3.15. kramânyatvaṃ pariṇāmânyatve hetuḥ.
Which transformation occurs is determined by differences in interval and sequence.[32]

3.16. pariṇāma-traya-saṃyamād atītânāgata-jñānam.
From *samyama* (conscious identification) with respect to the triad of transformations comes knowledge of the past and future.

3.17. śabdârtha-pratyayānām itaretarâdhyāsāt saṃkaras tat-pravibhāga-saṃyamāt sarva-bhūta-ruta-jñānam.
Because of wrong projections among objects, meanings, and ideas, there is (psychological) confusion. From *samyama* on their division comes knowledge of all creatures' cries (the language of beasts).[33]

3.18. saṃskāra-sākṣāt-karaṇāt pūrva-jāti-jñānam.
Through direct acquaintance with mental dispositions (*samskara*) comes knowledge of previous births.

3.19. pratyasya para-citta-jñānam.
From *samyama* on ideas (or ideative currents) comes knowledge of other minds (the *chitta* of others).

3.20. na ca tat sālambanaṃ tasya aviṣayībhūtatvāt.
That does not include the substratum or representational nature of the other's *chitta* (e.g., the language employed), since that is outside the range of *samyama*.

3.21. kāya-rūpa-saṃyamāt tad-grāhya-śakti-stambhe cakṣuḥ-prakāśâsaṃprayoge antar-dhānam.
By performing conscious identification (*samyama*) on the body's visible form, another's power to grasp it is suspended, there being a break between the light (necessary for perception) and the operation of the other's visual organ: (hence comes the *siddhi* of) invisibility.[34]

3.22. sopakramaṃ nirupakramaṃ ca karma tat-saṃyamād aparânta-jñānam ariṣṭebhyo vā.
Karma ranges from active to dormant. From *samyama* on it comes knowledge of (time of) death. Or, time of death may be known from unfavorable symptoms or signs.

3.23. maitry-âdiṣu balāni.
From *samyama* on friendliness and so on come powers (of friendliness and so on).

3.24. baleṣu hasti-balâdīni.
From *samyama* on powers come such powers as the strength of an elephant.

3.25. pravṛtty-āloka-nyāsāt sūkṣma-vyavahita-viprakṛṣṭa-jñānam.
From casting the higher light on any effort, the object of the effort is known, whether subtle, hidden, or distant.

3.26. bhuvana-jñānaṃ sūrye saṃyamāt.
Knowledge of the cosmic becoming comes from *samyama* on the sun.[35]

3.27. candre tārā-vyūha-jñānam.
From *samyama* on the moon (or lunar sphere) comes knowledge of (i.e., cognitive opening to) the multitudes of stars.[36]

3.28. dhruve tad-gati-jñānam.
From *samyama* on the pole star comes knowledge of their movement.

3.29. nābhi-cakre kāya-vyūha-jñānam.
From *samyama* on the navel *chakra* comes knowledge of the members of the body.

3.30. kaṇṭha-kūpe kṣut-pipāsā-nivṛttiḥ.
From *samyama* on the well in the throat come cessation of hunger and thirst.

3.31. kūrma-nāḍyāṃ sthairyam.
With it on the tortoise duct (*kurma-nadi* at the throat) comes steadiness.[37]

3.32. mūrdha-jyotiṣi siddha-darśanam.
With it on the light at the crown of the head comes vision of the perfected ones (*siddha*s).

3.33. pratibhād vā sarvam.[38]
Or, from luminous *samyama,* anything.

3.34. hṛdaye citta-saṃvit.
With it on the heart, awareness of the *chitta*.

3.35. sattva-puruṣayor atyantâsaṃkīrṇayoḥ pratyayâviśeṣo bhogaḥ parârthatvāt svârtha-saṃyamāt puruṣa-jñānam.
Enjoyment (everyday experience, *bhoga*) is constituted by no (awareness of) distinct ideative streams of *sattva* and the conscious being (*purusha*), which are (in reality) absolutely unmixed. Since *sattva* exists to serve the other (*purusha*), knowledge of the conscious being (the *purusha*) comes from *samyama* on that which is for its own sake (or, not for anything else).

3.36. tataḥ prātibha-śrāvaṇa-vedanā-darśâsvāda-vārtā jāyante.
From that come luminous (or supranormal) hearing, touch, sight, taste, and smelling.[39]

3.37. te samādhāv upasargā vyutthāne siddhayaḥ.
These powers or *siddhi*s (wonders or miracles), according to the ordinary human consciousness, are obstacles to *samadhi*.

3.38. bandha-kāraṇa-śaithilyāt pracāra-saṃvedanāc ca cittasya para-śarīrâveśaḥ.
From loosening the connecting causes along with awareness of the (subtle) passageways (of *chitta*), the *chitta* can enter another body.[40]

3.39. udāna-jayāj jala-paṅka-kaṇṭhakâdiṣv asaṇga utkrāntiś ca.
From mastery of the *udana* (a form of *prana* or psychic energy, up-breath) comes lack of (injurious) contact with water, mud, thorns, etc., as well as levitation.

3.40. samāna-jayāj jvalanam.
From mastery of the *samana* (abdominal or equalizing breath) comes kindling (of a psychic aura).[41]

3.41. śrotrâkāśayoḥ saṃbandha-saṃyamād divyaṃ śrotram.
From *samyama* on the connection of the organ of hearing and the ether comes divine audition.[42]

3.42. kāyâkāśayoḥ saṃbandha-saṃyamāl laghu-tūla-samāpatteś ca ākāśâgamanam.
From *samyama* on the connection of the body and the ether, and from the yogic balance (*samapatti*) called light cotton as well, there is traveling in the ether.

3.43. bahir akalpitā vṛttir mahā-videhā tataḥ prakāśâvaraṇa-kṣayaḥ.
Outside (the range of the body), a fluctuation, which is not imagined, is the "Great Bodiless" (state of mind) whereby the covering blocking the light (above the head) is diminished.

3.44. sthūla-sva-rūpa-sūkṣmânvayârthavattva-saṃyamād bhūta-jayaḥ.
From *samyama* on the gross, essential, subtle, connecting, and purposive comes mastery of the elements.

3.45. tato aṇimâdi-prādurbhāvaḥ kāya-sampat tad-dharmânabhighātaś ca.
From that, there is manifest the *siddhi*s of minuteness (or, atomization) and so on (the eight *siddhi*s of special bodily powers) as well as perfection of the body and nonobstruction of its functions.[43]

3.46. rūpa-lāvaṇya-bala-vajra-saṃhananatvāni kāya-sampat.
Perfection of the body means beauty, grace, strength, and adamantine hardness.

3.47. grahaṇa-sva-rūpâsmitânvayârthavattva-saṃyamād indriya-jayaḥ.
From *samyama* on the essence of grasping, egoity, connectedness, and purposefulness comes mastery of the sense organs.

3.48. tato mano-javitvaṃ vikaraṇa-bhāvaḥ pradhāna-jayaś ca.
Thence come speed like that of the internal organ (*manas*), freedom from the cognitive instruments, and mastery of the root form of nature (*pradhana*).[44]

3.49. sattva-puruṣânyatā-khyāti-mātrasya sarva-bhāvâdhiṣṭhātṛtvaṃ sarva-jñātṛtvaṃ ca.
The yogin whose awareness is restricted to perception of the difference between (the strand of nature called) intelligence (*sattva*) and the conscious being achieves mastery over all states of (inner) being and knowledge of it all as well.

3.50. tad-vairāgyād api doṣa-bīja-kṣaye kaivalyam.
Through disinterest in that achievement arises aloneness (*kaivalya*) in the attenuation of the seeds of defects.

3.51. sthāny-upanımantraṇe saṅga-smayâkaraṇaṃ punar aniṣṭa-prasaṅgāt.
On being called by divinities, a yogin should not let the attention give rise to pride or attachment, since that could lead again to unwanted consequences.

3.52. kṣaṇa-tat-kramayoḥ saṃyamād viveka-jaṃ jñānam.
From *samyama* on moments (the units of time) and their succession (in the flow of fluctuations of *chitta*) comes cognition born of discrimination (of the conscious being from nature), *viveka*.

3.53. jāti-lakṣaṇa-deśair anyatâvacchedāt tulyayos tataḥ pratipattiḥ.
From that comes understanding by differentiation of each though identical with another with respect to type, characteristics, and place.[45]

3.54. tārakaṃ sarva-viṣayaṃ sarvathā-viṣayam akramaṃ ca iti viveka-jaṃ jñānam.
The cognition born of discrimination (*viveka*) carries to the farther shore with everything as its object in every fashion and nonsequentially.

3.55. sattva-puruṣayoḥ śuddhi-sāmye kaivalyam iti.
When the intelligence (strand, i.e., *sattva*) and the conscious being are equal in purity, aloneness (*kaivalya*) ensues.

4.1. janma-auśadhi-mantra-tapaḥ-samādhi-jāḥ siddhayaḥ.
Powers, *siddhis*, come by birth, from herbs, mantras, asceticism, and *samadhi.*[46]

4.2. jāty-antara-pariṇāmaḥ prakṛty-āpūrāt.
Transformation into a different type of being (or, into another birth) comes about from a superabundance of natural potentiality.

4.3. nimittam aprayojakaṃ prakṛtīṇāṃ varaṇa-bhedas tu tataḥ kṣetrika-vat.
Practicing yoga does not impel transformations of nature. Rather, like a farmer (irrigating, weeding, etc., to let plants grow), yoga practices break up coverings or obstacles (so that one's true nature can become manifest).

4.4. nirmāṇa-cittāny asmitā-mātrāt.
Thought and emotion (*chitta*) are shaped solely from egoity.

4.5. pravṛtti-bhede prayojakaṃ cittam ekam anekeṣām.
For all the great diversity of effort and action, there is *chitta* that directs it. That is a single (type of) thing belonging to many (people).[47]

4.6. tatra dhyāna-jam anāśayam.
Among these (individuated *chitta*s belonging to different people), that born of meditation is without stores of ripening karma.

4.7. karmâśuklâkṛṣṇaṃ yoginas tri-vidham itareṣām.
Karma is neither good nor bad that belongs to the yogin. For others, it is of three types (good, bad, or a mix).[48]

4.8. tatas tad-vipākânuguṇānām eva abhivyaktir vāsanānām.
Mental dispositions (across births), *vasana,* manifest just according to the ripening (in good or bad deeds as well as in moral payback) that results from the (moral) types of karma.[49]

4.9. jāti-deśa-kāla-vyavahitānām apy ānantaryaṃ smṛti-saṃskārayor eka-rūpatvāt.
Since remembering conforms to mental dispositions, *samskaras*, causal sequences of *samskaras* occur despite divisions of type (or birth), place, and time.

4.10. tāsām anāditvaṃ ca āśiṣo nityatvāt.
And these *vasana* have no beginning, since desiring is permanent.[50]

4.11. hetu-phalâśrayâlambanaiḥ saṃgṛhītatvād eṣām abhāve tad-abhāvaḥ.
Since desiring and *vasana* are connected as cause and effect, as mutual support and dependence, in the absence of the one there is the absence of the other.[51]

4.12. atītânāgataṃ sva-rūpato 'sty adhva-bhedād dharmāṇām.
In essence, the past and the future exist. Particular events and properties (are objects of consciousness and real) according to the different modalities or pathways (of past, present, and future).[52]

4.13. te vyakta-sūkṣmā guṇâtmanaḥ.
Particulars are manifest or subtle. They are of the nature (of combinations) of the strands (the three *gunas*).[53]

4.14. pariṇāma-ekatvād vastu-tattvam.
The truth or particularity of a thing is due to a unique transformation (of nature, a unique combination of *gunas*).

4.15. vastu-sāmye citta-bhedāt tayor vibhaktaḥ panthāḥ.
Since with regard to one and the same thing, *chitta* differs (on different occasions of perception, or from the perspectives of two different perceivers), the two (*chitta* and objects) have a distinct mode of being.[54]

4.16. na ca eka-citta-tantraṃ vastu tad apramāṇakaṃ tadā kiṃ syāt.
And (to exist) a thing does not depend on a single mind or awareness (*chitta*). Were it not cognized by that mind, what then would it be?[55]

4.17. tad-uparāgâpekṣitvāc cittasya vastu jñātâjñātam.
Something remains known or unknown to a particular mind, according to its conditioning or expectations.[56]

4.18. sadā jñātāś citta-vṛttayas tat-prabhoḥ puruṣasya apariṇāmitvāt.
The fluctuations of mind are always known to their lord, the conscious being, the *purusha,* inasmuch as the *purusha* is unchanging.[57]

4.19. na tat svâbhāsaṃ dṛśyatvāt.
That (the *chitta*) is not self-luminous, because it is something to be perceived.[58]

4.20. eka-samaye ca ubhayânavadhāraṇam.
And there is no possibility of (*chitta*) cognizing both (objects and itself) at the same time.[59]

4.21. cittântara-dṛśye buddhi-buddher atiprasaṅgaḥ smṛti-saṃkaraś ca.
It would be absurd to assume that different *chitta* is required to grasp *chitta,* because of an impossible regress of one cognition after another being required

(in order that any be known). This would also mean memory's (impossibility because of) confusion.[60]

4.22. citer apratisaṃkramāyās tad-ākārâpattau sva-buddhi-saṃvedanam.
Self-awareness—consciousness of self and of cognition—occurs when the *chitta* (*citi* = *chitta*), (now) unfluctuating, assumes the form of that (the conscious being).[61]

4.23. draṣṭṛ-dṛśya-uparakte cittaṃ sarvârtham.
Chitta that is conditioned by both awareness of the seer and that to be seen is capable of cognizing anything.

4.24. tad-asaṃkhyeya-vāsanābhiś citram api parârthaṃ saṃhatya-kāritvāt.
Although the *chitta* is moved by countless deep mental dispositions (*vasana*), it works by unifying (diversities) for the sake of the other (the conscious being).[62]

4.25. viśeṣa-darśina ātma-bhāva-bhāvanā-vinivṛttiḥ.
For one who sees the distinction (between nature and the conscious being), the projection of sense of self in nature ceases.[63]

4.26. tadā viveka-nimnaṃ kaivalya-prāgbhāraṃ cittam.
Then the *chitta*, settling into deep discrimination, is carried on toward (reflecting) the aloneness, *kaivalya* (of the conscious being).[64]

4.27. tac-chidreṣu pratyayântarāṇi saṃskārebhyaḥ.
In the gaps (or weaknesses) of discrimination, other ideational presentations (i.e., distractions) may arise by force of (unexhausted) mental dispositions (*samskara*).

4.28. hānam eṣāṃ kleśa-vad uktam.
These are to be banished, like the afflictions, in the ways explained.

4.29. prasaṃkhyāne 'py akusīdasya sarvathā viveka-khyāter dharma-meghaḥ samādhiḥ.
The *samadhi* called Cloud of Dharma occurs for a person who has no interest even in elevated awareness, whose awareness is in every way directed to discrimination (of the conscious being from nature).[65]

4.30. tataḥ kleśa-karma-nivṛttiḥ.
Thence afflictions and karma cease.

4.31. tadā sarvâvaraṇa-malâpetasya cittasya anantyāj jñeyam alpam.
Then, since awareness is unlimited when parted from coverings and impurities, what remains to be known is trivial.[66]

4.32. tataḥ kṛtârthānāṃ pariṇāma-krama-parisamāptir guṇānām.
Thence the completion of processes of transformation on the part of the strands (*guna*s), their purpose fulfilled.[67]

4.33. kṣaṇa-pratiyogī pariṇāmâparânta-nirgrāhyaḥ kramaḥ.
Process, which is relative to the units of time, is apprehensible at the end of a transformation.[68]

4.34. puruṣârtha-śūnyānāṃ guṇānāṃ pratiprasavaḥ kaivalyam sva-rūpa-pratiṣṭhā vā citi-śaktir iti.
Aloneness (*kaivalya,* the *summum bonum*) entails the reversal of the course of the strands of nature (*guna*s), now empty of meaning and value for the conscious being. Or, it may be understood as the power of consciousness returned and established in its own true self.[69]

Here ends the *Yoga Sutra* of Patanjali.

om shantih shantih shantih.

APPENDIX D

Selections from (Tantric) Kashmiri Shaivite Texts

The history and core themes of tantra are introduced in the third section of chapter 1. Let me again emphasize its richness and complexity. A chronology for tantric literature has been determined by scholars only roughly.[1]

There is Hindu, Buddhist, and Jaina tantra, and complex interactions and dependences among authors with a tantric perspective. In practically all yoga traditions, there is what I call the tantric turn. Although today there are sects of Vaishnavism and Shaivism that perform *puja*s (rites of worship), etc., grounded in old scriptures called Tantras and Agamas, the texts mention many rituals and alchemical practices that researchers have looked for but not found.[2] There is little that is distinctively tantric, as perhaps is fitting given its spirit of inclusivism. Tantric scriptures do not reject the authority of the Upanishads or the *Gita* or even the *Yoga Sutra,* for that matter (although Abhinava Gupta, for one, is very critical of the *Yoga Sutra*). The distinctively tantric line is that these teachings are incomplete or too difficult or in another way inappropriate for our day, the Dark Age, the Kali Yuga—or, in modern tantric teachings, inappropriate for our complex and noisy homes and workplaces—at least compared to tantric teachings and practices that are appropriate for our times.

Here our focus must be mainly arbitrary. We shall sample the work of the great yoga master and Kula philosopher, Abhinava Gupta, who lived in Kashmir in the tenth and eleventh centuries. With Abhinava in particular, aesthetics, spiritual metaphysics/theology, ethics within yoga teachings, and professional exegesis and epistemology all reach high points not only within tantra as a movement but also within classical literature as a whole. The tantric development that has probably the profoundest overall cultural impact, the occult psychology, is not much addressed by him, though it is present in many of the sacred texts he recognizes. A yogic or "subtle" or occult body comprised of "canals," *nadi*s for *prana* and *shakti,* along with *chakra*s, "wheels" or centers of occult consciousness and energy exchanges, became systematized in tantra, though hardly at a stroke. I shall discuss the tantric psychology in the next section, in connection with the *Hatha Yoga Pradipika* (c. 1400, which, by the way, quotes Abhinava). This ordering of topics is mainly for convenience; one should not think that earlier tantric literature—pre-Abhinava—contains no expressions of the distinctively tantric psychological or physiological system. In this appendix, I shall try to take more of a philosophic overview, with a tilt toward the Kaulism of Abhinava.

According to scholar Alexis Sanderson, in tantra's early history in Kashmir rituals were reformed and "aestheticized" in Kaulism.[3] This judgment is broadly in accord with that of the scholar of classical aesthetics Edwin Gerow, who finds the Vedantic philosophy of Brahman to be "aestheticized" in the case of Abhinava.[4] This, the premier Kaula philosopher, brought together at least three prominent streams of tantric practice and ritual, the early Kaula (the "Familial," from *kula,* "family") with two other Shaivite groups, the Trika (the "Triadic") and the Krama (the "Sequential").[5] These "streams" are not really sects but rather traditions of practice and teaching. Abhinava also synthesized these views with two further textual and philosophic lines (in texts not associated with particular rituals and pratices), the Spanda, the "Vibration" view (the world is a tremor in the divine consciousness) and the Pratyabhijna, "Recognitive" view (liberation is like recognizing something from your past, the self, *atman,* that you have forgotten).

Abhinava wrote prolifically in aesthetics and metaphysics, but not so prolifically about yogic practices. Perhaps, as some have surmised, he considered certain Tantras to be sufficiently clear in that regard.[6] Still, he was influential as a guru as well as a writer. He is a prime source for the yoga of art and beauty discussed in chapter 5, although he hardly makes what we said explicit. The little he says explicitly about practices centers not on *rasa* but on four ways, *upaya,* to experience the unitive consciousness.[7] But my claim in chapter 5 was not that Abhinava lays out a *rasa* yoga but rather that one is implicit in much of what he says—as well as in the practices of countless artists offering their performances to the divine, in the spirit of karma yoga.[8]

Moreover, we cannot do justice to all the many dimensions of Abhinava's contributions—more than twenty-six major compositions, including a commentary on the *Gita* that is terrifically subtle along with philosophic works such as the *Tantraloka,* "Light on Tantra," that are terrifically long.[9] We shall try to flush out the convergence of aesthetics and yoga (or Yoga) in Kaulism and Abhinava.

First let us look at verses from the *Kularnava Tantra,* the tantra of "The Surge of the Kula, the Family, the All," the title of which is more commonly rendered "Ocean of the Kula." This text allows an overview before turning to Abhinava's work. This popular Agama may have been contemporaneous with Abhinava or more probably appeared a century or so later (c. 1100). He does not mention it among the scriptural sources of his philosophy (more than twenty Agamas, according to the count of K.C. Pandey).[10]

Like many other Agamas, the *Kularnava Tantra* (*KT*) is structured as a dialogue between Shiva and the Goddess, with the Great God teaching the Devi principles and methods of yoga, and enjoining her to teach them herself to help human beings of good will and resolve. The *KT* has been said to be "without doubt the most important of its class,"[11] that is, of the later Agamas that are in this way dialogically structured. It is often quoted in still later literature, the experts tells us, and its style and language are clear and crisp but also light and cheerful, with many simple symbols and analogies. Some of it has been translated, and almost the entire text nicely summarized by M. P. Pandit.[12] Of the text's seventeen chapters, I present below verses from the first two. In the notes, some interpretive problems are addressed and further background given.

From the *Kularnava Tantra*

1.1. Seated on the peak of Mount Kailasa, the God of Gods, the World Guru, the Supreme Lord, whose bliss is transcendent, was approached and questioned by Parvati (the Goddess).

Shri Devi said:

1.2. O Blessed, O God of Gods, O Lord, who have ordained the five ritual acts, all-knowing, you whom it is easy to love, you who love as loves a mother all who in you take refuge!

1.3. O Lord of the Family (*kula*), Supreme Ruler, O Ocean of the nectar of compassion, in what is not your essence, in wild transmigratory existence, there are those fouled by every kind of pain and suffering.

1.4. In various types of embodiment, endless living hosts are born and die. For them, there is no freedom (no *moksha,* no "spiritual liberation").

1.5. They are afflicted by pains and sufferings continually; there is never anywhere a truly happy person. O Deva, tell me by what means, Lord of Lords, by what method (*upāya*) can a person be free?

Shri Ishvara (the "Blessed Lord," Shiva) said:

1.6. Listen, Goddess (Devi), I will tell you, I will answer the question you ask. Merely from hearing what I have to say, a person can be liberated from *samsara,* from transmigration.

1.7. There is, Devi, the Auspicious (*shiva,* "kind," "agreeable"), the status of the Highest that is Whole, Integral, whose own form is the Supreme Brahman (the Absolute)—all-knowing, all-doing, Lord of all, pure, without a second.

1.8. Self-luminous, without beginning or end, without flaw, changeless, beyond the beyond, transcendent of the *guna*s, (in itself) being, consciousness, bliss. Every living thing is a part of That.

1.9. Living things are characterized by beginningless (spiritual) ignorance, like sparks (thrown away) from a fire (forgetful of the whole, their origin). They are differentiated by circumstances of birth determined by karma, talents, and so on.

1.10. Controlled by their own good and bad deeds that result in pleasures and pains, they obtain a body connected to this and that kind or species, a life span, and enjoyment born of karma.

1.11. Every rebirth they get this, coming to be humans of dull consciousness. Beloved, the subtle body is imperishable up to liberation.

1.12. Plants, worms and lotuses, birds, wild beasts, humans of thirteen different characteristics, and then, in order, like that, there are those who are seeking liberation.

1.13. Having held and held—restraining a thousand times—the bodies of four types (physical, breath, lower-mind, and higher-mind), from good action having become a human being, liberation would be got if one has Knowledge (of the Whole).

1.14. Among the eighty-four-hundred-thousand bodies that are possible for the embodied, Knowledge of reality is not had by any without a human birth.

1.15. O Parvati, here among thousands of (types of) births taken by even more thousands, occasionally a creature attains the human level from accumulation of merit (by action).

1.16. Having attained the difficult to obtain, the human status, step by step, one who does not carry himself across (to the further shore of liberation), well, who is worse than he?

1.17. Therefore, having obtained the best birth as well as excellence of talents and faculties, if you do not know what is good for yourself, you are going to harm yourself. (By listening to what is being revealed, you can learn what is good for yourself.)

1.110. Some want the Advaita (Nondual view), and others prefer the Dvaita (Dual view). Neither group knows my truth, which goes beyond both.

1.111. There are two paths, to bondage and to liberation. One is the path of "It's mine," and one is the path of not-"It's mine," the nonpossessive. By the path of "It's mine" a creature is bound. It is not the case that one becomes liberated by the path of "It's mine."

1.112. That karma which is not for bondage is the Knowledge that liberates. Karma, action, that is other than that leads to exhaustion. Knowledge that is other than that is nothing but skillful craftsmanship.

1.113. So long as desire and the like burn, so long as there are (untoward) mental dispositions, vectors of transmigration, so long as the faculties are unsteady, what is the point of telling the truth of things?

1.114. So long as you have to try very hard, so long as the effort is intense, forced, or impulsive, so long as you are thinking about what you are going to do, thinking about your resolve, so long as your mind is not steady, what is the point of a telling of the truth?

1.115. So long as there is identification with the body, so long as there is myness, so long as there is not the compassion of the guru, why then a telling of the truth?

1.116. So long as the truth has not been found, people do *tapas,* make pilgrimages, chant, sing praises, and so on, and the stories of the Vedas, the Shastras, and the Agamas are necessary.

1.117. Therefore, with every effort, in every state of consciousness, at all times, be one, Devi, who takes her stand in the truth, if you would desire self-realization, the liberation of the self.

The blessed Devi said:

2.1. O Lord of the Family (Kula), you who for every living being are the ocean of compassion, yes, indeed, I do desire to hear. The Dharma of the Kula, the Way of the Family that you have indicated has not by you been made clear.

2.2. Speak to me the Mahatmya (the "Importance," a succinct statement of the essence) of this Dharma that you say is the supreme way. Speak to me the Mahatmya, as conceived by you, of (the text named) the "Upper Road of the High Tradition."[13] If you care about me, Supreme Ruler, tell me about this.

 The blessed Lord said:

2.3. Listen, Devi, I will explain what you of me implore. By merely hearing this, one will become dear to the yoginis.[14]

2.4. I didn't tell this to Brahma, Vishnu, or Guha, the royal seer. I say it to you because I love you. You are a person whose mind is one-pointed, exclusively intent on listening.

2.5. What I am about to say has come down in a sequence (of teachers), a lineage, firmly established (originating) in (one of) my "five mouths."[15] In its deepest sense it is unsayable. Even so, I am going to tell you.

2.6. By you too this must be kept protected. It is not to be given to just anyone. It is to be given to a practitioner of *bhakti* yoga or a devoted student. Otherwise, a falling away will occur. (You will lose the secret, if you tell it to just anyone.)

2.7. The Vedas are superior to all other teachings (about ordinary life), better than the Vedas is the Vaishnava teaching, the Shaivite is better than the Vaishnaiva, and better than the Shaivite is the Right-handed tantric.

2.8. The Left-handed is superior to the Right-handed, the Siddhanta better than the Left-handed. The Kaula is better than the Siddhanta. Nothing is better than the Kaula.[16]

2.9. O Goddess, this is more secret than secret. This is the essence of the essence. This is better than the best. O Goddess, it is the Kula (the Family), the word of Shiva, come down directly from ear to ear, hearer to hearer.[17]

2.10. The Kula Dharma has been extracted by me stirring with the staff of Knowledge the ocean of the Vedas and Agamas, stirred by me who knows their essence, Devi.

2.11. The Dharmas (the teachings, paths), sacrifices, pilgrimages, vows and the like (undertaken in spiritual endeavors) in all their diverse portions are unified (in the end sought). (Similarly) because of its unity, the Kaula Dharma, among these, is the best, O dear one.

2.12. For, as rivers (all) enter the ocean whether they go straight or wind, just like that all observances enter the Kula.

2.13. As you can put the footprint of any living creature into the footprint of an elephant, so, dear one, all the (spiritual) philosophies (*darshana*) fit into the Kula.

2.14. And insofar as copper is similar to gold, in that way another observance is similar to the Kula Dharma.

2.15. As of all rivers there is no equal to the Ganga, just so there are no observances equal to the Kula Dharma.

2.23. If a yogin, then not at all could one enjoy the world. If enjoying the world, then not at all could one be skilled in yoga. The Kaula is of the nature of enjoyment and yoga. Therefore, dear one, it is universal.[18]

2.24. If one follows the Dharma of the Kula, O Queen of the Family, enjoyment becomes yoga immediately, misbehavior art (the good deed), and transmigratory existence (all of life) liberation.[19]

2.33. Knowledge of the Kula (the Family, the Whole, the All) shines forth for a person whose thought and emotion (*chitta*) have been purified, for the one of spiritual peace who serves the guru in action, for the zealous devotee, for the one who lives in secret.

2.34. The person whose love and devotion (*bhakti*) stays firm, for the blessed guru, for the Kula teachings, for Kaulas, for the Kula's supports, that person is one for whom Knowledge of the Kula comes to shine.

2.35. Through faith, culture, joy, and the like, right behavior and vows that are firm, by righteous acts protecting the guru's instructions, Knowledge of the Kula is obtained.

2.36. For the unfit, for one yet unready for deep Knowledge of the Kula, it (*bhakti*) won't stand long at all (even if he or she seems to grasp what I am saying). Therefore, consider carefully what's to be said, the Knowledge of the Kula by me presented (in words).

2.52. The Way, the Dharma, of the Kula, dear one, if harmed harms (the offender), if protected protects. If honored, it will make honored in an instant. Therefore, don't reject it.

2.61. Mere trees live. Deer and birds live. The person whose mind is based in the Kula Dharma, well, that person (really) lives (in the fullest sense of the word).

2.62. Days come and go for one unmindful of the Kula Dharma. Like the bellows of an ironsmith, though breathing he doesn't (really) live.

2.70. People who are wealthy and fortunate, whose karma is meritorious, good people, as well as yogins and yoginis, well, Devi, the Knowledge of the Kula (the Whole) can shine forth for them too, by (your) grace.

2.71. People who are the best of the human lot, venerable, generous, content in their accomplishments, in the hearts and minds of such people I make Knowledge of the Kula appear.

2.72. All (contemplative) visiting of places of light, all plunging into mysteries at holy crossings (*tirtha*) brings one into the Kula Dharma as well as any sacrificial performance or ritual.

2.77. For a person who knows the Kula (the "All") knows everything (worth knowing), even if he has left the Vedas and the Shastras behind. A person may know the Vedas, the Shastras, and the Agamas, but if he does not know the Kula he doesn't know anything.

2.78. Only those who are your *bhakta*s, your devotees, know the greatness of the Kula, not others. Only the chakora bird (singing to the moon in love with it), not others, knows the moonbeam.

2.83. The world is made of Shiva and Shakti. The Kaula teaching is founded on the world. Therefore, it is the best of all. What a universal, comprehensive teaching!

2.84. The six philosophies (Nyaya, Vaisheshika, Samkhya, Yoga, Mimamsa, and Vedanta) are limbs of my body, feet, belly, hands, head. He who carves divisions in them breaks my body.

2.85. Just these are also six limbs of the Kula. Therefore, know the Vedic Shastras to be Kaula in character.

2.86. According to all the philosophies (properly interpreted), there is a single Divine who grants results. Dear one, the Divine grants enjoyment and liberation within this family (*kula*) of human beings.

2.87. The Kula teaching may run against the wisdom of the world, O Queen of Siddhas, O Queen of accomplished yogins and yoginis. But, dearest, it is a knowledge source because it is the result of (yogic) perception.

2.88. And perception is directed to the generation of knowledge in the case of all beings with breath, dear. All bad reasoners ("bad" in opposing Kula teachings) are defeated by the force of perceptual evidence.

2.89. Who indeed knows what is not perceived, what will be, or to whom it will occur? Verily only that which is the fruit of perception is the best philosophy.

2.113. Such a vision of the Kula (the Whole) is obtainable through the guru's grace. Your *bhakta*s alone, not others, have it, know it, know that which gives enjoyment and liberation.

2.117. If a human could really attain perfection (*siddhi*) through wine drinking, then let all the riffraff get perfection who'd love to do nothing but drink wine.

2.118. If by merely eating meat (spiritual) merit would accrue, then all the meat eaters in the world would enjoy (spiritual) merit.

2.119. O Queen of the Gods, if liberation could really be had by sexual enjoyment, then just any creature could be liberated by having sex.

2.120. In no case is the path to be blamed, the path of the Kula, Great Goddess. It's those lacking good behavior that are to be blamed here, not others (practitioners of Kaula rituals whose behavior is good).

2.121. Otherwise is the behavior described by me (above) of one who is on the Way of the Kula. Goddess, deluded people thinking themselves learned are wayward when acting otherwise (than acts the true Kaulika as described).

2.122. You may walk on the edge of a sword, you may hang on to the neck of a tiger, you may hold a (poisonous) snake and carry it—these are all easier than living (in the right way) in the Kula.[20]

The selections now from Abhinava Gupta belong to two different genres of literature. The first is a type of poem, a *stotra,* hymn of praise, followed by a remarkable prose passage on aesthetics. A similar poem translated by Paul Mueller-Ortega comes from the same collection of nine poems edited by K.C. Pandey and reproduced in Devanagari characters.[21] My translation and understanding, I should like to acknowledge, benefit from both Mueller-Ortega's and Pandey's work, as well as from a French translation and commentary by Lilian Silburn.

Professor Silburn explains the poem in lucid detail in her commentary, uncovering multiple senses and interpretations as well as echoes of earlier tantric literature.[22] In notes, I mention several points of hers. She also identifies an overall theme of alignment of the microcosm of the human individual with the macrocosm of the reality of Shiva/Shakti. Shakti engages in creative, supportive, and ecstatically reabsorptive activities (see in particular verse 6). Silburn brings out the image of the thousand-petaled lotus that is indeed there, suggested pretty explicitly though not in so many words: the infinitely petaled "wheel," or *chakra,* namely, the lotus above the head that spreads in all directions from a central axis or hub where sits Shiva/Shakti, Bhairava/Bhairavi. Note, however, in verse 3, "Bhairava-Bliss" (*bhairavananda*) is said to be "seated in the lotus of the heart." Combining the images, one would have Bhairava illumining the central channel, *sushumna,* or perhaps raining down from the outside, penetrating the heart center.

Concerning the word *deha* in the title, which means body, clearly it is not just the body made of matter (*annamaya kosha*) that is intended by Abhinava, who stations divinities in the pranic, mental, and occult bodies as well as associated parts of the physical frame.

Finally, whether or not there is a secondary sense of the word *chakra,* wheel, in the title (and I agree with Silburn that there is), the primary sense is the ritual act of saluting a *circle* of divinities, turning to address each in turn. Although all our experience and all factors in and causes of experience are, in the philosophic conception, included in the eight goddesses' offerings, the particular forms those offerings take are in the language of the poem the best of whatever factor, a distilled essence or finest example (see, e.g., verse 6, 10, 11, 12, or 13).

Dehastha-devata-chakra-stotra: The Wheel (Chakra) Hymn to the (Circle of) Divinities Seated in the Body

1. (Shiva's elephant-headed son, Ganesha, god of beginnings) the Leader of the Assembly (of Shiva and Shakti's retinue), honored by the multitudes divine and undivine, delighted in the bestowal of what one regards as a boon, and worshipped at the outset of hundreds of treatises of philosophy, him I salute who is manifest in (up-)breath (energy, *prana*).[23]

2. Vatuka (Shiva's other son, Karttikeya, the young ascetic), whose feet are touched by real heroes, yoginis, *siddha*s in (all) lineages, by whom the troubles of the well-behaved are taken away, him I salute who is picked out in down-breath (energy, *apana*).

3. (The fearsome form of Shiva) Bhairava-Bliss (*ananda*), who is made of consciousness, whom, seated in the lotus of the heart, the goddesses of the senses worship always with (offerings of) objects experienced internally, I salute him.

4. The true Guru (*sad-guru*), who takes the form of vigilance, unsullied (no matter what the activity), who by the force of intelligence (*dhi*) reveals to *bhakta*s the whole universe as the path of Shiva, constantly I salute him.

5. (The fearsome form of Shakti) Bhairavi-Bliss, who in the form of self-consciousness (*vimarsha*) plays (*lilam karoti*) ceaselessly bringing up, appearing as, and chewing up the universe, I salute her.[24]

6. Brahmani (the Divine), seated on the petals of (Indra) the lord of the gods, saluting Bhairava with flowers of certitude, constantly I bow before her who is the rational mind (*buddhi*).[25]

7. Shambhavi (the Kind, Parvati), seated on the petals of Agni (Fire), worshipping Bhairava with flowers of pride, forever I salute her who is egoism, the Mother.[26]

8. Kaumari (the Young Woman), roaming the southern petals (of Yama, Death), forever expressing adoration for Bhairava with flowers of imagined possibilities, whose essence is the lower mind (*manas,* the sensuous mind), I salute her.[27]

9. I forever bow before Vaishnavi (Vishnu's feminine side), the Shakti, who takes the form of sound (words and music); roaming the petals of the southwest (i.e., of Nirriti, goddess of destruction), with flowers of sound she adores Bhairava.

10. I honor Varahi (the Female Boar) who assumes the form of the organ of touch; making her station the westerly petals (of Varuna, god of waters), she delights Bhairava with flowers of touch, heart-stealing flowers of touch.

11. Indrani (wife of Indra and the right pupil), who, in a body sitting on the petals of the Maruts (the Winds), worships Bhairava with flowers of the color spectrum, the very best, I salute her in her body of sight.

12. I honor Chamunda (Durga with the terrifying tongue dangling down from her mouth), who is picked out in the tongue as the organ of taste; abiding in the (lotus) buds of (Kubera) master of wealth, she worships Bhairava with foods of all the combinations of the six flavors.

13. At every moment I bow before the Great Lakshmi (goddess of beauty and fortune), who, seated on the petals of the Lord, adores Bhairava spreading diverse fragrances, Great Lakshmi, who is named in the nose as the organ of smell.

14. I salute the one named the self (*atman*), honored in the six philosophies, infusing the thirty-six categories, granting *siddhi*s, the proprietor of the field (the witness).[28]

15. The wheel of divinities roaming my own body thus I sing, the wheel (*chakra*) pulsating as the essence of experience, settled in everywhere (but) forever (absolutely) near, arising (and talked about) continually.

The second selection is from Abhinava's famous commentary on the *Natya Shastra,* which has been edited in Sanskrit and translated by J. L. Masson and M. V. Patwardhan in their book, *Shantarasa.*[29] The translation below is thus doubly indebted to their work. But it is a fresh effort, hopefully more accessible than theirs, with which I have compared it almost word by word. For background, see the second section of chapter 5. Further background is provided in some of the notes. The immediate context is examination of the thesis, endorsed by Abhinava, that there are not only eight *rasa*s, or kinds of aesthetic relishing, but nine, to include *shanta rasa,* the relishing of the spiritual peace (*shanti*) that is the result of discovery of the *atman,* the primordial self.

(Opponent:) What, then, is the (corresponding) ordinary, abiding emotion (for the *rasa* of spiritual peace, *shanta-rasa*)?

We answer: It is just knowledge of reality (i.e., the self, *atman*). Insofar as this is the means to liberation (*moksha*), it is appropriately thought of as enduring (spiritual realization is not transitory, unlike other "knowledges," *jnana*). And knowledge of reality is just knowledge of the self (*atman*).

And this is knowledge of the self as an object, as it were, that is distinct (from other objects).[30] For otherwise the self as something else would *ipso facto* be the same as the not-self (which is absurd). . . . Just the self is here the (corresponding) ordinary, abiding emotion (*sthayin* for *sthayi-bhava,* implying the self can be felt as an emotion, *bhava,* literally, "state"), the self, i.e., who is (intrinsically) connected to unsullied characteristics of knowledge, bliss, and so on. . . .

If it is asked why the self should be counted separately (from the other abiding emotional states, since, as already argued, it is implicated in every emotional state), we answer that it is separately and distinctly enjoyed when it is (enjoyed in itself) not in connection with tasting (other *bhava*s and corresponding *rasa*s).[31] . . .

. . . Therefore, knowledge of reality is simply the true nature of the self (its native state), which is tranquility (*shanti*). Further, sexual feeling and the rest (of the ordinary abiding emotions) are thus just particulars of (relative) sullying coloration. Admittedly, the self is understood as pure, of unmixed character. On the strength of the evidence of *samadhi* (yogic trance), one understands it as homogeneous. Nevertheless, upon returning to everyday consciousness, a person is tranquil, at peace. As it has been said (*Yoga Sutra* 3.10), "That transformation is borne along *tranquilly* because of (restriction-causing) *samskara*s (becoming dominant)."[32]

Furthermore, the whole range of ordinary and extraordinary states of mind (states and fluctuations of thought and emotion, *chitta*) can be used dramatically as subordinate transitory emotions supporting (the aesthetic transformation of) this abiding emotion characterized by knowledge of reality. And dramatically it does have symptoms (indications), those fostered by such things as practice of the *yamas* and the *niyamas* (of the *Yoga Sutra*). . . . It does dramatically have stimulants too, the grace of God and so on. . . .

Furthermore, the person (who knows the self), for whom what has to be done has been done with regard to the person's own self-interest, well, such a person makes effort solely in the furtherance of others' welfare. Therefore, being energetic (which is the abiding emotion transformed dramatically into the heroic *rasa*) with such a person (depicted dramatically) would take the form of a wishing, along with effort on his or her part that has helping others as goal. An additional subsidiary (dramatically considered) is the (enlightened) person's being focused on others through compassion.

Just for this reason, some (philosophers) identify (a *rasa* of) compassionate heroism, on the strength of compassion being (dramatically) a transitory supporting emotion (for the *rasa* of spiritual peace, *shanta rasa*); others identify it as dharmic (righteous) heroism.

Objection: Being energetic lives on egoism, but being at peace has the character of relaxing, loosening egoism.

(Abhinava:) Wrong. For using even a (diametrically) opposed emotion (dramatically) as a transitory supporting emotion (as, for example, disgust supporting the *rasa* of love) is not unsuitable (depending on the plot). . . . There is no psychological state whatsoever without energy. To think there could be one without desire, effort (etc.) would invite citing a stone as the untoward consequence.

And it is for this reason that insofar as a person has, with respect to his or her own self, truly fathomed it, both high and low (both in its universal nature and in particular), there would be nothing left to be done (and still the person would act). It follows from this that giving on the part of those whose hearts are at spiritual peace, such giving as proceeds wholeheartedly, holding nothing back, not the body (or even life), in order to help someone else, is not opposed (dramatically) to *shanta rasa*. . . .

. . . Vedic scriptures and "sacred memory" (e.g., the *Bhagavad Gita*) say alike that liberation can occur in all the (prescribed) stages (*ashrama*) of life for those who know (the self). So it has been declared, "If delighted in honoring the gods and goddesses and grounded in knowledge of reality (i.e., the self), fond of guests (treating them graciously), even a (benighted) householder making ceremonial offerings to ancestors is liberated."

{ 240 } Not only this but also (there is the following evidence:) bodhisattvas, who are persons who know reality (i.e., know the self though it is conceived as *nirvana,* who thus according to Buddhist doctrine are souls who could disappear), appear again even after (their enlightenment) in a body that is perfectly appropriate for them in their intention, dharmic (righteous) and born out of concern for others' welfare, whose only consequence would be others actually being helped.

APPENDIX E
Selections from the *Hatha Yoga Pradipika*

This amazing work outlining yoga practices with only a little metaphysics but lots of occult psychology is by a fifteenth-century author, Svatmarama. One achieves "mental silence," the goal of the yoga of the *Yoga Sutra,* by mastering the violent (*hatha*), strenuous practices of asana, breath control, and sequenced movements, learning to move the prana in occult paths. Unlike in mainstream tantra, action by God or one's higher self is, if necessary for liberation in some sense (see below, verse 3.2), not the focus. One takes heaven by storm. Although, as with Abhinava and company, yoga may be thought of as a matter of preparation, getting oneself ready for grace, the road-building goes on at a furious pace in hatha yoga. God and the guru's grace are mentioned in a verse or two, but *bhakti* is not prominent. Philosophically, the *HYP* is notable for its claim that mental and vital energy are inseparable and that control and redirection of *prana* is essential to achieving a quiet mind.

The *HYP,* whose title means light on hatha yoga, is a late tantric text that borrows from many philosophic predecessors.[1] But it is first of all a yoga handbook, in this way much like the *Yoga Sutra,* a text that it often echoes. Its closest predecessors, however, are the *Goraksha-paddhati* and other works by Goraksha (c. 1150), who is traditionally viewed as the founder of Swatmarama's lineage. Swatmarama in several places borrows verses from Goraksha, who himself uses, we may note, the tantric chakric psychology. And like a few other texts that also stand in the tradition of Goraksha, the *HYP* breaks with the *YS* not only in metaphysics but also, most importantly, in the practices it teaches, especially in emphasis and in matters of asserted efficiency. Even meditation is ineffective without the difficult practices of hatha yoga (2.76 and elsewhere)—*pranayama,* in particular, coupled with mastery of psychic locks, *bandhas* (see chapter 1) and the know-how and skill to perform difficult sequences involving asanas, breath, and locks (called *mudra;* see below). However, meditation is hardly ignored. The last chapter has a long excursion on nada yoga, the yoga of listening to inner sounds, where interesting references to the chakras are made, according to the classical commentator Brahmananda as well as to the Bihar School.

The *HYP* has been translated into English several times. I have consulted two translations, both of which I can recommend. First, an 1893 Sanskrit edition and English translation by Srinivasa Iyengar (with an introduction by Tookaram Tatya), re-edited by A. A. Ramanathan and S. V. Subrahmanya Sastri, in an Adyar Library publication (1972), but "thoroughly revised . . . so as to conform more closely to the text and yet be readable" (vi). The book includes an easy and helpful Sanskrit commentary by the nineteenth-century pundit Brahmananda, bits of which appear in occasional comments by the editors in English. In second place, I have consulted the Bihar School of Yoga's translation and commentary by Swami Muktibodhananda (1993), a book that includes diagrams of asanas and sets of instructions.[2] The transliteration here follows the edition by Pandit Iyengar as re-edited by Ramanathan and Shastri. (The verses in Sanskrit are metrically regular, melodious, and easy to memorize.)

Since practicewise so much explanation is called for and so much of the *HYP* concerns practice, I have chosen only three passages, all of which seem particularly accessible as well as salient to the projects of this book, the philosophical and psychological theses here encountered. Comments are interspersed.

The *HYP* has four chapters of different lengths, a total of just under four hundred verses. The first chapter is about asanas. The second is on breath control and preliminary cleansing practices. The third is on *mudra*—a word that in some contexts means sacred gestures (and seals of yoga-generated energy) but here means something else. For the *HYP,* a *mudra* is an attitude made manifest in a sequence of asanas along with *bandha* engagement (engagings and releasings of the psychic locks). The fourth, the most philosophic chapter, discusses *samadhi,* yogic trance, as well as nada yoga, the yoga of sound.

Among postures, *siddhasana,* Perfection Pose, is preferred apparently for its stimulating effect on occult energies and the central channel, *sushumna.* Several others are listed along with general benefits.[3] The message of the first chapter is: master the asanas because they—and control of the body and breath in general—are presupposed by more vigorous practices, called *mudra,* which directly lead to *samadhi.* For example, the *mudra* called *viparita-karani,* which involves wholesale "reversal" of psychic energies, begins with Headstand, *shirshasana.*

Despite some interesting advice about yoga practice in general, there is less in chapter 1 concerning Yoga philosophy and psychology than in later chapters. We shall skip directly to chapter 2 and verses in praise of *pranayama* and breath retention (*kumbhaka*) in particular.

Proper breath control along with use of the psychic locks, *bandha,* can by themselves secure the goal of mental silence, which is the goal of raja yoga (the yoga of the *YS*), we are told repeatedly (e.g., in 2.75 echoing 1.67). In chapter 3, we are introduced to *mudra,* which are complicated practices sometimes called *kriya,* actions, along with their occult underpinnings in *kundalini,* the mystic serpent power. Finally, in chapter 4 we have a remarkable passage on the results of the yoga of sound (*nada*), of listening to internal sounds to the exclusion of all other available objects. Here the occult psychology is in high relief.

The text opens with a *mangala* verse of "auspiciousness." Thus it signals itself not as a scripture reporting a dialogue of Shiva and Shakti but rather as a textbook within a Shaivite tantric tradition that does indeed hold Shiva to be the source of yoga instruction in dialogue with Parvati (Devi). There are 67 verses in chapter 1, 78 in chapter 2, 130 in chapter 3, and 114 in chapter 4. Ellipses are filled in following the commentary of Brahmananda.

2.39. brahmâdayo 'pi tri-daśāḥ pavanâbhyāsa-tat-parāḥ
abhūvann antaka-bhayāt tasmāt pavanam abhyāset.
Even the thirty gods, Brahma and the rest, practice yoga with wind (breath energy), intent on it. They do so out of fear of its end. Therefore, one should practice with wind (the "purifier," *pavana,* i.e., breath energy, *prana*).

2.40. yāvad baddho marud dehe yāvac cittaṃ nirākulam
yāvad dṛṣṭir bhruvo madhye kāla-bhayam kutaḥ.
How can there be fear of time (death) so long as the wind is tied to the body (by yogic breath control), the thought and emotion (*chitta*) empty and steady, the gaze (*drishti*) set (on the *chakra*) between the eyebrows?

2.41. vidhivat saṃyāmair nāḍī-cakre viśodhite
suṣumnā-vadanaṃ bhittvā sukhād viśati mārutaḥ.
Through proper regulation (awareness becoming identified with) breath energy (*prana*), the (subtle) canals, *nadis,* and chakras become cleansed. Easily then the mouth of the central channel opens, the *sushumna* opens, and the wind (the breath energy) enters in.

2.42. mārute madhya-saṃcāre manaḥ-sthairyaṃ prajāyate
yo manaḥ-susthirībhāvaḥ saivâvasthāmanônmanī
When the wind (*maruta* = *prana*) is moving through the central channel, mental steadiness is born. That state of consciousness is known as *manonmani,* "(eager) intentional absence of mind," which is a state of extraordinary steadiness of the *manas,* the thought-mind.

2.43. tat-siddhaye vidhāna-jñāś citrān kurvanti kumbhakān
vicitra-kumbhakâbhyāsād vicitrāṃ siddhim āpnuyāt.
To accomplish this, those who know the rules (of proper practice) perform

various kinds of breath retention, *kumbhaka*. (As a side benefit) various kinds of *siddhi* are obtained from practice of the various kinds of *kumbhaka*.

atha kumbhaka-bhedāḥ
2.44. sūrya-bhedanam ujjāyī-sītkārī śītalī tathā
bhastrikā bhrāmarī mūrcchā plāviny aṣṭa-kumbhakāḥ.
Here are the varieties of breath retention: *surya-bhedana* ("splitting the sun-channel": inhalation through the right nostril, the "sun," *pingala,* and exhalation through the left, the "moon" and "earth," *ida*), *ujjayi* ("victorious": deep breathing with contraction of the epiglottis), *sitkari* ("hissing": breathing through the mouth and teeth making the sound "seet," which expresses pleasure), *shitali* ("cooling": breathing through the rolled tongue), *bhastrika* ("bellowslike": rapid breathing), *bhramari* ("humming": exhaling with sound like a bee), *murchchha* ("swoon": holding the breath almost to the point of fainting), and *plavini* ("floating": swallowing air into the stomach) are the eight *kumbhaka*s.

2.45. pūrakânte tu kartavyo bandho jālaṃdharâbhidhaḥ
kumbhakânte recakâdau kartavyas tu uḍḍīyānakaḥ.
Then at the end of the inhalation the lock should be done called *jalamdhara* (throat lock). But *uddiyana* lock (stomach lock) should be done at the end of retention when beginning the exhalation.

2.46. adhastāt kuñcanena āśu kaṇṭha-saṃkocane kṛte
madhye paścima-tānena syāt prāṇo brahma-nāḍi-gaḥ.
The throat contraction in place (*jalamdhara-bandha,* throat lock), then through quick contraction from below (*mula-bandha,* root lock), (and at the same time) by stretching the belly back (and engaging *uddiyana-bandha,* stomach lock), the *prana* is forced into the channel of Brahman (*sushumna,* the central channel).

2.47. apānam ūrdhvam utthāpya prāṇaṃ kaṇṭhād adho nayet
yogī jarā-vimuktaḥ san ṣodaśâbda-vayā bhavet.
Making the apana (downward breath) come up (reversing its normal flow through engaging root and stomach locks), one can lead the *prana* down from the throat (with the throat lock engaged). (Thus) the yogin becoming free from old age comes to look like someone sixteen years of age.

atha sūrya-bhedanam
2.48. āsane sukha-de yogī baddhvā caivâsanaṃ tataḥ
dakṣa-nāḍyā samākṛṣya bahiḥ-sthaṃ pavanaṃ śanaiḥ.
Now *surya-bhedana* (is described in the next three verses):
Taking a comfortable seat and making it an asana, the yogin, drawing in through the right nostril (*pingala*) air outside the body, slowly—

2.49. ā keśād ā nakhâgrāc ca nirodhâvadhi kumbhayet
tataḥ śanaiḥ savya-nāḍyā recayet pavanam śanaiḥ.
—should retain it up to the limit of cessation (of breathing), up to the hair on the head and the nails of the fingers and toes (feeling pressure). Then slowly, through the left nostril (*ida*), one should empty the air, slowly.

2.50. kapāla-śodhanaṃ vāta-doṣa-ghnaṃ kṛmi-doṣa-hṛt
punaḥ punar idam kāryaṃ sūrya-bhedanam uttamam.
The *surya-bhedana* type of breath control is the best for clearing and cleansing the cranium, destroying disorders (*dosha*) of *vata* (vital air), dispelling disorders caused by worms. Again and again should it be practiced.

. . .

2.75. rāja-yoga-padaṃ câpi labhate nâtra saṃśayaḥ
kumbhakāt kuṇḍalī-bodhaḥ kuṇḍalī-bodhato bhavet
anargalā suṣumnā ca haṭha-siddhiś ca jāyate.
In addition (to the benefit of the power just described), from mastery of breath retention the state of raja yoga (a silent mind) is gained, no doubt about it. From mastery of breath retention, the serpent power (*kundalini*) is awakened. And there would be, from the awakening of the serpent power, unbolting of the central channel (*sushumna*), and perfection (*siddhi*) would be born, the goal of hatha yoga.

Even the gods and goddesses practice *pranayama,* "extension and control of the breath energy"! This extends and iconizes the thesis that *prana* and *chitta,* the *YS*'s "thought stuff," are inextricably intertwined. There is no perfection in yoga without control or redirection of the life energy. The word used in verse 2.39 is *pavana,* which means purifier and is used to refer to air as the fourth of the five elements.[4] The element aside, it's as though divine individuality is maintained by perfect breathing. The gods and goddesses are conceived as occult energies, as in tantra generally but here without the emphasis on *bhakti*. Divine beings traverse subtle elements corresponding with the five gross elements, earth and the rest, and are thought to have connections with particular types of subtle energies that pass through our various chakras and subtle bodies.

It seems that surely the Immortals would not fear death, but how is their individuality sustained through time? Verse 2.40 answers that it is through particular yoga practices. No one is exempt from practice. Then verses 2.41 and 2.42 describe *prana* entering the central channel connecting all the major chakras and eliciting the "thousand-petaled" enlightment or self-realization visualized at the high end.

Verse 2.43 lays forth breath retention as the means to that end, underscoring the connection between prana and mental silence, *chitta-vritti-nirodha,* in the conception of the *YS*. Thought follows desire and emotion, and so no mental silence is possible without a yoga that addresses these factors. Implicitly, however, our text hints that breath-control practices are superior—in accordance, we may remark, with the order of limbs of the *ashtanga yoga* of the *YS* (*yama, niyama, asana, pranayama, pratyahara, dharana, dhyana,* and *samadhi*).

Verse 2.44 names eight varieties of breath retention. Most of the rest of the chapter consists in description and elaboration of the eight, touting benefits for health and the acquisition of *siddhi*s. The first of these, *surya-bhedana,* is taken up in 2.48. Verses 2.45 through 2.47 preview the *mudra*s that are the subject of chapter 3. Introducing the locks, the psychic *bandha,* the passage tells us how to make the *prana* flow consciously into the central channel. Verse 2.47 appears to characterize the same exercise in different terminology, talking about the usually downward, eliminative "air" or "breath," the *apana* (which is also mentioned at 1.48), made to flow up and the normally upward energy of breathing with the lungs and diaphram made to flow down. This action apparently occurs in the pranic body (figure 4A).[5]

The chapter continues with detailed description of the remaining types of breath retention along with benefits—until a final handful of verses, including 2.75, about the serpent power (*kundalini*). The divine energy asleep in the lower chakras is the central topic of the opening passage of chapter 3. The last verse of chapter 2, 2.78, lists slimness, freedom from illness, brightness of complexion, and clear eyes as among the signs of perfection in hatha yoga.

3.1. saśaila-vana-dhātrīṇāṃ yathâdhāro 'hi-nāyakaḥ
sarveṣāṃ yoga-tantrāṇāṃ tathâdhāro hi kuṇḍalī.
As the chief of serpents (Ananta, the Infinite, on whose back Vishnu reclines) is the support of Mother Earth with her craggy mountains and forests, / so indeed is Kundali (*kundalini,* the serpent power) the support of the principles of yoga.

3.2. suptā guru-prasādena yadā jāgarti kuṇḍalī
tadā sarvāṇi padmāni bhidyante granthayo 'pi ca.
Asleep, Kundali awakens through the grace of the guru. Then the lotuses (the chakras of the occult body) are all pierced and all the psychic knots (*granthi*) cut.

3.3.prāṇasya śūnya-padavī tadā rāja-pathāyate
tadā cittaṃ nirālambaṃ tadā kālasya vañcanam.
Then the trail to the Void comes to be the royal road for *prana.* Then the thought and emotion (*chitta*) disconnect from their objects (i.e., become still). Then time (death) is cheated.

3.4. suṣumṇā śūnya-padavī brahma-randhraṃ mahā-pathaḥ
śmaśānaṃ śāmbhavī madhya-mārgaś cêty eka-vācakāḥ.
There is a single referent of the expressions, "Sushumna" (the Gracious),

"trail to the void," "cleft of Brahman" (at the back of the head), the "Great Path," / "Cremation Ground," "Shambhavi" (the Kind Mother), and the "Middle Way" (the central channel).

3.5. tasmāt sarva-prayatnena prabodhayitum īśvarīm
brahma-dvāra-mukhe suptāṃ mudrâbhāsaṃ samācaret.
Therefore, with all effort one should act to arouse this the Female Lord, / who is asleep at the mouth of the door to Brahman, through practice of *mudra* (i.e., *kriya,* actions, to be listed).

3.6. mahā-mudrā mahā-bandho mahā-vedhaś ca khecarī
uḍḍīyānaṃ mūla-bandhaś ca bandho jālaṃdharâbhidhaḥ.

3.7. karaṇī viparītâkhyā vajrolī śakti-cālanam
idam hi mudrā-daśakaṃ jarā-maraṇa-nāśanam.
For there is, destructive of agedness and wasting away, this group of ten *mudra*s (attitudes or *kriya*): (1) the Great *mudra* (with one heel tucked in below the sexual organs, the other leg outstretched, retention of breath after an inhale, engagement of throat lock, and, to end the round, very slow exhalation), (2) the Great Lock (Root Lock, Stomach Lock, and Throat Lock engaged simultaneously), (3) the Great-Piercing Attitude (Lotus Pose combined with a lift of the buttocks and a beating of them, gently, against the ground along with Throat Lock), (4) *khechari* (tongue curled back to touch the palate, eyes rolled back with all attention directed to the third eye), (5) Stomach Lock, (6) Root Lock, (7) Throat Lock, (8) the Reversing Attitude (low shoulder stand with *ujjayi* breath), (9) *vajroli* (retention of sexual fluids and energy, *saholi* for women), and (10) Coursing the Shakti (in the central channel).

3.8. ādi-nāthôditaṃ divyam aṣṭaiśvarya-pradāyakam
vallabhaṃ sarva-siddhānāṃ durlabhaṃ marutām api.
These were taught by the original teacher (Shiva, the founder of yoga). They belong to our higher nature. They bring the eight powers, the eight *siddhi*s. / They are the practices preferred by all the *siddha*s (the perfected ones), though they are difficult even for the *marut*s (the highly flexible wind gods).

These verses provide an overview of practices said to be especially effective in arousing the serpent power.

The eight *siddhi*s, which are commonly attributed to the *Yoga Sutra* but are not spelled out there explicitly, are, according to *HYP* commentator Brahmananda: *animan,* shrinking; *mahiman,* extension; *gariman,* immovability; *laghiman,* lightness; *prapti,* cognition at a distance; *prakamya,* irresistible will; *ishita,* mastery of the body and the *manas* (thought mind); and *vashita,* dominion over external elements. This list is closer to the list in the *YS* commentary by King Bhoja than it is to Vyasa's in his comments on *YS* 3.45 (see that sutra as well as note 43 to appendix C).[6] Brahmananda provides a little elaboration for each, although some of his examples are highly implausible.[7]

The serpent power is not the same as the *jivatman,* the individual soul that survives death. The *jivatman* becomes liberated through Kundalini's awakening, splitting the psychic knots (*granthi*), and rising to the thousand-petaled lotus or chakra through the central channel, which in these verses is deified. The *sushumna* is the Royal Road, etc. It's as though the spark soul can now roam freely throughout the system newly alive with shakti, the facilitating divine energy that now flows freely.

The chapter continues to the very end by elaborating and describing the benefits of each of the ten *mudras*. Although the *HYP* is not a good example of the theme we have been calling the tantric turn, one of the verses on the ninth *mudra, vajroli,* which involves sex, is remarkable. The tantric sex prescribed involves both partners trying to withhold fluids as well as, upon release of fluids, to siphon them back up into one's own sexual organ, whether male or female (a kind of yogic competition!). After listing the practice's benefits (including a perfect body), verse 3.103 says in effect that here enjoyment (*bhoga*) and making progress towards liberation (*mukti-da*) are compatible.

All these methods of yoga are said at the end of chapter 3, as at the end of chapter 2, to confer *siddhi*s. The list of eight (see above) is indicated by mention of the first, *anima,* shrinking. Death too is overcome, the last verse says (3.130).

Chapter 4 begins with a round of salutations to Shiva, suggesting a fresh beginning if not interpolation. There is a lot of repetition of ideas previously introduced. Yogic trance, *samadhi,* is the main topic, which, although hardly described in terms of worldly action, is said to protect the yogin or yogini from harm from anything outside (conferring immunity from weapons, etc.). There is nevertheless much reference to the tantric psychology of chakras and so on, in particular in the midst of a long tract elaborating an additional yogic method, nada yoga, some verses of which are translated below. Two *mudra*s are also discussed at length, one, *khechari,* which was also listed and discussed in the third chapter, along with *shambhavi mudra,* which is not on the earlier list of ten. The word *shambhavi* is derivative from *shambhu*, "kind, peaceful," which is a common epithet for Shiva. The *mudra* is not as complex as any of the ten, involving simply fixing the vision or *drishti,* with eyes open or closed, at a spot just beyond the middle of the eyebrows, i.e., on the *ajna chakra,* says Brahmananda.

In chapter 4—as also in chapter 3 with respect to *sushumna* (3.4)—the *HYP* appears itself to acknowledge the legitimacy of a worry about objectivity. As might be expected given that it is a late text with respect to the whole of yoga literature (fourteenth century), it evinces awareness of a pluralism of conceptions concerning, in particular, *samadhi* as yogic goal. Verse 4.3–4 lists appellations of the yogic goal and supreme personal good (*parama-purushartha*) across a wide range of yogic and religious traditions. To my mind, this move helps to alleviate the historicist worry that occult teachings are particularly culture-bound. The problem of partial intersubjectivity is answered by the fact of the difficulty of the yogic prerequisites.

The section on nada yoga begins with verse 66 and runs for thirty-seven verses almost to the end of the chapter. Below are eight verses listing four advanced stages that presuppose *pratyahara,* withdrawal of the senses from their objects. Verse 68 says that not only the eyes but also the ears, the nose, and the mouth should be closed, meaning that the associated sensory organs should be withdrawn. Then one begins to hear sounds in the central channel that apparently have the power to split the psychic knots and usher in other, similarly puissant sounds as well as bliss and eventually enlightenment.

4.70. brahma-granther bhaved bhedo hy ānandaḥ śūnya-sambhavaḥ
vicitraḥ kvaṇako dehe 'nāhataḥ śrūyate dhvaniḥ.
For should the "knot of Brahma" (*brahma granthi*) be cut, *ananda* (bliss) arises out of nothing (out of the void, *shunya*). / Wondrous buzzing in the body is heard; the "unstruck" (*anahata*) sound is heard (in the *anahata* or heart chakra).

4.71. divya-dehaś ca tejasvī divya-gandhas tv arogavān
saṃpūrṇa-hṛdayaḥ śūnya ārambhe yogavān bhavet.
A divine body too is his, splendid (full of *tejas,* spiritual energy), with a supernatural scent, free of disease, / his heart full (of shakti), if the yoga practitioner enters into the beginning stage of "living in the void" (*shunya*).

4.72. dvitīyāyāṃ ghaṭīkṛtya vāyur bhavati madhya-gaḥ
dṛḍhâsano bhaved yogī jñānī deva-samas tadā.
In the second stage, the yogin becoming a vessel (*ghata*), the wind (*prana*) enters the central channel. / Then the yogin comes to be settled in his consciousness, a knower, equal then to a god.

4.73. viṣṇu-granthes tato bhedāt paramânanda-sūcakaḥ
atiśūnye vimardaś ca bherī-śabdas tadā bhavet.
And then upon the splitting of the knot of Vishnu (in the throat chakra), which is indicated by supernal bliss, / there is in the "over-void" (*atishunya*) the rumbling sound of a kettle drum.

4.74. tṛtīyāyāṃ tu vijñeyo vihāyo-mardala-dhvaniḥ
mahā-śūnyaṃ tadā yāti sarva-siddhi-samāśrayam.
But in the third stage, what is to be known is a drum's sound in the space (of the *ajna chakra*). / The "Great Void" (*maha-shunya*) at that time arises. The yogin attains the full availability of every kind of *siddhi.*

4.75. cittânandaṃ tadā jitvā sahajânanda-saṃbhavaḥ
doṣa-duḥkha-jarā-vyādhi-kṣudhā-nidrā-vivarjitaḥ.
Then mastering the bliss of the *chitta* (thought and emotion), he knows (another) bliss that is spontaneously born. / From flaws and imperfections, pain and suffering, aging, hunger, and sleep he becomes free.

4.76. rudra-granthiṃ yadā bhittvā śarva-pītha-gato 'nilaḥ
niṣpattau vaiṇavaḥ śabdaḥ kvaṇad-vīṇā-kvāṇo bhavet.
When the knot of Rudra has been cut, the wind (*prana*) is absorbed into Shiva's province (the *ajna chakra*). / That accomplished, a flutelike sound occurs, a ring resonating like a vina (a large guitar).

4.77. ekībhūtaṃ tadā cittaṃ rāja-yogâbhidhānakam
sṛṣṭi-saṃhāra-kartasau yogîśvara-samo bhavet.
Then the *chitta* comes to be single-pointed, (in a state) designated *raja yoga* (the royal yoga). / Such a yogin comes to be like the Lord (*ishvara*), capable of (creative) emanation and (destructive) retraction.

The passage continues with advice not to rest content even with this fourth stage of "living in the void" called raja yoga (which is usually taken to be a name for the yoga of the *YS*), albeit what has been achieved is extremely enjoyable (4.78–80). The section on nada yoga concludes with verse 102, and the book ends with verse 114.

The last thirteen verses again extol *samadhi*. The commentator Brahmananda is apparently so offended by the ending's lack of *bhakti* that he launches a long (five-page) excursion on the compatibility of *bhakti* with the methods described, and, in the words of the editors Ramanathan and Subrahmanya Sastri, concludes that "*bhakti,* in its most transcendental aspect, is included in . . . *samadhi.*"[8]

GLOSSARY

Sanskrit Words and Sanskrit-Derived Anglicizations

Guide to Pronunciation

Sanskrit words are spelled throughout this book without diacritical marks but otherwise in the standard indological fashion—with the following exceptions, made in the interest of better pronunciation:

ṛ	becomes ri (pronounced like "rea" in "real")
c	ch (pronounced like "ch" in "such")
ch	chh (aspirated "ch," i.e., with slightly more breath)
ś	sh (like "sh" in "hush")
ṣ	sh (also like "sh" in "hush")

Vowels are pronounced in standard ways, except:

i	ee (like "ee" in "feed")
e	a (like "a" in "cake")
ai	i (like "i" in "bike")
au	ow (like "ow" in "cow")

Consonants are also pronounced in standard ways, except:

ph	p (aspirated "p" as in "part," not "f").

Whole Sanskrit sentences transliterated in the notes and in some of the appendices do employ the standard system, and here in this glossary both styles are used. Words appear first in our simplified, anglicized way in boldface and then in the indological manner italicized and in parentheses. Quotation marks are used to indicate a comparatively literal rendering.

Transliterated Words with Diacritics

Vowels (omitting two that rarely occur):

a like "u" in "mum": *manas* (both vowels: muhnuhs)
ā like "a" in "father": Nāgārjuna (naa-gaar-joo-nuh)
i like "y" in "baby": *mukti*
ī like "ee" in "feed": Śrī (shree)
u like "u" in "pull": *mukti*
ū like "oo" in "moon": *sva-rūpa* (svuh-roo-puh)
ṛ like "rea" in "really" (while turning the tip of the tongue up to touch the palate): *Ṛg Veda*
e like "a" in "maze": *tejas* (tay-juhs)
ai like "i" in "mine": Jaina
o like "o" in "go": *yoga*
au like "ow" in "cow": *yaugika* (yow-gee-kuh)

Consonants and semivowels (which are best understood as a particular class of consonants) are pronounced roughly as in English. A few special cases are worth noting:

kh exactly like "k" in Sanskrit—that is, like the "k" in "kite"—except aspirated, that is, breath out, as with "keel": *mukha*
All other aspirated consonants follow the same principle: "gh" like "g" except aspirated, "th" like "t," and so on.
c like "ch" in "churn"
ch is another aspirate, same principle: *sac-chid-ānanda*
ñ like "n" in canyon
ṭ There is no English equivalent: a "t" sound (as in "tough") but with the tip of the tongue touching the roof of the mouth.
ṭh aspirated "ṭ"
ḍ like "d" in "deer" but "lingualized" as with "ṭ"
ḍh aspirated "ḍ"
ṇ lingualized "n" sound

There are three sibilants:

ś like "sh" in "shove"
ṣ lingualized "sh" sound
s like "s" in "sun": *sūrya*

ḥ calls for breath following a vowel. For example, *duḥkha* ("pain") is pronounced as follows: "du" and then breath (very short) and then "kha."

ṃ This is shorthand for all nasals, the particular type determined by the class of the following consonant: "ṅ" is guttural, "ñ" palatal, "ṇ" lingual, and "n" dental. For example, the "ṃ" in "Sāṃkhya" is equivalent to "ṅ," since "kh" belongs to the guttural class.

Euphonic Combination, Sandhi

The "hat" symbol (ˆ) is used for vowel *sandhi* or "combination" when two words are compounded (e.g., *tāḍa*, "mountain," compounded with *āsana*, "pose, posture," results in *tāḍâsana*, Mountain Pose). The hat (ˆ) designates that a vowel so marked is long (or is the dipthong *e* or *o*) because of *sandhi* in the bringing together of the two separate words. For example:

tāḍâsana (*tāḍa* + *āsana*)
jñānêndriya (*jñāna* + *indriya*)
śāmbhavôpāya (*śāmbhava* + *upāya*)

abhyasa (*abhyāsa*) repeated exercise or practice

adhikara (*adhikāra*) prerequisite, yogic prerequisite

adhikarin (*adhikārin*) person who is qualified, entitled, "fit" (by yogic practice, etc., for yogic experience, God's grace, etc.)

adho-mukha shvanasana (*adho-mukha-śvanâsana*) "Downward-Facing Dog," an important asana for basic conditioning

adhyasa (*adhyāsa*) superimposition

adrishta (*adṛṣṭa*) unseen (moral) force, impersonal cosmic force of karmic payback

Advaita Vedanta (*advaita-vedānta*) a prominent school of classical philosophy subscribing to an Upanishadic monism ("All is Brahman," including—and especially—the seemingly individual consciousness or self)

agni (*agni*) fire, psychic fire

ahamkara (*ahaṃkāra*) egoism; the individuating principle (*tattva*) in Samkhya

ahimsa (*ahiṃsā*) nonharmfulness; see note 17 to chapter 3

ahimsika (*ahiṃsika*) one who practices *ahimsa* (q.v.)

ajna chakra (*ājñā-cakra*) third eye, the "command" chakra where tantrics say is heard the "directive" of the divine or one's highest self

akasha (*ākāśa*) ether, the medium of sound, one of five material elements, according to almost all classical views; sometimes "space"

alankara shastra (*alaṃkāra-śāstra*) aesthetics, the "science of ornament," the classical tradition of literary criticism in particular

alaya vijnana (*ālaya-vijñāna*) "storehouse consciousness"; a principal concept in early Yogacara Buddhism

amrita (*amṛta*) nectar of immortality

anahata chakra (*anāhata cakra*) the "heart" center, where tantrics say the "unstruck" sound can be heard, the chakra where *bhakti* is felt

ananda (*ānanda*) bliss, spiritual ecstasy; the nature of Brahman considered affectively, according to Vedanta

anandamaya kosha (*ānandamaya-kośa*) body made of bliss, *ananda,* the *kosha* nearest the intrinsic nature of the self, *atman*

anatman (*anātman*) "no self" or "no soul," an important Buddhist doctrine

anavopaya (*aṇavôpāya*) the Kaula way of the minute, for those of coarse natures

anekanta-vada (*anekânta-vāda*) nonabsolutism, positive perspectivalism, the "doctrine of many-sidedness"; the metaphysical stance of Jaina philosophers

anga (*aṅga*) limb, subordinate part

animan (*aṇiman*) thinness; *siddhi* of shrinking

anirvachaniya (*anirvacanīya*) "impossible to say"; the Advaita view of the ontological status of the everyday world in relation to Brahman

anjali mudra (*añjali-mudrā*) "hands cupped in offering," prayer position

anjaneyasana (*añjaneyâsana*) Crescent Moon Pose—a matronymic for Hanuman, the monkey king, who is a great *bhakta*

annamaya kosha (*annamaya-kośa*) body made of matter, "food," *anna,* the physical body

anta (*anta*) end, extreme

anubhava (*anubhava*) experience, awareness (perceptual, inferential, and other veridical awarenesses)

anumana (*anumāna*) (cogent) inference; a knowledge source or *pramana* (q.v.) according to practically all classical schools

anusara (*anusāra*) alignment

anuvyayasaya (*anuvyavasāya*) apperception, cognition of cognition, according to Nyaya

anyatha khyati (*anyathā-khyāti*) "presentation of something as other than what it is," the view of perceptual error that stresses the reality of the thing misperceived and the reality of the thing which the presented object is misperceived *as*

aparigraha (*aparigraha*) nonpossessiveness, the fifth *yama* (q.v.) according to the *Yoga Sutra*

apta (*āpta*) expert; a person whose testimony is reliable

apurvaka (*apūrvaka*) without causal intermediary

ardha uttanasana (*ardha uttānâsana*) "half" *uttanasana*

artha (*artha*) wealth; goal, object

arthapatti (*arthâpatti*) postulation, presumption; circumstantial implication—deemed an independent *pramana* by Mimamsa and some other classical philosophers, but a form of inference (inference to the best explanation), according to Nyaya

asamprajnata samadhi (*asamprajñāta-samādhi*) yogic trance without any meditational prop according to the *Yoga Sutra;* utter yogic self-absorption; equivalent to enlightenment and *brahma vidya* according to some Vedantins

asana (*āsana*) poses and meditational postures taught as part of disciplines of yoga

asat (*asat*) nonbeing, bad

ashrama (*aśrama*) spiritual and yogic retreat; stage of life

ashtanga namaskara (*aṣṭâṅga-namaskāra*) "eight-points bowing"

ashtanga yoga (*aṣṭâṅga-yoga*) "eight-limbed yoga" of the *Yoga Sutra:* (1) *yama,* (2) *niyama,* (3) *asana,* (4) *pranayama,* (5) *pratyahara,* (6) *dharana,* (7) *dhyana,* and (8) *samadhi*

asmita (*asmitā*) egoity, the principle of individuation in Samkhya; egoism

asteya (*asteya*) nonstealing, the third *yama* (q.v.) according to the *Yoga Sutra*

atman (*ātman*) self; the Upanishadic term for our truest or most basic consciousness; universal Self

avadhuti (*avadhūti*) central channel; see *sushumna*

avatara (*avatāra*) divine incarnation, e.g., Krishna and Rama

avidya (*avidyā*) spiritual ignorance; in much Vedanta, lack of direct awareness of Brahman, the true self, or God

ayur-veda (*āyur-veda*) medicine ("knowledge of life")

avyakta (*avyakta*) unmanifest

badha (*bādha*) epistemic defeating or "blocking," e.g., experiential sublation, as a veridical perception of a rope correcting an illusory perception of a snake; epistemic or justificational defeating

bandha (*bandha*) "bond," binding, lock; a muscular lock that redirects pranic energy

bhagavad (*bhagavad*) blessed, divine

bhakta (*bhakta*) devotee

bhakti (*bhakti*) devotional love

bhakti yoga (*bhakti-yoga*) yoga of love and devotion

bhashya (*bhāṣya*) commentary

bhastrika (*bhastrikā*) "bellowslike" rapid breathing, a form of *pranayama*

bhava (*bhāva*) natural emotion: see *sthayi bhava*

bhava chakra (*bhāva-cakra*) wheel of birth, death, and rebirth, according to Buddhism

bhavana (*bhāvanā*) enlivening or re-enlivening (as of an intention, *samkalpa*)

bhoga (*bhoga*) enjoyment

bhramari (*bhramarī*) "humming," exhaling with sound like a bee (*bhramara*), a form of *pranayama*

bhuta (*bhūta*) gross element (earth, water, fire, air, and ether)

bodhisattva (*bodhisattva*) one who is capable of a final extinction of individual personality in an ultimate nirvana but who retains form out of compassion for sentient beings; the yogic ideal of Mahayana Buddhism

brahmacharya (*brahma-carya*) sexual restraint, celibacy, the fourth *yama* (q.v.) according to the *Yoga Sutra*

brahma randhra (*brahma-randhra*) the cranial cleft through which runs the "central channel," *sushumna* (q.v.)

brahma sakshatkara (*brahma-sākṣātkāra*) immediate awareness of Brahman; *brahma-vidya* (q.v.)

brahma vidya (*brahma-vidyā*) yogic knowledge of Brahman, the Absolute (or God); the *summum bonum*, according to Vedanta

Brahman (*brahman*) the Divine Absolute; the One; the God, *ishvara* (q.v.); the key concept of the Upanishads and all Vedanta (q.v.) philosophy

Buddha (*buddha*) "the Awakened"; an epithet of Siddhartha Gautama, the founder of Buddhism, after his enlightenment or *nirvana* (q.v.)

buddhi (*buddhi*) rational intelligence

Buddhism (*bauddha-darśana*) world religion founded by Siddhartha Gautama, the Buddha or "Awakened One," who taught that a supreme felicity and end to suffering occur in a special experience called nirvana and who laid out a way or ways to attain it

buddhi yoga (*buddhi-yoga*) discipline for the higher intelligence

chakra (*cakra*) occult center of consciousness, "wheel" of occult energy

chandra namaskara (*candra-namaskāra*) Moon Salutations, a series of asanas

Charvaka (*cārvāka*) the classical Indian philosophic school of materialism, religious skepticism, and hedonism

chaturangasana (*catur-aṅgâsana*) Four-Limbs Pose, a planklike asana with elbows in under the ribs

chikirsha (*cikīrṣā*) "desire to do"

chin mudra (*cin-mudrā*) the "consciousness seal (or gesture)"

chitta (*citta*) thought and emotion, mind stuff

chitta-vritti-nirodha (*citta-vṛtti-nirodha*) stilling of the fluctuations of thought and emotion; the definition of *yoga* given by the *Yoga Sutra*

darshana (*darśana*) world view or philosophy, a "viewing"

deha (*deha*) body

devi (*devī*) female divinity, "goddess"; superconscient power of one's higher self

dharana (*dhāraṇā*) concentrated perseverance; meditation or concentration (especially in movement)

dharma (*dharma*) (1) duty, right way of action; (2) quality or state of awareness; (3) property

dharma kaya (*dharma-kāya*) Dharma body of the Buddha (see *dharma*)

dhyana (*dhyāna*) meditation (proper)

dosha (*doṣa*) fault, disorder

drishti (*dṛṣṭi*) gaze, sight

duhkha (*duḥkha*) pain and suffering

ekagrata (*ekâgratā*) one-pointedness of mind, "exclusive concentration"

gariman (*gariman*) weight; dignity; *siddhi* of immovability

gita (*gītā*) song

gopi (*gopī*) cowgirl (*gopi*s are famously beloved of Krishna, symbolizing individual souls)

granthi (*granthi*) psychic "knot" blocking the flow of *shakti* in the chakras and central channel

guna (*guṇa*) quality, property; twenty-four are enumerated in the early Nyaya–Vaisheshika literature, including cognition (*jnana*), which is a quality resting in the self (*atman*); mode or strand of nature, according to Samkhya (see *sattva, rajas,* and *tamas*)

guru (*guru*) teacher, venerable person

hamsa (*haṃsa*) (Siberian) crane, swan, goose; the symbol of the transmigrating self or soul (*jivatman*)

hatha (*haṭha*) force, obstinancy, necessity

hatha yoga (*haṭha-yoga*) type of self-discipline emphasizing postures, *pranayama,* and *mudra* (q.v.) as means to pierce occult *granthi,* open chakras, and awaken *kundalini* (q.v.)

hetu (*reason*) reason, inferential mark or sign

hetvabhasa (*hetv-ābhāsa*) "pseudo-reason," fallacy

hita (*hita*) "favorable"; an Upanishadic word for subtle connections or canals of subtle energies (see *nadi*)

ida (*iḍā*) earth; moon; devotion as goddess; channel or *nadi* that runs from the left nostril, pranic channel

indriya (*indriya*) sense organ or faculty

ishita (*iṣita*) "desired," wanted; *siddhi* of mastery of the body and the *manas* (thought mind and focus)

ishta-devata (*iṣṭa-devatā*) "preferred divinity"

ishvara (*īśvara*) God, the "Lord"; viewed as the equivalent of Brahman in theistic Vedanta

ishvara-pranidhana (*īśvara-praṇidhāna*) "concentration on God," "surrender to the Lord" (a term appearing in the *Yoga Sutra* that has been variously interpreted)

Jainism (*jaina-darśana*) an ancient Indian religion founded by Mahavira, c. 500 B.C.E., who, like the Buddha, propounded a "supreme personal good"; in later periods, Jaina philosophers addressed a broad range of issues

jalandhara bandha (*jālandhara-bandha*) throat lock, the "netting" lock (see *bandha*)

japa (*japa*) yoga of repetition of mantras such as *om*

Jataka (*jāṭaka*) stories of the Buddha's previous incarnations, a portion of the Pali or southern canon

jivan mukti (*jīvan-mukti*) "living liberation," a living person's attainment of spiritual enlightenment

jivatman (*jīvâtman, jīva*) individual, living person, transmigrating self

jnana (*jñāna*) cognition, consciousness

jnana yoga (*jñāna-yoga*) yoga of meditation

jnanendriya (*jñānêndriya*) sense organ, any of the five faculties of sense perception and knowledge

kaivalya (*kaivalya*) aloneness or independence: the *summum bonum* according to Samkhya and the Yoga of the *Yoga Sutra*

kama (*kāma*) pleasure, especially sexual pleasure; sensory gratification

kama-vasaya (*kāma-vāsaya*) the *siddhi* of dwelling wherever desired

karma (*karman*) (1) "action"; (2) habit; the psychological law that every act creates a psychic valency to repeat the act; (3) sacrifice, ritual

karma yoga (*karma-yoga*) yoga of action and sacrifice or giving

karmendriya (*karmêndriya*) organ of action, such as locomotion as an ability

karuna (*karuṇā*) compasssion

Kaulism (*kula-marga*) "Way of the Family" (*kula*), an important stream of Kashmiri Shaivism

kaya (*kāya*) body

khechara (*khecara*) *mudra* with the tongue curled back to touch the palate, eyes rolled back with all attention on the *ajna chakra* (q.v.)

klesha (*kleśa*) affliction; five are listed in the *Yoga Sutra* (sutra 2.3: see appendix C) as obstructing spiritual accomplishment

kosha (*kośa*) sheath, body

Krama (*krama*) "sequence"; a stream of Kashmiri Shaivism (see note 5 to appendix D)

kriya (*kriyā*) action; series and combinations of asanas and movements with breath, outlined in the *Hatha Yoga Pradipika* and other yoga manuals

krodha (*krodha*) anger

kshana (*kṣaṇa*) moment, point-instant

kula (*kula*) "family" (see notes 5 and 12 to appendix D)

kumbhaka (*kumbhaka*) breath retention or halting, on either the inhale or the exhale; a technical term of *pranayama* practice

kundalini (*kuṇḍalī, kuṇḍalinī*) occult serpent power; divine energy said to be asleep in the lowest or *mula* chakra, the awakening of which is in tantra taken to be equivalent to enlightenment and *jivan mukti* (q.v.)

kusha (*kuśa*) grass or straw said to be suitable for covering the ground for asana practice and meditation

ku-yogin (*ku-yogin*) bad yogin

laghiman (*laghiman*) lightness; *siddhi* of lightness

lila (*līlā*) play, sport; as a concept belonging to Vedanta, the world as Divine play

linga-sharira (*liṅga-śarīra*) subtle body comprised of sense data or subtle elements transmigrating with the *jiva* or individual soul

loka (*loka*) world, field of vision

Madhyamika (*mādhyamika*) Buddhist "school of the Middle" (avoidance of extremes) founded by Nagarjuna

maha bandha (*mahā-bandha*) "great lock" comprised of the simultaneous performance of *mula, uddiyana,* and *jalandhara bandhas* (q.v.)

maha vakya (*mahā-vākya*) "great statement"; one of eighteen or so Upanishadic statements taken by Shankara and other Vedantins to have special import for Vedanta philosophy

Mahayana (*mahāyāna*) northern Buddhism; the "Great Vehicle"

maitri (*maitrī*) friendliness, loving-kindness

manas (*manas*) sense mind, the inner sense, the internal organ, the conduit of sensory information to the perceiving self, soul, or consciousness, according to several classical schools

mandala (*maṇḍala*) cosmic circle, graphic representation of the universe

mangala (*maṅgala*) "doing something auspicious," such as chanting *om,* making a flower offering, etc.

manipura (*maṇi-pura*) the navel chakra, the "city of jewels"

manomaya kosha (*manomaya-kośa*) body or *kośa* made of lower or sensuous intelligence, *manas*

manonmani (*manonmanī*) "mind without mind," a name for *samadhi* or the supreme state accessible through yoga according to the *Hatha Yoga Pradipika*

mantra (*mantra*) verse of the Veda; words or sound with occult power to aid meditation, open chakras, etc.

marga (*marga*) way, path

matsyasana (*matsyâsana*) Fish Pose

maya (*māyā*) illusion, cosmic illusion, according to Advaita Vedanta; according to Vedantic theists, "(self)-delimitation" (from the root *ma,* to measure or delimit: see note 14 to chapter 5)

Mimamsa (*mīmāṃsā*) "Exegesis"; long-running school of classical philosophy devoted to defending the scriptural revelation of the Veda

mudra (*mudrā*) "seal," gesture; attitude; form imitating that of an enlightened guru, channel to yogic experience

mukti (= *mokṣa*) "liberation," enlightenment

mula bandha (*mūla-bandha*) root lock

muladhara chakra (*mūlâdhāra-cakra*) the lotus center at the base of the spine where the *kundalini* serpent power rests (normally) asleep

murchchha (*mūrcchā*) fainting, swooning; type of *pranayama* in which the breath is retained for an extended period

nada (*nāda*) sound, in particular occult or internal sounds

nada-yoga (*nāda yoga*) the yoga of concentrating on internal sounds

nadi (*nāḍī*) pathway for *prana* and *shakti* (q.v.)

namas te (*namas te*) "salutations to thee"; see note 26 to chapter 1

naya (*naya*) perspective

nirbija samadhi (*nirbīja-samādhi*) "trance without any seed (of a *samskara* that would force one back to the waking state)"—*Yoga Sutra* 1.51 and 3.8

nirguna (*nirguṇa*) without attributes

nirvana (*nirvāṇa*) extinction (of suffering); enlightenment; the experience of the "void" (of desire and attachment); the *summum bonum* in Buddhism (although in Mahāyāna the goal is to become a bodhisattva [q.v.])

nirvikalpaka jnana (*nirvikalpaka-jñāna*) indeterminate awareness, "concept-free" awareness, nonpropositional awareness

niyama (*niyama*) (personal) restraints, the second limb of *ashtanga-yoga*, comprising: (1) *shaucha*, (2) *santosha*, (3) *tapas*, (4) *svadhyaya*, and (5) *ishvara-pranidhana* (q.v.)

Nyaya (*nyāya-darśana*) "Logic"; a school of realism and common sense prominent throughout the classical period, from the *Nyaya Sutra* (c. 200) on, developing out of canons of debate and informal logic; explicitly combined with Vaisheshika in the later centuries beginning with Udayana (c. 1000); focused on issues in epistemology but also defending yoga practice

padmasana (*padmâsana*) Lotus Pose

parama-purushartha (*parama-puruṣârtha*) "supreme personal good"

paramita (*pāramitā*) perfection; six moral and spiritual perfections are exhibited by a bodhisattva (q.v.), according to Mahayana Buddhism: (1) charity, (2) uprightness, (3) energy, (4) patience, (5) concentration (*samadhi*), and (6) wisdom (*prajñā*)

parampara (*param-parā*) lineage of teachers or gurus

parshvottanasana (*parśvôttānâsana*) Side Stretch

pingala (*piṅgala*) channel or *nadi* that runs from the right nostril, pranic channel; "Sun"

plavini (*plāvinī*) "floating"; type of *pranayama* in which the breath is swallowed into the stomach

pradhana (*pradhāna*) root form of nature or *prakriti* according to Samkhya

prajna (*prajñā*) wisdom; spiritual insight; one of the "perfections," *paramita* (q.v.) or marks of a bodhisattva (q.v.), according to Mahayana Buddhism

prakamya (*prākāmya*) *siddhi* of irresistible will

prakara (*prakāra*) predicate content, the "way" something appears

prakriti (*prakṛti*) nature conceived as operating mechanically, without intrinsic consciousness; a principal Samkhya concept

pramana (*pramāṇa*) source of knowledge; justifier; according to Nyaya, there are four: perception, inference, anology, and testimony

prana (*prāṇa*) breath; inhalation; type of wind or vital air or energy animating certain bodily functions; life or vital energy (see note 15 to appendix A)

pranamaya kosha (*prāṇamaya-kośa*) body made of life energy, *prana*

pranayama (*prāṇâyāma*) breath control

pranidhana (*praṇidhāna*) devotion, meditation, devotional surrender

prapanca (*prapañca*) worldly display

prapatti (*prapatti*) surrender (to God)

prapti (*prāpti*) "obtaining"; *siddhi* of cognition at a distance

prasarita padottanasana (*prasārita-pādôttānâsana*) Widespread Forward Fold

prasanga (*prasaṅga*) a form of philosophic argument: reductio ad absurdum, dialectical difficulty; Nagarjuna's refutational method

pratibandhaka (*pratibandhaka*) "blocker," obstruction; epistemic defeater

pratitya samutpada (*pratītya-samutpāda*) interdependent origination; the Buddhist doctrine that each event comes to be in interdependence with all other events

pratyabhijna (*pratyabhijñā*) recognition

pratyahara (*pratyāhāra*) "withdrawal" from the sense organs to cognize only sense data, or, in some interpretations, external objects directly through the *manas* (q.v.)

pratyaksha (*pratyakṣa*) perception; a source of knowledge, *pramana* (q.v.), according to Nyaya and practically all classical philosophy

puja (*pūja*) ceremony of worship

purusha (*puruṣa*) individual conscious being, person

rajas (*rajas*) *guna* of passion and activity

rasa (*rasa*) aesthetic "flavor," "juice"; aesthetic experience, relishing; see the list on p. 153

rishi (*ṛṣi*) seer-poet, author of mantras of the *Rig Veda;* enlightened seer who, with other seers in some instances, originates a tradition of yoga or a skill or craft

rupa skandha (*rūpa-skandha*) sense data, form, and matter as comprising a "band" of an individual (see *skandha*)

sachchidananda (*sac-cid-ānanda*) Existence-Consciousness-Bliss, a popular Vedantic characterization of Brahman in itself; *sat* = pure being, the self-existent, *chit* = consciousness or consciousness force, *ananda* = delight, bliss, self-delight

saguna (*saguṇa*) with attributes

sahasradala (*sahasra-dala*) "thousand-petaled (lotus)," divine center or chakra connectioning occultly with the *brahma-randhra* and *sushumna* (q.v.), four fingers above the head

sahasrara (*sahasrâra*) "thousand-spoked (wheel)"; see *sahasra-dala*

saholi (*saholī*) retention of sexual fluids and energy (for women, *vajroli* for men)

sahridya (*sahṛdaya*) the aesthetic expert or connoisseur, "like-hearted" member of an audience

sakshatkartavya (*sākṣāt-kartavya*) to be made immediate in experience

sakshin (*sākṣin*) witness

sama sthiti (*sama-sthiti*) Equipose Stance, the starting and finishing position of a series or flow of asanas

samadhi (*samādhi*) yogic trance, "enstacy," the ability to shut off mental fluctuations (see note 1 to chapter 5)

samagri (*sāmagrī*) collection of causal factors together sufficient for an effect

samana (*samāna*) "equalizing breath," one of five *prana*s mentioned in the Upanishads and manipulated in *pranayama*

samapatti (*samāpatti*) "yogic balance"; see note 13 to appendix C

samatva (*samatva*) balance, equinimity
samjna skandha (*saṃjña-skandha*) *skandha* (q.v.) of cognition, thought
samkalpa (*saṃkalpa*) intention
Samkhya (*sāṃkhya-darśana*) "Analysis"; an early school of Indian philosophy according to which the "supreme personal good" is achieved through psychological disidentification
samnyasa (*saṃnyāsa*) renunciation
sampradaya (*sampradāya*) yogic lineage
samprajnata samadhi (*samprajñāta-samādhi*) *samadhi* "with prop"; the penultimate stage of yogic accomplishment according the *Yoga Sutra;* see *asamprajnata-samadhi*
samsara (*saṃsāra*) transmigratory existence, the wheel of birth and rebirth, worldly existence
samskara (*saṃskāra*) disposition; mental disposition, memory or subliminal impression
samskara skandha (*saṃskāra-skandha*) *skandha* (q.v.) of mental connectives, rationality
samyama (*saṃyama*) control through conscious identification and extension of self
sandhi (*sandhi*) euphonic combination
santana (*santāna*) stream of psychological elements (*dharma*) said by Buddhist philosophers to comprise personal identity
santosha (*santoṣa*) contentment, self-acceptance; the second *niyama* (q.v.) according to the *Yoga Sutra*
sapta bhangi (*sapta-bhaṅgi*) seven styles or truth values, according to Jaina philosophers, i.e., seven combinations of three truth values, truth, falsity, and indeterminacy
sarga (*sarga*) creation, emanation
sarvangasana (*sarvâṅgâsana*) Shoulder Stand ("All-Limbs Pose")
sat (*sat*) being; good
sat-karya-vada (*sat-kārya-vāda*) theory that the effect in some sense preexists in the cause; view of causality appearing in Samkhya and Vedanta
satta (*sattā*) beingness
sattva (*sattva*) *guna* (q.v.) of intelligence and purity
satya (*satya*) truth; telling the truth, the second *yama* (q.v.) according to the *Yoga Sutra*
savikalpa jnana (*savikalpaka-jñāna*) determinate awareness, propositional awareness, verbalizable awareness
setu bandhasana (*setu-bandhâsana*) Bridge Pose
seva (*sevā*) service
shabda brahman (*śabda-brahman*) Brahman as the Creative "Word"
shakha (*śākhā*) branch of Vedic recension
shakti (*śakti*) divine energy, power of God; the Goddess
shakti pata (*śakti-pāta*) descent of shakti; divine grace

shaktopaya (*śāktôpāya*) way of the Shakta, the devotee of divine energy (*shakti*)
shambhavopaya (*śāmbhavôpāya*) way of Shambhu, Shiva
shanta rasa (*śānta-rasa*) relish of spiritual peace
shanti (*śānti*) spiritual tranquility, peace
shastra (*śāstra*) an individual science or craft; a scientific textbook
shaucha (*śauca*) cleanliness; the first *niyama* (q.v.) according to the *Yoga Sutra*
shavasana (*śavâśana*) Corpse Pose
shirshasana (*śīrṣâsana*) Head Stand
shishya (*śiṣya*) "fit to be instructed," student
shitali (*śītalī*) Cooling Breath, inhaling through the rolled tongue, a form of *pranayama*
shiva (*śiva*) kind, agreeable; Shiva, the Great God (*maha-deva*)
shlesha (*śleṣa*) pun, double meaning
shoka (*śoka*) grief
shri (*śrī*) beauty, divine beauty; an honorific used in the sense of "blessed" or "revered," e.g., "Shree Ramakrishna"
shruti (*śruti*) "hearing"; scripture; the Veda, including the Upanishads, according to Vedanta and other schools
shunyata (*śūnyatā*) emptiness; void vibrant with compassion, according to Mahayana Buddhism
siddhanta (*siddhânta*) established view, proven position
siddhasana (*siddhâsana*) Perfection Pose
siddhi (*siddhi*) occult power, perfection
sitkari (*sītkārī*) Hissing Breath, inhaling through the teeth, a form of *pranayama*
skandha (*skandha*) band, aggregate of psychological elements, i.e., grouping of qualities (*dharma*), according to Buddhist philosophies (see figure 4B)
spanda (*spanda*) pulsation
sthayi bhava (*sthāyi-bhāva*) abiding emotional state; see the list on p. 153
stotra (*stotra*) hymn
sukhasana (*sukhâsana*) Easy Seat
sukshma sharira (*sūkṣma-śarīra*) subtle body, astral body, pranic body to include the mental *kośa*s
surya bhedana (*sūrya-bhedana*) Splitting the Sun Channel, inhaling through the right nostril and exhaling through the left, a kind of *pranayama*
surya namaskara (*sūrya-namas-kāra*) Sun Salutations, a series or flow sequence of asanas
sushumna (*suṣumnā*) centralmost *nadi* connecting the *muladhara* and *sahasrara* (q.v.) centers or chakras, the central channel
sutra (*sūtra*) "thread"; a philosophic or another type of aphorism
svadharma (*sva-dharma*) a person's individual *dharma* (q.v.)
svadhishthana (*svâdhiṣṭhāna*) "self-established," self-support; second chakric center (counting from the bottom or *muladhara*) said to be related to sexual and "lower-life" energies; location of the *kundalini* serpent power, according to a minority

svadhyaya (*svâdhyāya*) self-study (in the light of a yogic text), the fourth on the *Yoga-sutra*'s list of *niyamas* (q.v.)

svaprakasha (*sva-prakāśa*) "self-illuminating," self-lit; an Upanishadic doctrine of self-consciousness

svarupa (*sva-rūpa*) own nature, own form

svasamvedana (*sva-samvedanā*) self-reflexively perceiving; cognition as self-cognizing, a Buddhist view of consciousness

syad-vada (*syād-vāda*) "maybe"ism, perspectivism; the view that each opposing philosophic position has some validity, championed by Jaina philosophers

syat (*syāt*) maybe

tadasana (*tāḍâsana*) Mountain Pose

tamas (*tamas*) *guna* (q.v.) of dullness and inactivity

tanha (*tanhā*) thirst, desire

tanmatra (*tan-mātra*) subtle element; sense data

tantra (*tantra*) systematic instruction; "web" or (more literally) "woven fabric" of belief; family of related religious and philosophic systems using feminine imagery in ceremonies and stories, a movement valuing nature as an expression of *shakti* (q.v.) or the Goddess (*shri*, q.v.)

tapas (*tapas*) asceticism, yogic "heat," yoga in general

tapasya (*tapasyā*) asceticism, yoga in general

tarka (*tarka*) hypothetical reasoning, drawing out implications; spiritual or metaphysical reasoning, according to Abhinava Gupta, the most important "limb" (*anga*) of yoga

tattva (*tattva*) reality, "that-ness"; principle of being or reality

tejas (*tejas*) heat and warmth; enthusiasm, energy; spiritual energy

tirtha (*tīrtha*) holy place, "crossing" (between worlds)

Trika (*trika*) "Triad," stream of Kashmiri Shaivite tantra; see note 5 to appendix D

tvam (*tvam*) "you," second-person personal pronoun

udana (*udāna*) "up-breath," one of five *pranas* mentioned in the Upanishads and manipulated in *pranayama*

uddiyana bandha (*uḍḍīyāna-bandha*) stomach lock

ujjayi (*ujjāyī*) "victorious breath," deep breathing with contraction of the epiglottis, a form of *pranayama*

upalakshana (*upalakṣana*) (conversational) indicator, e.g., "hovering crows" in the conversation pointing out Devadatta's house, "It's the one where the crows are hovering"

Upanishad (*upaniṣat*) "secret doctrine"; various prose and verse texts (appended to the Vedas, q.v.) with mystical themes centered on an understanding of the self and its relation to the Absolute or God, called Brahman; the primary sources for classical Vedanta philosophy and the first texts advocating yoga practices

upaya (*upāya*) way, means; yogic means (for Abhinava Gupta on four *upaya:* see note 7 to appendix D)

urdhva hastasana (*ūrdhva-hastâsana*) Raised-Hands Pose
urdhva-mukha shvanasana (*ūrdhva-mukha-śvānâsana*) Upward-Facing Dog
uttanasana (*uttānâsana*) Standing Forward Fold
vada (*vāda*) theory or perspective of interlocking beliefs
vairagya (*vairāgya*) dispassion, disinterestedness
Vaisheshika (*vaiśeṣika*) Atomism; a classical philosophy focusing on ontological issues, sister to Nyaya
vaishishtya (*vaiśiṣṭya*) relationality, typically the relation between a property and its bearer or locus
Vajrayana (*vajra-yāna*) the "Lightning-Bolt Vehicle," a stream of Buddhist tantrism (see note 7 to chapter 5)
vajroli (*vajrolī*) retention of sexual fluids and energy (for men, *saholi* for women)
vama marga (*vāma-marga*) the left-hand path
vasana (*vāsanā*) mental disposition or *samskara* that spans lifetimes, generalized subliminal impression and force; *karma*
vashita (*vāśitā*) *siddhi* of dominion over external elements
vata (*vāta*) vital air, form of *prana*
Veda (*veda*) "(revealed) knowledge"; the four Vedas, comprising principally hymns to gods and goddesses; the oldest texts in Sanskrit
vedana skandha (*vedanā-skandha*) *skandha* (q.v.) of sensation, feeling
Vedanta (*vedânta*) originally an epithet for the Upanishads ("end of the Veda"); school of classical Indian philosophy based on the Upanishads and the *Brahma Sutra* and centered on a concept of Brahman, comprising several subschools, Advaita (q.v.) and theistic Vedanta in particular
vidya (*vidyā*) spiritual knowledge
vijnanamaya kosha (*vijñānamaya-kośa*) sheath or body made of higher intelligence, *vijnana*
vijnana skandha (*vijñāna-skandha*) *skandha* (q.v.) of consciousness
vijnapti matra (*vijñapti-mātra*) "consciousness only"; a central doctrine of Yogacara Buddhism
vikalpa (*vikalpa*) possibility, imagination
vimarsha (*vimarśa*) self-consciousness; reflection
viparita-karani (*viparīta-karaṇī*) *mudra* or *kriya* that involves wholesale "reversal" of psychic energies
vira-bhadrasana-ka (*vīra-bhadrâsana-ka*) Warrior One
virasana (*vīrâsana*) Hero's Pose
visheshana (*viśeṣana*) qualifier, property; adjective
vishuddhi (*viśuddhi*) the "pure," the throat chakra, center of inspiration
vishayata (*viṣayatā*) objecthood, intentionality
viveka (*viveka*) "discrimination," especially of *purusha* from *prakriti* according to Samkhya
vritti (*vṛtti*) modification (of awareness)
vyavahara (*vyavahāra*) conventional discourse; everyday speech; taken by classical philosophers as *prima facie* evidence

yajna (*yajña*) sacrifice, ritual
yama (*yama*) (ethical) restraints, the first limb of *ashtanga-yoga:* (1) *ahimsa,* (2) *satya,* (3) *asteya,* (4) *brahmacarya,* (5) *aparigraha* (q.v.)
yana (*yāna*) religious career, vehicle for salvation
yantra (*yantra*) diagrams the contemplation of which is said to absorb attention
yaugika pratyaksha (*yaugika-pratyakṣa*) yogic perception
yoga (*yoga*) connection, relation; self-discipline; "union" with higher self or God
Yoga (*yoga-darśana*) the philosophy of the *Yoga Sutra;* a philosophy that advocates and defends yoga practices
Yogachara (*yogâcāra*) Buddhist idealism

Notes

Introduction: Setting an Intention

1. Sanskrit words are transliterated without diacritical marks except within sentences of Sanskrit text (which occur mainly in the appendices) and terms in the glossary. The first page of the glossary spells out the conventions utilized in this book (changing, for example, indological ś to sh), and gives all Sanskrit words used here both in the standard way with diacritics and in our anglicized fashion.

2. The *Yoga Sutra*, which belongs to the fourth or fifth century C.E., says that *om* designates the *ishvara,* the "Lord" (*YS* 1.27: "The Lord is indicated by the syllable *om*"). In this way it joins much earlier Upanishads, theistic Upanishads—the fourth or fifth century B.C.E.—and the very early *Mandukya,* sixth century B.C.E. or earlier, which is not theistic (see appendix A). The *ishvara* in the *YS* is at a minimum the archetypal yogin, self-rapt, self-illuminating, if not also, as understood by some, the creator of the universe (*YS* 1.23–29). Some view the *YS*'s *ishvara* as the impersonal self, *atman,* which would be, then, the sense of *om*. But Buddhists chant *om* while rejecting all notions of *atman* and *ishvara*. Suffice it to say that *om* means traditionally whatever the chanter takes to be the highest and best in herself or the universe.

3. Henry Clarke Warren, *Buddhism in Translations* (1896), "The Story of Sumedha," 5–31.

4. At *Yoga Sutra* (*YS*) 1.20 (see appendix C), we get inclusivism about ways to *samadhi,* the mystic trance or mental silence considered the goal of yoga (see section 5.1): "*Others* attain it (*samadhi*) through faith, energy, remembering (i.e.,

 meditation), and wisdom deriving from (previous) *samadhi.*" That there is more than one way to attain the goal is also stated at *YS* 1.24 with the use of the word "or" (*va*): the sutra specifies devotional yoga. The little word *va* appears again at *YS* 1.34 and again in each of the following five sutras. It of course functions as a sentence connective, but it carries the sense of a certain methodological pluralism. At *YS* 1.33, the method is *pranayama,* which apparently by itself can carry one to mental silence. Yogic sleep is another method mentioned. Analogously, different philosophies support yoga practices. The explanation why distinct methods of yoga work to achieve mental silence is that different people face different difficulties while each of us has a core consciousness that is silent and thought-transcendent. Once the obstacles are removed (*YS* 4.2 and 4.3), our true nature stands revealed. The analogy to pluralism in Yoga philosophy is that philosophy removes intellectual blocks that are different for different people and in general provides intellectual support for the practices in distinct ways.

5. Warren, *Buddhism in Translations* (1896), "Questions Which Tend Not to Edification," 117–28.

1. Theory and Practice

1. Swami Satyananda of the Bihar School of Yoga in a manual: "Try to feel the different parts of your body in contact with the floor. This is important for it starts to develop your awareness of the different parts of the body." Swami Satyananda Saraswati, *A Systematic Course in the Ancient Tantric Techniques of Yoga and Kriya* (1989), 27.

2. Charles MacInerney, *Shavasana, the Art of Relaxation* (1995). *Shavasana* is traditionally a very important posture. It is expressly mentioned, for instance, in the *Ḥatha Yoga Pradipika,* verse 1.32.

3. H. David Coulter, *Anatomy of Hatha Yoga* (2001), 62.

4. B.K.S. Iyengar, *Light on Yoga* (1979), 423–24.

5. Some of Iyengar's usages appear a lot more abstract and theoretical than others. Traditional theory of "breaths" and vital energies is itself quite complex. See the range of usages in particular in Iyengar's presentation in *Light on Pranayama* (1987), 12–14.

6. Swami Satyananda Saraswati, *Asana Pranayama Mudra Bandha* (1989), 27.

7. The term *chitta* (*Yoga Sutra* 1.2 and throughout the text) is used to frame the goal of yoga: stilling of the fluctuations of *chitta.* The word is a nominalized past passive participle of *chit,* to be aware. The "mind"—*chitta*—connects the world and consciousness. "Mind" is also okay to translate the Sanskrit word, although *chitta* includes emotion as well as thought and perceptual experience. With respect to consciousness, *chitta* is object, like the things of the world. But with respect to the world, it is subject, having an object directedness, or intentionality, among other features. In relation to consciousness, the "mind" can be controlled, in meditation. But objects determine its intentionality, in veridical

perception, for example, the objects perceived, which the perceptions in turn indicate, according to *YS* 1.8 and the classical commentaries. Similarly, a person can check remembering (remembering is a form that *chitta* takes), but any remembering would be *about* something or other experienced previously.

In the *YS, chitta* comprises thought, emotion, and perception, including internal perception, as well as dreaming. Perhaps the conscious being has a native perception, but all conceptualized perception, *savikalpaka-pratyaksha,* would be a formation of *chitta.* Emotion is thought to color *chitta* in common classical conception, but there are few explicit statements about emotion in the *YS.* Patanjali himself lists five types of fluctuation of *chitta* (*YS* 1.6). From *YS* 1.15, we might expand the idea to include desire. (See also *YS* 4.10.) Controlling desire is in any case considered necessary to still the mind, since desire is given voice by the mind.

For more on *chitta,* see in particular notes 48, 51, 55, and 56 to appendix C. For a modern account, see, e.g., J. Krishnamurti, *Talks and Dialogues* (1970).

8. For more on *ajna chakra* and references, see: Sir John Woodroffe, *The Serpent Power* (1928), and Hiroshi Motoyama, *Theories of the Chakras* (1981). Books from the Bihar School of Yoga generally include talk of chakras, as does Iyengar (e.g., in his *YS* translation: *Light on the Yoga Sutras of Patanjali,* 1993).

9. Swami Satyananda, *Asana Pranayama Mudra Bandha* (1989), 407–08.

10. Iyengar, *Light on Yoga* (1979), 437.

11. Coulter, *Anatomy of Hatha Yoga* (2001), 184.

12. The *Hatha Yoga Pradipika* (*HYP*) is not the earliest text we know of where chakras are mentioned explicitly. Several are earlier, e.g., the *Goraksha Paditi* of the eleventh century, from which the *HYP* borrows, and there are bits of much earlier texts that can be interpreted as mentioning, or presupposing, the tantric system, e.g., *YS* 3.29–34. See also note 30 to chapter 4.

13. The contemporary philosophic literature on testimony has begun to criticize an inferentialist account (we have to know that the testifier is trustworthy and infer that what she says is true on that basis). And it has begun to understand testimony similarly to Nyaya (to wit, that acceptance and understanding are normally fused, and that in practice we give the benefit of the doubt). H. H. Price, in *Belief* (1969), long ago moved in this direction (112–29). A paper by Arindam Chakrabarti, "Telling as Letting Know," in *Knowing from Words,* ed. A. Chakrabarti and B. K. Matilal (1994), presents a cogent case in favor of a noninferentialist theory (99–124). We could not understand one another were acceptance not the epistemic default. Then in a summary judgment about the whole area of contemporary philosophy, Peter Graham says: "The testimony debate is largely over whether testimony-based beliefs are epistemically inferential or, like perception, memory, and introspection-based beliefs, epistemically direct" ("Liberal Fundamentalism and Its Rivals," in *The Epistemology of Testimony,* ed. J. Lackey and E. Sosa, 2006, 93). Graham lists eleven leading philosophers who argue the "direct" thesis in a couple of dozen books and papers, and cites the Scottish philosopher Thomas Reid (1710–96) as the classical (Western) source of the thesis.

14. Nyaya's epistemology of testimony begins with the *Nyaya Sutra* (c. 200 C.E.), which suggests (in sutras 1.1.7 and 2.1.49–56) that the speech act of the expert who knows and wants to communicate without deceit is the proximate cause of acquisition of knowledge through testimony. Later Nyaya philosophers say that it is the statement under the interpretation of the hearer that is the proximate cause, the trigger of the knowledge acquisition, given that other conditions are in place.

15. Pattabhi Jois and his Power Yoga teachers famously use a form of *pranayama* (called *ujjayi,* Victorious Breath: see below, note 20) in their hatha flow series, but they too would say proper *pranayama* is done sitting or lying down. Among other yoga teachers tying this type of breathing to a series of asanas is Gary Kraftsow, who also follows the convention of distinguishing right breathing in asana flow from genuine *pranayama;* see *Yoga for Wellness* (1999) and *Yoga for Transformation* (2002).

16. The ones mentioned in the fifteenth-century manual *HYP* are nicely presented in English by B.K.S. Iyengar, *Light on Pranayama* (1987), as well as in various publications of the Bihar School of Yoga.

17. Among Web sites giving instructions for Moon Salutations, *chandra namaskara,* is http://odin.himinbi.org/moon_salutation. The following comes from Austin yoga teacher Cary Choate (to whom apologies for the modifications).

The origins of Sun Salutations, *surya namaskara,* are said to lie with Hanuman, the Monkey King of *Ramayana* legend, specifically in Hanuman's gratitude to his guru, the Sun (*surya*), for teaching him asanas—which he learned, so goes the story, backpedaling across the sky to face his guru and his chariot on their daily journey. The Moon Salutations series is said to have been developed in the Kripalu Yoga Center in Stockbridge, Massachusetts, but I could find no information on the center's Web site to verify this. There is traditionally no story comparable to Hanuman's and Sun Salutations. (Someone should invent one.)

The sequence: 1. Mountain Pose (*tadasana*) with hands at the heart in *anjali mudra* (see note 18 following). 2. Inhale to Raised-Hands Pose, *urdhva hastasana.* 3. Exhale and bend to the left. 4. Inhale to center. 5. Exhale and bend to the right. 6. Inhale to center. 7. Exhale to a small backbend. 8. Inhale to center. 9. Exhale to (1) Mountain Pose, etc., called *sama-sthiti,* the Original Position, hands in prayer position. 10. Inhale and jump to legs spread wide, arms shoulder height, palms above ankles. 11. Exhale to Widespread Forward Fold, *prasarita padottanasana,* hands on shins. 12. Inhale and look up. 13. Exhale and fold. 14. Inhale to vertical, hands joined in prayer above the head, elbows by ears. 15. Exhale and turn to the left for a version of Side Stretch, *parshvottanasana,* hands in prayer in front of the left foot or on the shin, head over the knee, which is bent at first and then slowly straightened. 16. Inhale to vertical, hands above head. 17. Exhale and turn to the right for Side Stretch on the right side. 18. Inhale to vertical. 19. Exhale to face forward and inhale, bringing in the feet to Raised-Hands Pose. 20. Exhale in a swan dive to Forward Fold, *uttanasana.* 21. Inhale, place the fingertips on the floor or on the shins. 22. Exhale, turn left, and step a large step back with the right leg into preparation for Crescent Moon Pose, *anjaneyasana*—a matronymic for Hanuman—getting ready to lift the heart or sternum (in imitation of Hanuman's devotion to the Divine Mother, Sita, who is also the Moon). 23. Inhale to Crescent Moon, slight backbend, remaining on toes, right knee to the floor, hands above head, elbows by ears, hands folded, fingertips touching. 24. Exhale and crouch, bringing the right leg up even with the left, on tiptoes with both feet, fingertips on the floor, hands under the shoulders and shoulder-width apart, weight on the toes, thighs parallel to the floor. 25. Inhale to Crescent Moon on the other side, stepping the left foot back. 26. Exhale and hold. 27. Inhale and exhale to Downward Dog, *adho-mukha shvanasana*. 28. Inhale, raising the left leg as high as possible, pushing back through the heel. (Variation: Tilt back right, opening the torso.) 29. Exhale to Downward Dog. 30. Inhale, raising the right leg in the same fashion as the left. 31. Exhale to Downward Dog. 32. Inhale, moving through Four-Limbs Pose, *chaturangasana,* to *urdhva-mukha shvanasana,* "Up-Dog." 33. Exhale and hold, look up. 34. Inhale and jump, step, or walk to squat on tiptoes, torso upright, crown of the head in line with the tailbone, chest up, thighs parallel to the floor. 35. Exhale and inhale to raise the arms to the ears, fingertips touching above the head, Upward Salute. 36. Exhale and inhale to stand up slowly back to the Original Position, *sama sthiti,* which is Mountain Pose with hands folded in *anjali mudra*.

18. "Hands Cupped in Offering" renders *anjali mudra*. The word *mudra* means (sacred) gesture expressing a particular attitude (here devotion), also seal, both tokening the meaning of the gesture and firmly securing it, "sealing it off," in the consciousness.

19. The reference is to *Gita* 2.48, *samatvam yoga ucyate,* "Yoga is defined as equanimity [balance, *samatva*]."

20. Almost all yoga manuals include instructions for *ujjayi pranayama,* Victorious Breath, which is mentioned in the *HYP* (2.51–53). Notably, it is practiced in Power Yoga, the Ashtanga Yoga of K. Pattabhi Jois (see: http://www.ayri.org). (Jois, Iyengar, and two other great modern hatha yoga gurus, T.K.V. Desikachar and Srivatsa Ramaswami, were all students of Tirumalai Krishnamacharya [1888–1989] in Bangalore and Mysore in South India.) Particularly clear on this form of breath control is Iyengar, *Light on Yoga* (1979), 441–43, whom I follow. The technique involves full inhalations and exhalations but no retentions. The distinctive trick is to sound like Darth Vader, slightly contracting the larynx as air runs through the throat.

21. The word *kumbhaka* is a technical term of *pranayama* or breath-control practice: "retention," i.e., a moment of stillness, of not breathing in or out. The word connotes the base of a pillar, and breath retention is commonly said to be a foundation of *pranayama*.

22. For *chin mudra,* the consciousness seal (or gesture), which involves, in one variation, the tip of the forefinger touching the tip of the thumb, forming a circle, with the other fingers extended straight, palms up, and the hands on the thighs or knees, see Swami Satyananda, *Asana Pranayama Mudra Bandha* (1989), 427–29.

23. The *HYP* lays out the practice in four verses, 2.7–10. Iyengar, *Light on Pranayama* (1987), has a long section on *nadi shodhana* (209–20), and my rendition of course ignores many fine points covered by him and in other standard manuals. Indeed, Iyengar discourages this practice until, as he says (210), "your nasal membranes develop sensitivity and your fingers dexterity by practicing the Pranayamas described earlier [i.e., in the preceding 200 pages of the book!]." H. Maheshwari of the Sri Aurobindo Ashram in Pondicherry taught me the technique in 1972 or 1973.

24. That yoga teachers use the term "sit-bones"—which does not occur in the professional medical lexicon—proves again my point of the first section that yoga teaching is from a first-person point of view. Sit-bones are easily identified in asana practice (they are phenomenological), but anatomical charts are drawn from an externalist point of view, as though the bones were not ours.

25. A *kriya* is an action combining a series of asana, breath-control practices, and/or locks. The particular *kriya* here is described at *HYP* 2.46 (see appendix E): "The throat contraction in place [*jalamdhara bandha,* Throat Lock], then through quick contraction from below [*mula bandha,* Root Lock], [and at the same time] by stretching the belly back [and engaging *uddiyana bandha,* Stomach Lock], the *prana* is forced into the channel of Brahman [*sushumna,* the central channel]."

26. The pragmatic meaning of *namas te*—literally, salutations to thee (or you)—is salutations to the (divine) child (in your heart). In proper Sanskrit usage, no one says *te* or any form of *tvam* to an adult, *tvam* being the familiar "you" reserved for children mostly, and *te* being the dative form of *tvam*. When such a pragmatic rule is broken, we understand a secondary or metaphorical sense, as we do in a yoga class with *namas te*.

27. Louis Renou in "Études Védiques: *Yoga*" (1953) delineates the meaning in the *Rig Veda*, which is the oldest Sanskrit text. The dictionary by Hermann Grassmann, *Worterbuch zum Rig-Veda* (1873), lists all occurrences of root *yunj* and its derivatives for the *Rig Veda*. K. S. Joshi, "On the Meaning of Yoga" (1965), surveys a dozen classical usages as well as usages within the early literature.

28. For instance, *Taittiriya Samhita* 4.1.1–5, verses that are repeated at the beginning of the second chapter of the *Shvetashvatara Upanishad*: (4.1.1) *yunjanah prathamam manas,* "Disciplining the mind first." The word *yunjanah* is a form of the verbal root, *yunj,* from which the noun, *yoga,* is also derived.

29. See note 2 to appendix A for comments by the great scholar and philosopher Sarvepalli Radhakrishnan on the controversy about importance and originality.

30. An excellent introduction to the history and multiple developments of classical Vedanta remains Surendranath Dasgupta, *A History of Indian Philosophy* (1922–1955), in five volumes. Volumes II through V are dominated by expositions of varieties of classical Vedanta; volume I includes a discussion of the thought of early Upanishads as well as Shankara's Advaita Vedanta. I shall say a few words in overview later in the main text.

Then there is neo-Vedanta, whose relationship to yoga practices and teachings is so rich and complex that it would take at least another book to do it justice. See, for example, works by K. C. Bhattacharyya, who takes an Advaita perspective—*Studies in Philosophy* (1956, 1958) and *Search for the Absolute in Neo-Vedanta* (1976). There is also most notably T.M.P. Mahadevan, *The Philosophy of Beauty* (1969), who at once endorses the classical Advaita understanding of Brahman and a criterion of beauty as reflection of Brahman in terms of temporality and finitude. Neo-Vedantins include the scholar and philosopher Sarvepalli Radhakrishnan, who in *An Idealist View of Life* (1937), among many books and papers, blends Vedanta with Western idealism. Further, Swami Vivekananda and Sri Aurobindo, among other yoga masters, are called neo-Vedantins. I shall have several occasions to refer to Vivekananda's and Aurobindo's teachings.

31. I explore Nagarjuna's influence on philosophy in my *Classical Indian Metaphysics* (1995).

32. Teun Goudrian and Sanjukta Gupta, *Hindu Tantric and Shakta Literature* (1981), 224–31.

2. Yoga and Metaphysics

1. See (in appendix C) *Yoga Sutra* 1.4 in particular.

2. *YS* 2.5. Bliss in Vedanta, including Advaita, is supposed to be intrinsic to our truest self or Brahman. This is a old Upanishadic theme, or megatheme, that is made dramatic in several passages, e.g., *Brihadaranyaka Upanishad* 4.3.33:

> If among humans one is accomplished and prosperous, in charge of others, best provided with all human enjoyments—that is, to consider human beings, (said to be) the highest bliss. Now a hundred times that bliss, a hundred of the blisses of humans, equals one bliss of . . . the Pitris' world and a hundred times that bliss equals one bliss of . . . the Gandharvas' world and a hundred times that bliss equals one bliss of . . . the gods-by-works' world and a hundred times that bliss equals one bliss of . . . the gods-by-births' world and a hundred times that bliss equals one bliss of . . . Prajapati's world and a hundred times that bliss equals one bliss in the world of the Absolute Brahman—and of one who has heard the sacred teaching, is not devious, and not afflicted by desire. Now this is truly the highest bliss.

3. *Brihadaranyaka Upanishad* 4.3.9.

4. Shankara, *Brahma-sutra-bhashya,* introduction to 1.1.1 (tr. G. Thibaut, *The Brahma Sutra of Badarayana,* 1890), gives us a definition of sublatable consciousness, which has a dualistic structure permitting what the translator renders "superimposition" (the appearance of one thing as another):

> But what have we to understand by the term "superimposition?" The apparent presentation, in the form of remembrance, to consciousness of something

> previously observed, in some other thing. Some indeed define the term "superimposition" as the superimposition of the attributes of one thing on another thing. Others, again, define superimposition as the error founded on the non-apprehension of the difference of that which is superimposed from that on which it is superimposed. Others, again, define it as the fictitious assumption of attributes contrary to the nature of that thing on which something else is superimposed. But all these definitions agree in so far as they represent superimposition as the apparent presentation of the attributes of one thing in another thing. And therewith agrees also the popular view which is exemplified by expressions such as the following: "Mother-of-pearl appears like silver," "The moon although one only appears as if she were double."

5. Shankara and his most able interpreters grasp what Western philosophers call the Kantian notion of the transcendental unity of apperception, and they distinguish the pure witness, *sakshin,* as a presupposition of all experience, from the self, *atman.* (Kant, by the way, conflates the two.) When it comes to the self, there is really neither the witnessed nor witnessing, since self-illuminating consciousness is nondual. So we have to keep mind, Advaitins would warn, that the "witness" is a concept of everyday life and experience, and that what we are after is the self. Bina Gupta has made these points especially clear in two books, *The Disinterested Witness* (1998) and *Perceiving in Advaita Vedanta* (1991).

6. It is a commonplace among Advaita authors that yoga removes obstacles (a dominant theme of, e.g., Shankara's *Upadesha-sahasri* [Mayeda 1979]), as do Vedic sacrifices with respect to bad karma. No action, Shankara stresses, directly brings about the supreme good, since the self is something already accomplished. See, e.g., *Brahma-sutra-bhashya* 1.1.4. The *Yoga Sutra* takes a similar position, discussed here at the beginning of chapter 5.

7. *Kena Upanishad* 1.3 (tr. R. Hume, 1921, 335):

> There the eye goes not; / Speech goes not, nor the mind. / We know not, we understand not / How one would teach It.

Here is a quotation from the eleventh-century Advaitin Shriharsha that I discuss in my *Classical Indian Metaphysics* (1995), 82 and 347, note 35.

> Indeed this (awareness as self-illumining) is made known by scripture, which is a source of knowledge (*pramana*) for it. (Scripture does not make it known directly, since—as I have already argued—it cannot, by its very nature, be known directly through words, but scripture) *indirectly indicates it* through its general purport (i.e., in considering the general purport of Upanishadic texts). Thus, although as it is it cannot be directly denoted, from the perspective of spiritual ignorance, in contrast, scripture in its general purport is to be taken as the knowledge source (*pramana*) after the manner of our opponents. In reality, however, it is self-certified in the form of consciousness.

2. YOGA AND METAPHYSICS

Indirect indication is discussed by the great New Nyaya philosopher Gangesha (c. 1300) in an entire section of his *Tattva-cinta-mani,* translated by myself and N. S. Ramanuja Tatacharya, *Epistemology of Perception* (2004), 641–57. The point is that expressions can fix a referent without having the remotest relevance to what the thing is by nature, its structure and necessary properties. "Devadatta's house is the one where the crows are hovering" tells someone where to find the house through an indicator, the hovering crows, that have nothing to do with a house—this is one of several stock examples.

8. Like Yoga philosophy, Yoga psychology is not monolithic. There are several overlapping schema, all of which are at odds with materialist assumptions. The "sheath" conception according to which consciousness has five types of embodiment—physical, vital (or "breath-made," pranic), lower mental, higher mental, and blissful *kosha*s—first appears in the *Taittiriya Upanishad,* c. sixth century B.C.E. (Brahmanandavalli 2ff.); see figure 4A. The idea has been picked up by centuries of commentators, including Buddhists in the idea of *skandha;* see figure 4B. While famously antimetaphysical, Buddhist philosophy, like almost all forms of Yoga, assumes a subtle body that survives death.

9. Here are the major theories. Property dualists say that, contra Descartes, consciousness is not itself stuff. It is a property, like an object's color or shape. Consciousness is a property of the living body. There is only one kind of stuff, but there are two kinds of property, physical and mental. (Compare classical Indian Charvaka: "From the material elements, earth, etc., consciousness is produced, like the intoxicating power of grain fermented.") Others, called functionalists, claim that consciousness is an event. It is something that happens, a bodily process or function, like digestion or sleep. (Certain Buddhists might be called functionalists by this mark, but Western functionalists, unlike the philosophers of the Eastern religion, see mental events as physically caused.)

Hard materialists, called reductionists, hold that all description, including description of the mental and consciousness, is reducible to scientific language. The reason—according to "type-type-identity" theorists—is that types of brain event correlate with types of mental event. Others argue that mind-body correlations connect nonrepeating particulars that stand as either the mental or physical terms. All mind-body generalizations are, to this group, suspicious: these are "token-identity" materialists. Another faction holds that our ordinary ways of speaking are misguided. What we say about consciousness and its objects phenomenologically is false, and, according to some, can be eliminated. Eventually everyone will learn to speak in technical terms. Words like "consciousness," "desire," and "intention" belong to a "folk psychology" that will be replaced by proper science, the terms disappearing, like "phlogiston." Other nonreductive materialists are "mysterians": consciousness is a natural phenomenon but human concepts are, for various reasons, inadequate to the explanatory task.

Functionalism and other nonidentity materialist views developed out of an epiphenomenalism in vogue a hundred years ago. Consciousness is an epiphenomenon that while distinct from things physical is caused by them. Consciousness has no causal power itself. The physical universe is causally closed. Consciousness is, then, in the current jargon, supervenient, like the faces in a photograph whose appearance depends on the colors and patterns of pixels on the paper, or the computer screen, on which they are seen. Any self or person, on this view, would have an all-determining material substratum, riding piggyback on its material cause. Functionalists say that supervenience occurs not on static physical entities but rather on processes. The correlates of consciousness are functions that physical things assume. An analogy to computer programs has become familiar: steps in programs do not reduce to states of electrons, since they might be realized in different ways on different machines. Computers made by one company of silver and by another of lead can all run UNIX. Programs are nevertheless entitywise simply physical.

10. Explanations have a structure: propositions that explain—the *explanans*—and propositions that are explained—the *explananda*. According to materialism, brain science would do the explaining; descriptions of consciousness and mental events would be explained. To state the point a little differently: materialists debate among themselves about the ontology of things mentioned in the sentences that comprise the *explananda* of brain science without abandoning the supposition that consciousness is physically caused.

11. Among the more dramatic and reputable of documented cases where there is little or no measurable brain activity is: L. K. Kothari, A. Bordia, and O. P. Gupta (all at the time professors in Indian medical schools), "Studies on a Yogi During an Eight-Day Confinement in a Sealed Underground Pit" (1973).

12. Actually, this view of later Nyaya was pioneered in its sister Vaisheshika school, in particular by Prashastapada (c. 550), *Padarthadharmasangraha* (tr. Jha, 1916, 1985), 570–74. Compare C. J. Ducasse, *Nature, Mind, and Death* (1951), 402–04.

13. Technically, only "indeterminate perception," *nirvikalpaka pratyaksha,* is the end result of the triggering of a person's physico-psychological dispositions, since "determinate cognition," *savikalpaka pratyaksha*, is fed its "predication content" (*prakara,* the way something appears) by an immediately prior indeterminate perception. At least this is the view of the New Nyaya school. The earliest commentators on the *Nyaya Sutra* (until Vachaspati, c. 950) do not distinguish the two types of perception.

14. Some of these reverse dependences are dramatic. Learning language, for example, fashions the brain in a very deep way, not just the face. The "wild child" called Genie did not learn language because of abuse, and her brain did not develop in the normal way: Susan Curtiss, *Genie: A Psycholinguistic Study of a Modern-Day "Wild Child"* (1977). Note also how a group of language speakers, e.g., the French, have facial resemblances in virtue of the facial movements required to speak the particular language.

15. David Chalmers, *The Conscious Mind* (1996), 94–99 and 120–21.

16. For other arguments, see Chalmers, *The Conscious Mind* (1996). Chalmers is rhetorically efficient in showing what is wrong with a materialist view of the mind, arranging the difficulties to mount a convincing case.

2. YOGA AND METAPHYSICS

There are several further refutations and motivating considerations identified in the papers of *The Case for Dualism*, ed. John Smythies and John Beloff (1989), among which is an asymmetry that many point out: our world is imaginable on (let us say) idealist premises that accede no reality to "matter," whereas it is not imaginable on materialist premises that accede no reality to "consciousness."

There are several who claim that one or another materialist theory of the mind resolves these difficulties, and there are now hundreds of books and papers by professionals in now perhaps the hottest subject area in academic philosophy. The reason for the excitement would seem to be, from the Yoga vantage point, that materialism is wrong and the fact of consciousness shows it.

17. L. Wittgenstein, *Philosophical Investigations* (1951).

18. Of course, we should not concede that literal meaning is in all contexts restricted to physical referents. Linguistic requirements targeting mystics' communicating with nonmystics are discussed in my "Mystic Analogizing and the 'Peculiarly Mystical,'" in *Mysticism and Language*, ed. Steven Katz (1992). The upshot is that mystics successfully communicate, although later experience may bring deepened understanding in an intellectual sense as well as experientially. In the classic discussion of Nyaya and other schools, being told that a water buffalo (*gavaya*) is like a cow in certain respects and unlike it in others, one learns, even without water-buffalo experience, what a water buffalo is. But after encountering a real water buffalo, even one's intellectual understanding is firmed up, while of course the experience is itself something richer. Yogic experience is, like an immediate perception of a water buffalo, a rather different mode of knowledge in the first place.

19. A famous chariot metaphor in the *Katha Upanishad* (3.3–9) has the body as the carriage, the sense organs as the horses, the thought-mind (*manas*) as the reins, the rational intelligence (*buddhi*) as the driver, and the self (*atman*) as passenger. But the point of the passage is that if the passenger would reach "the highest place of Vishnu," he has to give the orders and take the reins. The chief has to take better control of her subordinates, integrating the instruments into a spiritual journey.

20. Many Upanishads present dualist Samkhya conceptions. This is doubtless the reason the *Brahma Sutra* (c. 200 B.C.E.)—the founding document of classical Vedanta as a philosophic school—is at such pains to dispute the claim that Samkhya captures the teaching of the Upanishads. The *Bhagavad Gita* also uses some Samkhya terminology, and is generally counted as an important precursor for classical Samkhya. For the history of the major Samkhya texts, see Gerald Larson, *Classical Samkhya* (1969).

21. Gerald Larson, voicing scholarly consensus, puts Patanjali's *YS* as contemporaneous with Ishvarakrishna's *Samkhya-karika*, that is, around 400 C.E.: *Samkhya*, Vol. IV of *The Encyclopedia of Indian Philosophies* (1987), 165–67.

22. Among scholars, I hardly stand alone in viewing Patanjali as opposed here to the practicing mainstream. See, e.g., David White, "Yoga in Early Hindu Tantra," in *Yoga: The Indian Tradition* (2003), ed. Ian Whicher and David Carpenter,

 for example, 143, as well as, in the same book, David Lorenzen, "Kapalikas and Kalamukhas: Two Lost Shaivite Sects," 93–94.

23. There is also an internal inconsistency, since the *YS* conceives of *samadhi,* mystic trance (or the ability to enter trance), to be included in the nature of what it calls *samyama* (conscious identification), *YS* 3.4. How can *samadhi* be part of what *samyama* is and also be transcendent to all "powers?" That powers flow from *samyama* is the central theme of *YS* chapter 3, occupying thus almost a fourth of the sutras of the entire text.

24. Surendranath Dasgupta long ago in his classic *A History of Indian Philosophy* (1922) argued that Patanjali was a compiler and editor. He claims that the classical commentators Vachaspati and Vijnana Bhikshu also looked at Patanjali this way, without, however, citing textual evidence. My own sense is that this is right, though it is not said in so many words. The internal evidence, however, does make the case for Dasgupta's reading, which seems to me warranted on the whole. From Dasgupta (1922), I:229:

> Patanjali was probably the most notable person [of a certain school of Samkhya] for he not only collected the different forms of yoga practice, and gleaned the diverse ideas which were or could be associated with the yoga, but grafted them all on the Samkhya metaphysics, and gave them the form in which they have been handed down to us. Vachaspati and Vijnana Bhikshu . . . agree with us in holding that Patanjali was not the founder of the Yoga, but an editor.

25. Probably, however, a convergence of evidence (*pramana samplava*) should be viewed as Patanjali's official position, though this does seem the argument of *YS* 2.22 and 4.16. Accepted "knowledge sources," *pramana,* are listed at *YS* 1.7.

26. Classical Indian philosophers writing in Sanskrit were aware of the problems of the *YS*'s dualism, and, indeed, the view is not nearly as prominent as others in late classical times, so far as we can judge from philosophic texts. The *Nyaya Sutra* (*NyS*) itself contains a refutation of the Samkhya approach to consciousness (3.2.1–9), and Nyaya philosophers think of the philosophy of the *YS* as a brand of Samkhya without saying it in so many words.

And then there is an argument by Uddyotakara (c. 600), elucidating Vatsyayana's commentary on *NyS* 1.1.2. If the yogins responsible for the *shastra* (science) on the topic of meditation and other practices leading to the supreme personal good were lost to the world and incapable of communication, that *shastra* would be bogus—an outrageous possibility that Uddyotakara dismisses without further argument. In other words, if there were an entire disconnection of consciousness and matter in the liberation experience, then there could be no yogin "liberated in life" who could tell us about it. However, we are told.

27. *Yoga Sutra* 1.50: "The dispositions (*samskara*) created by this state (yogic trance) block the firings of other dispositions."

2. YOGA AND METAPHYSICS

In case some may think that Nyaya is not a Yoga philosophy since it is motivated mainly by epistemological questions concerning knowledge of everyday facts, let me point out that to accept yogic perception, *yaugika pratyaksha,* as a genuine knowledge source, *pramana,* is the mainstream Nyaya position. And the *YS* is often quoted by Nyaya philosophers as a psychological authority.

28. I mentioned the Buddha's parable of the arrow in the introduction. Nagarjuna taught what is famed as the "Four-Cornered Negation." From his *Mulamadhyamaka-karika,* 18:8 (tr. Jay Garfield, 1995, 102): "Everything is real and not real. Both real and not real. Neither real nor not real. That is Lord Buddha's teaching."

Within the secondary literature on Nagarjuna and his school, I recommend the overview of David Ruegg, *The Literature of the Madhyamaka School of Philosophy in India* (1981), and Christian Lindtner, *Nagarjuniana* (1986). For the logic of Nagarjuna's method, please see Graham Priest and Jay Garfield's "Nagarjuna and the Limits of Thought" in Priest, *Beyond the Limits of Thought* (2002), 249–70. Lindtner, however, seems to my mind to better capture the spirit of Nagarjuna's Buddhism since Priest and Garfield provide a decidedly intellectual as opposed to a mystic reading: Nagarjuna discovered true contradictions (a position they call dialethism).

We should note further that the mainstream Mahayana view seems to be that those who have direct (yogic) perception of emptiness do know something about the connections between the realms, albeit they cannot be expressed in ways easily understood by us. Nagarjuna, moreover, in addition to his more famous treatises, wrote letters of advice on yoga practice and indeed devotional poetry.

29. Advaita, despite its laudable silence about nature, is not so silent about the self. Like the metaphysics of the *YS,* the view strips will and action away from consciousness. The only value, and indeed the only true reality (to take these words in an imaginative sense), is self-absorption, the self's self-illumining consciousness. This leaves out our abilities; the self neither acts nor refrains from action. Extraordinary powers, *siddhis*, are a trap, Advaita avers (at least does one faction of Advaita, that following Padmapada, c. 800 C.E.), just as Patanjali asserted. Indeed, most of the same reasons that were given why Patanjali's dualism is unsatisfactory show that Advaita is not the Yoga philosophy for us. At least, it cannot be for those who are "experience seekers" or "*siddhi* seekers" (terms of derision that I have heard from contemporary Advaitins in conversation). Note, finally, that for Advaita the "mind" does not include the self. Indeed, it is open to Advaita to take a materialist position on mentality. The self transcends all science, as we learned in the first section, and cannot be correlated with anything.

30. Recognition of psychosomatic phenemona is no longer controversial within mainstream medicine. Imagery is a special instance, about which skeptics might consult the *Handbook of Therapeutic Imagery Techniques,* ed. Anees Sheik (2002), especially the introductory essay, 1–26, on the history of the technique in medicine by Carol McMahon and the editor, the latter a professor at the Medical College of Wisconsin and a past president of the American Association

 for the Study of Mental Imagery as well as the founder of *The Journal of Medical Imagery*.

Michael Murphy in *The Future of the Body* (1992) presents a veritable encyclopedia of "metanormal" capabilities, hundreds of pages of cataloging of dramatic determinations of consciousness. Murphy cites more than a dozen studies published in mainstream medical journals in a note to the following claim (372): "Many clinical and experimental studies have shown that imagery practice can facilitate relief from various afflictions, among them depression, anxiety, insomnia, obesity, sexual problems, chronic pain, phobias, psychosomatic illnesses, cancer, and other diseases." But some of the most notable examples of the power of imagery are in the Christian tradition of religious imagining, with well-documented cases of stigmata. See, in particular, 497–502.

31. The most dramatic yogic feat I know of through a modern scientific source, the yogic death of Haridas as recounted by the British Chief Medical Officer for Lahore and the Punjab, 1837, is highlighted by Murphy, *The Future of the Body* (1992), 472–74. This is a fantastic story, too long, unfortunately, to quote. The upshot is that CMO was convinced. Elaborate care had to be taken in reviving the entranced yogin, whose state may be compared to hibernation.

32. Ian Whicher is the first, so far as I am aware, to use the word "sattvafication." He also deserves credit for showing that this is the central transformational thesis of the *YS;* see *The Integrity of the Yoga Darshana* (1998).

33. An excellent survey is Michael Levine, *Pantheism* (1994).

34. The Indian theistic conception is developed in many of same texts that are the classic expositions of yoga; see appendix A. Of particular interest, however, is the "Inner Controller" passage from the *Brihadaranyaka Upanishad* (3.7.3–23), the first couple of lines of which are (R. Hume translation, 1921):

> 3.7.3. He who, dwelling in the earth, yet is other than the earth, whom the earth does not know, whose body the earth is, who controls the earth from within—He is your Soul [*atman*], the Inner Controller, the Immortal.
>
> 3.7.4. He who, dwelling in the waters, yet is other than the waters, whom the waters do not know, whose body the waters are, who controls the waters from within—He is your Soul [*atman*], the Inner Controller, the Immortal.
>
> . . . [and so through about twenty items: fire, wind, sun, moon, the visual organ, the rational intelligence, et cetera.]

For an overview and history of Indian theism, see E. W. Hopkins, *The Religions of India* (1970).

35. *Chandogya Upanisad* 3.14.1. Among many other Upanishadic passages that express the monistic idea is *Taittiriya* 2.1–9 (the Anandavalli), where the "sheath" theory is introduced (see figure 4A). Each of our bodies is discovered to be the Brahman.

That there is a single self that is everything is of course a centralmost Upanishadic theme. In the midst of punning and false etymologizing, the *Brihadaranyaka* brings out the logic with a light touch. From 1.4.1–2: "In the beginning the world was self (*atman*) alone . . . He was afraid. . . . Then this one thought to himself, 'Since there is nothing else than myself, of what I am afraid?' Thereupon, verily, his fear departed, for of what should he have been afraid?" In chapter 3, we shall explore the connection of this idea with the yogic practice of *ahimsa*, nonharmfulness.

36. Shankara, the Advaitin (c. 700 C.E.), says that although through yoga comes acquisition of extraordinary powers (*siddhi*s), "the highest beatitude is not to be attained . . . by the road of yoga" (*yoga marga*): in his *Brahma Sutra* commentary on sutra 2.1.3 (tr. Thibaut, 1890, 1962), 1:298 (translation slightly altered), and 223 on *siddhi*s ("that yoga does lead to extraordinary powers, such as subtlety of body and so on, cannot be set aside by a mere arbitrary denial"). Possibly Shankara means that the supreme good cannot be obtained by the road of the *philosophy* of Yoga, i.e., of the *Yoga Sutra,* for not only is this sutra, 2.1.3, and all the sutras in this stretch of text, focused on systems (*darshana*), often Shankara states that yogins know Brahman in their meditations, e.g., in his commentary on *Brahma Sutra* 3.2.22 (tr. Thibaut, 1890, 1962, 2:166). But more probably he is thinking about self-illumining consciousness, which indeed requires no instrumentation and thus no yoga practice (Thibaut translates *yoga marga* as "road of Yoga-*practice*"). But we should also note that, as Shankara says in his *Upadesha-sahasri* (Mayeda 1979), that to be "self-disciplined in peace, self-control, compassion, and the like (i.e., other yogic characteristics, *shama-dama-dayadi-yukta*)," is preparation for self-realization, the "highest beatitude," as discussed in the first section of this chapter.

Ramanuja (c. 1100) and theistic Vedantins in general take a positive view of yoga that is less qualified. Nevertheless, asana and other traditional yoga practices have to give way to *bhakti* and then "surrender" (*prapatti*) to God. In the course of this, the person is transformed, not so much in terms of *siddhi*s, personal powers that a yogini might exercise on her own, but *bhava*s and *rasa*, emotions and (spiritual) relishing, that do sometimes—it is commonly thought—have extraordinary bodily manifestations. Ramanuja's commentary on *Brahma Sutra* 1.2.23 is a particularly clear statement of his attitude about yoga and *bhakti* (tr. Thibaut, 1904, 284–85). The notion of surrender, *prapatti,* became central in the later tradition of Vishishtadvaita Vedanta that developed from Ramanuja and Yamuna (c. 1050).

37. Plato's theory of the self is discussed in chapter 4.

38. William James, "Does Consciousness Exist," *Essays in Radical Empiricism,* 1912.

39. David Chalmers, *The Conscious Mind* (1996).

40. Here we may mention that this is the Nyaya position, namely, that philosophy is a form of yoga; see *Nyaya-sutra* 4.2.42–48. Philosophic debate as yoga practice is striking in certain traditions even today, most notably Tibetan Buddhism.

41. William James, *The Varieties of Religious Experience* (1902, 1982).

42. From James, *The Varieties of Religious Experience* (1902, 1982) in the chapter entitled "Conclusions," 398–99:

> Although the religious question is primarily a question of life, of living or not living in the higher union which opens itself to us as a gift, yet the spiritual excitement in which the gift appears a real one will often fail to be aroused in an individual until certain particular intellectual beliefs or ideas which, as we say, come home to him, are touched. These ideas will thus be essential to that individual's religion—which is as much as to say that over-beliefs in various directions are absolutely indispensable, and that we should treat them with tenderness and tolerance so long as they are not intolerant themselves. . . .
>
> Disregarding the over-beliefs, and confining ourselves to what is common and generic, we have in *the fact that the conscious person is continuous with a wider self through which saving experiences come,* a positive content of religious experience which, it seems to me, *is literally and objectively true as far as it goes.* If I now proceed to state my own hypothesis about the farther limits of this extension of our personality, I shall be offering my own over-belief—though I know it will appear a sorry under-belief to some of you—for which I can only bespeak the same indulgence which in a converse case I should accord to yours.

In Hinduism, the idiosyncratic character of overbelief matches the arbitrariness of one's preference for a particular divinity, one's *ishta devata,* preferred divinity; see, in this book, p. 151.

43. Saint Teresa, "Prayer of Quiet," chapter 15, *The Autobiography of St. Teresa of Avila* (tr. E. Peers, 1960), 159 in particular: "In these periods of Quiet, then, let the soul repose in its rest; let them put their learning aside; . . . for, if the state of Quiet is intense, it becomes difficult to speak except with great distress."

44. Whether or not the person who wrote the famous commentary on the *Brahma Sutra* is really the author of the *bhakti* poetry is beside the point. That many have taken the *Brahma Sutra* positions to be compatible with *bhakti* is clear just because the poems are attributed to Shankara.

We may also note that the *ishta-devata* idea is prominent in Tibetan Buddhism, where it is stressed that the deity (*yidam*) is to be understood differently at different levels of practice.

45. Here, as mentioned, they join Nyaya.

46. *Bhagavata Purana* 10.29.47–48, tr. G. V. Tagare (1978), IV:1442:

> Recipients of such a high honor from the noble-souled Lord Krishna, the Gopis got puffed up with pride and . . . Lord Krishna disappeared then and there, for curing them of that pride and showering Grace on them.

2. YOGA AND METAPHYSICS

A similar parable is told by Apuleius in *The Golden Ass* (tr. Robert Graves, 1951). The beautiful Psyche has an occult lover, Cupid, who flies away when she, prompted by her curious sisters (two older sisters in whom she shouldn't have confided in the first place), tries to know too much, holding a lamp to see the sleeping Psyche.

3. Karma

1. Karl Potter distinguishes sharply between philosophical and transactional views of karma in "The Karma Theory and Its Interpretation in Some Indian Philosophical Systems," included in *Karma and Rebirth in Classical Indian Traditions,* ed. Wendy Doniger O'Flaherty (1980), 241–67, showing the difference between a philosophical theory and popular mythology.

2. Buddhists sometimes explain universals or natural kinds, such as being water, as collective karma. A weaker view is that collective karma produces an "environmental effect": we are reborn in worlds that we experience as having certain types of properties, and these properties extend to the *types* of entity we believe exist in these worlds, not just to particulars. Also, worlds are not necessarily spatiotemporally distinct. Apparently, collective karmically induced generation of certain object types correlates with types of subjectivity. For example, a *deva* (god), a *preta* (ghost), and a human can all see an object as liquid. But the *deva* sees ambrosia, the *preta* poison, and the human water. Here we have the seed of the idea of cultural relativity.

3. Tibetan Buddhists, for example, tend to view the "fully ripened" effect type of single action as determining type of rebirth in certain cases. Thus no matter how much good karma you have and how little bad karma, matricide, unpurified, leads to rebirth as a hell-being.

4. On the *YS*'s concept of *chitta,* see note 7 of chapter 1. In brief, the notion encompasses emotion as well as thought. A common Upanishadic theme is that the mind rests on pranic airs.

5. The Nyaya school takes over much of the ontology of a sister school, Vaisheshika. The great Vaisheshika author, Prashastapada (c. 575) lists *samskara* as one of twenty-four qualities, finding three subtypes, *vega* (impetus or speed), *bhavana* (the experiential, the mental), and *sthiti-sthapaka* (elasticity): *Padartha-dharma-samgraha* (tr. Ganganatha Jha, 1916, 1982), 570–74. Although there is debate about whether the overall category captures a true universal, a natural kind, as opposed to a mentally projected generality (see Gopinath Bhattacharya, *Tarka-samgraha by Annambhatta,* 1976, 361), it is not too difficult to see the commonality, the dispositional nature of all three as a kind of self-perpetuation.

6. David Hume, *A Treatise of Human Nature* (1888), 84–86.

7. When Yogachara idealists such as Asanga (c. 300 C.E.) and Vasubandhu (c. 350) talk of a "storehouse consciousness" (*alaya-vijnana*), they are thinking about things as webs of *samskara*s, more commonly called *bija,* seeds, and

 vasana, dispositions in the broadest sense—including, in this idealist perspective, not only internal objects but also material things as, to use J. S. Mill's phrase, "permanent possibilities of experience." Stefan Anacker writes in the introduction to his translation of Vasubandhu's *Vimshatika* (Set of Twenty Verses), *Seven Works of Vasubandhu* (1984), 159:

> What is observed directly are always only preceptions, colored by particular consciousness-"seeds." The very fact that these "seeds" are spoken of at all indicates a double influence. On the one hand, every consciousness-moment deposits a "seed"; on the other, each "seed" influences every subsequent consciousness-moment, until a "revolution at the basis of consciousness" is achieved.

See also, e.g., Vasubandhu, *Trimshika* (Set of Thirty Verses) 19: *karmano vasana,* the force of karma that provides continuity (K. N. Chatterjee, *Vijnapti-matrata-siddhi,* which contains translations of both the *Vimshatika* and the *Trimshika* along with a Sanskrit commentary, also translated, and the Sanskrit text, 1980, 107ff.). The commentator Sthiramati, c. 550, is quite explicit about all this: "[the *vasana*] is the seed (or force) deposited in the Alaya by the object and subject (subject-object aspect of a self-conscious idea) that had risen earlier and is capable of giving rise to the yet-to-be similar subject-object aspect (of a self-conscious idea)" (Chatterjee's translation, 108). Conceived of earlier as *dharma,* property quanta, they fall into bundles or aggregates, *skandha,* corresponding to, roughly, the sheaths of the Upanishads and Vedanta. See figures 4A and 4B in chapter 4.

8. Yoga epistemology of knowledge sources is carried out by commentators on the *YS,* and in particular by Vachaspati Mishra (c. 900), relying on Nyaya views. Sutra 1.7: "The knowledge sources (along with the veridical awarenesses to which they give rise) are perception, inference, and testimony." The testimony referred to is probably meant to include scriptural testimony, the Upanishads, for example, as well as what we learn from teachers and friends. However, if a chain of testimony does not orginate in veridical perception (or inference based on perception), it would be unreliable, the philosophers argue. Perception is the premier knowledge source, and presupposed in the working of inference and other knowledge sources.

As is elaborated in this book in chapter 4, yogic perception is one variety of perception, defended—but not normally appealed to—by Nyaya philosophers in support of their theses. Nyaya philosophers for the most part did not presume to be yogins, and have left us no mystic psychology. But philosophers sympathetic to yoga practices and psychology do not themselves have to be yogins, at least not master yogins or yoginis, and of course yogic perception (along with testimony) is all-important for Yoga's occult teachings.

Vachaspati, we might add, is a treasury of wisdom and sophistication: a tenth-century philosopher who wrote an important commentary on the *YS* but who was also a luminary in Nyaya as well as, strange to tell (given the disputes with Nyaya), Advaita Vedanta.

9. These ideas are elaborated by me in several publications, including the introduction to *Epistemology of Perception* (2004), 7–20.

10. Vachaspati and others call this the *anyatha-khyati* position, "perceptual presentation of something as other than it is." Though it is not universally accepted among Yoga contributors, there is equally a role for *samskara* on alternative views.

11. The olfactory organ is normally stimulated when tiny bits of odiferous substances are breathed in, coming into contact with it. This conception is common to both the early Nyaya and Vaisheshika literature. The Navya–Nyaya philosopher Gangesha repeatedly uses the sandalwood example; see my *Epistemology of Perception* (2004).

12. The idealist and grammarian philosopher Bhartrihari (c. 450), the Indian Plato, appears to have been an important influence on tantric views of creation, as pointed out by Howard Coward, *Bhartrihari* (1976), 111. Bhartrihari has a theory of perfectly ordered universals, a hierarchy in which the higher determines the lower all the way down to the particulars of our world.

13. *YS* 1.50–51 and 3.9–10. Instead of "firing," the term normally used is "awakening," and triggers are "awakeners," *udbodhaka.*

14. See Abhinava's *stotra,* translated in appendix D. See also Paul Mueller-Ortega's discussion, "On Subtle Knowledge and the Refinement of Thought in Abhinavagupta's Liberative Tantric Method," in Knut Jabobson, ed., *Theory and Practice of Yoga* (2005), 181–212. Abhinava's thesis of the *bhava* of the self matching the ninth *rasa* of *shanti* is discussed in chapter 5, the second section.

15. Translated by R. Hume, *The Thirteen Principal Upanishads* (1921), 110.

16. Compare Robert Nozick, *Philosophical Explanations* (1981), 409–11. Hitler couldn't just change his mind all of a sudden or change his character, as though just waking up one morning and deciding to be a good person.

17. The Sanskrit word *ahimsa* is a derivative of the verbal root *han,* kill, harm, in an irregular form of the desiderative—normally, "He/she/you/I *desire* to X." Thus the word *ahimsa* carries a desiderative sense: *himsa* is desire to harm and *ahimsa* desire not to harm. The desiderative form is also used for will and intention, thus "will to X," and *ahimsa* intention not to harm, i.e., nonharmfulness. The popular translations "noninjury" and "nonviolence" are satisfactory, but the etymological lesson is that the word connotes an attitude or personal policy. Nonharmfulness is an attitude one adopts, or tries to adopt. The idea suggests a rule, or set of rules, governing effort and action.

18. In Buddhism, the focus is instead on *karuna,* compassion, and *maitri,* friendliness or loving-kindness. But these are said to entail *ahimsa.*

19. Unless otherwise indicated, translations are my own. I take the Sanskrit text from the edition by J. L. Shastri, *Upanishads* (1970).

20. Perhaps the earliest occurrence of the idea is in the *Brihadaranyaka;* see note 35 of chapter 2.

21. I follow the Sanskrit of the edition by Gokhale (1950).

22. In Tibetan Buddhism, the doctrine is dramatically exemplified in a meditation (*toglen,* "taking and giving") that involves accepting the suffering of others. Those accomplished in it are said to be able to transfer disease from others to themselves where it can be purified. This is made possible by a fundamental interconnectedness.

23. There is a term for the "bad yogin," *ku-yogin,* and there are examples strewn throughout the epics and Puranas, perhaps most notably, Ravana in the *Ramayana.* That such a character is used as a villian for plot development does not undermine the standard meaning, which implies a kind of saintliness for the accomplished yogin and a striving for saintliness in the beginner. The concept of the deviant is common in classical philosophy; consider, e.g., the difference between the veritable knowledge-generating inferential indicator or mark, *hetu,* and the fallacious sign that resembles it, which is not a *hetu* but rather a "pseudo-reason," *hetvabhasa,* the common term for fallacy.

24. Translation by M. Kumar (1981).

25. From chapter 8 of *The Bodhicaryavatara,* which is full of arguments that hinge on likenesses among subjects (verses 90, 94, and 95): At first one should meditate intently on the equality of oneself and others as follows: "All equally experience suffering and happiness. I should look after them as I do myself. . . . I should dispel the suffering of others because it is suffering like my own suffering. I should help others too because of their nature as beings, which is like my own being. When happiness is liked by me and others equally, what is so special about me that I strive after happiness only for myself?" Shantideva endorses the Buddhist "no-self" theory: there is neither one's own self nor others' selves as enduring realities. Nevertheless, one should try to end all suffering (verses 101 and 102): "The continuum of consciousness, like a queue, and the combination of constituents, like an army, are not real. The person who experiences suffering does not exist. To whom will that suffering belong? Without exception, no sufferings belong to anyone. They must be warded off simply because they are suffering." Metaphysically, there is nothing special about oneself or others. The nonharm attitude we apply to ourselves for whatever reason ("just because suffering is what it is") we should apply to others equally (verse 103): "If it [suffering] must be prevented, then all of it must be. If not, then this goes for oneself as for everyone." Translations by K. Cosby and A. Skilton (1996).

26. In Vaishnavism, for example, this accords with *ahimsa* heading lists of virtues in the *Gita*—5.7, 6.29, and so on (see appendix B)—despite the martial context of the Kurukshetra war. The ethics of nonharmfulness is most probably Yoga's greatest contribution to moral philosophy as a whole. And it is, through Mahatma Gandhi and Martin Luther King Jr., a major contribution to a global political ethic.

27. Here are several subtle points in danger of getting mixed up. Self-sacrifice is surely both possible and commendable in the right circumstances. But it would

be the circumstances that justify assuming harm, and the presupposition stands that one would and should not harm oneself—without benefiting others.

In Buddhist ethics—to take up another apparently opposed position—the emphasis is on others. Though it is said that to achieve acceptance of the suffering of others one may start by accepting one's own future suffering, the ethical ideal targets others, not by any means oneself. All self-interest seems banished. Nevertheless, current suffering is seen as motivational, spurring one on or to take up the Buddhist path. Then again, meditation that causes a person physical suffering (within limits) is encouraged in some traditions (e.g., Zen). Moreover, surely mastering asanas is not easy, not accomplished without pain. But there is good pain and bad pain, and one must learn to tell the difference. Also, pain changes, as does thought and emotion, under the influence of self-monitoring consciousness.

28. This is emphasized by Arvind Sharma in his work on Jaina philosophy, *A Jaina Perspective on the Philosophy of Religion* (2001), 43: "while *himsa* has ordinarily been understood as harm to others; for Jainas, however, it refers primarily to injuring *oneself*—to behavior which inhibits the soul's ability to attain *moksha*."

29. An eloquent and complex defense of the proposition can be found in a chapter in Aurobindo, *The Synthesis of Yoga* (1973), "Standards of Conduct and Spiritual Freedom," 170–88.

30. Within the context of *bhakti yoga,* there is the recurrent theme of slipping away from one's daily duties to dally with God, like Radha to meet her divine lover, Krishna.

31. Personally I am persuaded by the arguments landing W. D. Ross in an ethical pluralism of a handful of basic duties (but only a handful), more or less the ones he identifies. Professor Ross recognizes a total of six basic duties, including self-development but also including "duties of fidelity (promise-keeping)," reparation, justice, benevolence, and noninjury. W. D. Ross, *The Right and the Good* (1930, 2002), chapter II, "What Makes Right Acts Right," 16–47. To appreciate Ross's view should mollify (by its breadth) the queasiness of those who sense in the notion of a duty of self-development a guise for "self-cherishing," rationalization of action done merely for the sake of self-interest. But self-development can be motivated by the interests of others (the yogini as heroine).

32. Of course, the point that one's first spiritual responsibility is oneself is not to be used as an excuse not to provide help to others (*seva,* service), protection, comfort, spiritual advice, and so on, as gurus are wont to point out.

33. This observation is made by J. N. Mohanty, *Classical Indian Philosophy* (2000), 108. On the pluralism of yogic methods according to the *Yoga Sutra,* see above, note 4 to the introduction.

34. Not only is this move made in the Jaina argument outlined above, it is implicit in Christianity's "Golden Rule," it seems to me, as well as in Confucius. See in particular *Analects* 15.23, where "likeness to self" is said to be the "single thread of morality."

Among Western ethicists, Kant perhaps makes the most convincing case in discussing applications of the categorical imperative where all hinges on our ability "to stand in the other's shoes," to see ourselves and others as alike as "ends in themselves" (*Groundwork of the Metaphysics of Morals* [tr. Paton, 1964]).

35. For example, Mohanty, *Classical Indian Philosophy* (2000), 91.

36. B. K. Matilal, "The Jaina Contribution to Indian Logic," in *The Character of Logic in India,* ed. Jonardon Ganeri (1998), 130.

37. Compare Kant's identification of antinomies of reason with respect to certain questions such as the eternity of the universe (*Critique of Pure Reason* [1965]).

38. Mohanty, *Classical Indian Philosophy* (2000), 91.

39. Translation by R. Hume (1921).

40. The Buddhist view is that harmonies arise naturally from beings with virtuous minds. Samkhya and Advaita Vedanta tend to take a negative view of nature.

41. Laurie Patton, "Nature Romanticism and Sacrifice in Rgvedic Interpretations," in *Hinduism and Ecology,* ed. Christopher Chappel and Mary Tucker (2002). This passage is quoted in Sridhar and Bilimoria (2007), 301.

42. That degree of value in general maps degree of organic unity is argued by Robert Nozick, *Philosophical Explanations* (1981), 415–22.

43. That karma yoga is not exclusively a Hindu teaching is shown by James R. Egge, *Religious Giving and the Invention of Karma in Theravada Buddhism* (2002).

44. The *Brihadaranyaka* opens by cosmicizing the sacrificial horse (tr. R. Hume, 1921):

> *Om!* Verily, the dawn is the head of the sacrificial horse; the sun, his eye; the wind, his breath; universal fire (Agni Vaisvanara), his open mouth. The year is the body of the sacrificial horse; the sky, his back; the atmosphere, his belly; the earth, the under part of his belly; the quarters, his flanks; the intermediate quarters, his ribs; the seasons, his limbs; the months and half-months, his joints; days and nights, his feet; the stars, his bones; the clouds, his flesh. Sand is the food in his stomach; rivers are his entrails. His liver and lungs are the mountains; plants and trees, his hair. The orient is his fore part; the occident, his hind part. When he yawns, then it lightens. When he shakes himself, then it thunders. When he urinates, then it rains. Voice, indeed, is his voice.

However, we might also label the theme "interiorization of the sacrifice," anticipating the *Gita*. See appendix A. The interiorization/cosmicization-of-the-sacrifice motif is brought out by scholar Mircea Eliade in connection with the Upanishads in *History of Religious Ideas,* Vol. I (1978), 238–41, and then with the karma yoga teaching of the *Gita* in *History of Religious Ideas,* Vol. II (1982), 241 (a few lines are worth quoting):

> It can be said that the *Bhagavad Gita* attempts to "save" all human acts, to "justify" every profane action; for, by the mere fact that he no longer enjoys their "fruits," *man transforms his acts into sacrifices,* that is, into transpersonal dynamisms that contribute to the maintenance of the cosmic order. Now, as Krisna declares, only acts whose object is sacrifice do not bind (3.9). Prajapati created sacrifice so that the cosmos could manifest itself and human beings could live and propagate (3.10ff.). But Krisna reveals that man, too, can collaborate in the perfection of the divine work not only by sacrifices properly speaking . . . but by *all his acts,* whatever their nature. When the various ascetics and yogins "sacrifice" their psychophysiological activities, they detach themselves from these activities, they give them a transpersonal value (4.25ff.), and, in so doing, they "all have the true idea of sacrifice and, by sacrifice, wipe out their impurities" (4.30). This transmutation of profane activites into rituals is made possible by Yoga. [Italics in the original.]

Eliade is in error here only with the "all" part of the idea of karma yoga embracing profane acts: not every activity is suitable for offering since not every activity can be offered in the spirit of *bhakti,* as I shall argue.

45. Aurobindo, *The Life Divine* (1973). The view is perhaps at odds with certain traditional ideas. For example, both Hindus and Buddhists have tended to see time in cycles, with temporal succession usually aligned with regression and tendency to evil, not progress. Thus the stories of the "Golden Age" (*satya yuga*). In contrast, enlightenment is usually viewed as a one-way transformation, so that—to take Mahayana for example—eventually the universe is full of bodhisattvas. Historicity is usually taken to be intrinsic to a Western perspective and foreign to the classical Indian, and Aurobindo, a "modern" thinker, received a Western education in the late nineteenth century (see below, note 42 to chapter 4). But I think the question of different cultures' views of time and history is not so simple as this, and the developmental strand of Aurobindo's conception is not just due to his "Westernness" but has at least something to do with his reading of the *Gita.*

46. Karmic confidence is dramatically exampled in Tibetan Buddhist stories of lamas planning their reincarnations and how they will be recognized.

47. Many views about *adrishta* are common across classical schools, but they are perhaps best developed in Mimamsa, Exegesis. Wilhelm Halbfass explains both the concept and its history with reference to Mimamsa and other systems in "Karma, *Apurva,* and 'Natural' Causes," in O'Flaherty (1980), 268–302.

In the Madhyamika Buddhist view, not only does karmic causation work without a temporal intermediary, it takes place without essentially existent entities. Moreover, almost all Buddhist philosophy eschews the idea of a substrate for karma to rest in. But in Hindu as well as Buddhist theories, karmic causation is something like action at a distance.

48. Warren (1896, 1973) collects many of the "life lessons" in Jataka tales. See also Speyer, *Gataka-Mala* (1895), which is a translation of a collection of

 stories by the Mayayana Buddhist Aryasura (c. 400, at best guess). There are similar collections outside Buddhism, such as the *Hitopadesha* (Wilkins 1886, 1968).

Note that generally in Buddhist theory one is not "punished" for being "bad," but rather has self-evaluating negative feeling tones accompanying experience as a psychic consequence of having engaged previously in actions of a certain type.

49. A classical source for the view that species continuity is usual is Krishna's assurance to Arjuna in the *Gita* (6.40–45) that as a yogin he is guaranteed a birth that will allow his practice to continue from the point achieved in the previous life. Admittedly, Krishna's statement does not itself entail that every human being is at death guaranteed a human future unless every human being is a yogin. But isn't everyone potentially a yogin or yogini?

In support of the possibility of cross-species continuity are such stories as Franz Kafka's "The Metamorphosis," where Gregor Samsa wakes up one morning as a cockroach lying on its back, as well as a famous passage from Chuang Tzu about dreaming being a butterfly ("Now I do not know whether I am Chuang Tzu who dreamed he was a butterfly or a butterfly dreaming he is Chuang Tzu"). My sense is that there is no mainstream position among the classical Yoga philosophies. Cross-species reincarnation is a common idea in the Puranas as well as, strikingly, in the Buddhist Jataka tales.

50. This notion, which goes way back to the Vedas (that Vedic clans reincarnate together is an idea that underlies the practice of certain sacrifices), was popularized by the American novelist Kurt Vonnegut in *Cat's Cradle* (1963).

51. Murphy, *The Future of the Body* (1992) lists more than fifty studies in support of the general thesis of reincarnation, but none, as far as I can tell, supports much more than the general thesis; see his appendix E, "Studies of Near-Death, Out-of-Body, Reincarnation-Type, and Otherword Experiences," 618–21.

52. Ian Stevenson, *Children Who Remember Previous Lives* (1987), speculates that adults are less capable of previous-life memories since they are much more occupied in the affairs of this one than children (54).

53. From the *Introduction to the Jataka,* tr. Henry Clark Warren (1896, 1973), 74–75.

54. The first section of the first chapter of Gangesha's massive *Tattva-chintamani* (Jewel of Reflection on the Truth of Epistemomology) is about the causal efficacy of *mangala,* doing something auspicious, such as chanting *om,* making a flower offering, etc. Some of his reasoning there seems playful, not serious. But in the last section of the inference chapter, on *mukti,* he argues that such actions can negate the payback effect of karma; see Ramanuja Tatacharya (1999), the *mukti vada,* 396–442.

55. The phrase "attraction of the future" is Aurobindo's: *The Future Poetry* (1973), 255: "the spirit is the master of the future, . . . in a profound sense it is the call and attraction of the future that makes the past and present."

56. The stock example of a *samagri* is the sprouting of a seed joined with water, sunlight, etc., a seed that by itself would stand as a necessary though not a

sufficient condition for a seedling. The bundle of causal factors sufficient for the sprout include the seed but also water and warmth and earthen nutriment.

Buddhists reject the notion of a bundle, but substitute similar complexity. The topic is discussed at length by me along with Joel Feldman in our forthcoming translation and explanation of the *Kshana-bhanga-siddhi,* "Proof of Momentariness," by the twelfth-century Buddhist philosopher Ratnakirti. Please check my Web site for publication particulars: http://asnic.utexas.edu/asnic/phillips.

57. Karl Potter, "The Naturalistic Principle of Karma" (1964).

58. Shankara's "Commentary" or *Bhashya* (c. 750) on the *Brahma Sutra* (c. 200 B.C.E.) 2.1.34, tr. G. Thibaut, *The Vedanta Sutras of Badarayana* (1890, 1962), part 1, 357–59.

59. Shankara, *Brahma-sutra-bhashya* 2.1.35–36 (tr. Thibaut, 1890, 1962, 359–61).

60. Johannes Bronkhorst, *Karma and Teleology* (2000), argues that the need to explain rebirth and the workings of *adrishta* moved the Nyaya school progressively toward theism. This may be true of Udayana and of others too, but late Nyaya is not as theistic as some think, being misled by Udayana's prominence in matters of natural theology.

61. Rebirth theodicy is in this way similar to the theory of Augustine (e.g., *Of True Religion*) that natural evil is payback for sin. The Indian theory has the advantage, however, of the punishment better fitting the crime than in the Western version, because there are lines of individual continuity as opposed to our paying for the sins of remote ancestors. However, then there must be continuity in the consciousness making choices and after-death awareness of the connection between payback and choice (compare C. J. Ducasse's reasoning, discussed at the beginning of chapter 4). Otherwise, there could be no moral lessons and the retributive nature of karma would make no sense.

4. Rebirth

1. C. J. Ducasse, *Nature, Mind, and Death* (1951), 491–502.

2. Twins born with a common hip that are separated by operation would both possess the memory of a pain that occurred in the shared body part before the separation. Other fission cases also show that identity does not track a particular psychological process or ability; see note 11 below.

3. The quote from Leibniz occurs in *Nature, Mind, and Death* (1951), 497, where Ducasse cites Leibniz's *Philosophische Scriften,* ed. Gerhardt, IV:300.

4. Ducasse, *Nature, Mind, and Death* (1951), 502. In a later book, the professor develops this plank of his thesis further, within an even more sympathetic treatment that combs through empirical evidence: *A Critical Examination of the Belief in a Life After Death* (1961).

5. See note 40 below for Udayana's version of the argument.

6. Abhinava, echoing a theme from the *Gita* ("one shouldn't disturb the minds

of ordinary people"), says that Nyaya is the philosophy for the masses, according to K. C. Pandey, *Abhinavagupta* (1963), 382. We, however, are interested in the secret findings of yogic experience.

7. Stephen Braude, *First-Person Plural: Multiple Personality and the Philosophy of Mind* (1991).

8. *YS* 3.38 describes the *siddhi* of what some have termed "possession." Supposedly, a yogin or yogini can direct more than one body at once. David White treats the power—questionably in my opinion—as a distinguishing mark of a yogin in "Ceci n'est pas un yogi" (2006).

9. Buddhaghosha, *Visuddhimagga,* "The Path of Purification," tr. Bhikku Nyanamol (1976), 2:521–22. The eighty-nine items all lie within the consciousness "band" or "aggregate," *skandha;* see figure 4B. Mahayana has a slightly different list of fifty-one mental factors.

10. Bernard Williams in a famous paper, "The Self and the Future" (1973), shows that what matters most is mind, not the body, by the following thought experiment. A future group of scientists, heartless but with the full authority of the State, have designed an experiment involving you and another person whom you know nothing about. In an operation during which you—we'll call you person A—will lose consciousness, your brain will be "wiped clean" and reprogrammed, so to say, with the exact content of the mind of person B. Body B preoperation will have your mind A postoperation, so that all your current memories, intentions, skills, dispositions to emotion, preferences, daydreams, etc., will be housed by current body B. You have to decide now (you are convinced that what you say will be decisive to the outcome) whether postoperation you would like the combination of body A and mind B (Y) or the combination of body B and mind A (Z) to receive $100,000. Which would you choose and why? (Let us stipulate no altruism.) Almost everyone chooses to be mind A and body B. We give mental factors greater weight.

Of course, the term "mind" hides many of the interesting questions. Too much is lumped together. Not everything mental is equal. My question: What about cross-life continuities? If there are some, as all Yoga supposes, wouldn't that change our opinion of what matters?

11. The Buddhist Shantideva denies that there is any such privileged relationship: see chapter 3, note 25, for some of his arguments that we should care about the suffering of others just as much as our own. But even if these are persuasive morally, they are still prudentially insufficient, it seems to me, concerning the rebirth possibility.

A fission thought experiment is supposed to show that personal identity is not what matters. Imagine that your only chance of survival is that your brain be bisected and each half transplanted to a body that has every one of your memories and abilities. Arguably, your personal identity does not transfer to both Lefty and Righty, since the concept of identity entails something single. But you surely would be happy that there are to be these continuers of you. Better that than no survival. Indeed, how much more work could I get done if I could double! (Lefty and Righty could amicably divide up chores.) Personal identity is, then, not what matters most, concludes Derek Parfit, *Reasons and Persons* (1984), 262, in particular, drawing a similar conclusion to Shantideva's. But this and other arguments against the rationality of self-interest are weak. (Parfit, by the way, who has a reductionist view of personal identity, himself claims that his is the Buddhist position: 273 and 502–3.) Personal identity may not be what matters most in the Lefty/Righty scenario, but this does not show that what separates persons—or, in the Buddhist view, consciousness streams—is not something to care about. Indeed, as argued in chapter 2, we have special responsibilities to our future selves, whether at any given time that be just a single future self (as presumably would be normal) or more, because our actions are special causal factors.

Note again that it is part of yogic lore that one self or soul or consciousness stream can divide or somehow live in more than one (physical) body at a time. Reincarnation presupposes that a consciousness factor is continuous through a series of physical lives, and multiple embodiments is a consonant notion.

12. Parfit, *Reasons and Persons* (1984). Despite the general excellence of this work, Parfit is wrong to claim that his is the Buddhist position. Buddhists on the person and continuity share quite little with him in broad overview, since I cannot imagine Parfit subscribing to any version of reincarnation theory and all classical Buddhist views embrace rebirth, with the possible exception of some varieties of (anti-intellectualist) Zen. Nevertheless, Parfit not only rejects, like the Buddhist, the sufficiency of physical criteria of identity, he proffers a reductionism, which can be read as opposition to any Nyaya-like view of an essential self, the possessor of properties. This is an idea that the Buddhist too attacks. And the real target of Parfit is self-interest, which, as we have noted, the Buddhist Shantideva also attacks.

The key idea in Parfit's analysis is overlapping continuity. I cannot remember the five-year-old birthday party but I can remember events in the life of the seven-year-old who could remember events at five. Personal identity is comprised of multiple psychological and physical processes. These, again, do seem to be like the *skandha*s of Buddhist theory; see figure 4B.

13. *Nyaya Sutra* 1.1.10 as interpreted by Vatsyayana, who begins his commentary by discussing recognition (*pratisandhana*). The sutra itself says only that cognition is one of several psychological properties that show the existence of a self by inference.

In the Yoga context, the importance of recognition, we should note, is not only argumentational in that the tantric Abhinava Gupta uses this type of cognition as a model of enlightenment, of the awakening of the individual to its identity with Shiva or Brahman. Similarly, some of the best evidence for reincarnation are translife memories and/or training (such as knowing a language not learned in the current lifetime, called xenoglossy). The possibility of these phenomena require, if not a self, translife lines of continuity of consciousness.

14. *Nyaya Sutra* 3.1.1 and commentaries. See also Jonardon Ganeri, "Cross-Modality and the Self" (2000).

15. Udayana's reasoning is in his famous treatise defending the view of an enduring self, the *Atma-tattva-viveka* (Discrimination of Truth [from Falsehood] Concerning the Self), where this is one of a barrage of arguments put against the Buddhist stream theory, though also one of the most important.

16. This is at least what Udayana thinks, voicing what he takes to be the standard position in late Yogachara philosophy. We may note that another explanation open to Buddhists would be a rather common yogic thesis about sleep: consciousness of objects or properties very alien to our ordinary, waking awareness cannot be remembered without special training.

17. Udayana, *Atma-tattva-viveka,* ed. V. Dvivedhin and L. S. Dravida (1986), 808–9.

18. The position that every moment of consciousness is self-conscious is termed in Sanskrit *sva-samvedana*, and is prominent in particular in the Yogachara school of Vasubandhu (c. 350), Dignaga (c. 500), Dharmakirti (c. 625), and followers. However, it is work by Ratnakirti (*Kshana-bhanga-siddhi*), who seems to have been Udayana's contemporary, that appears targeted by the Nyaya philosopher. Ratnakirti combines Yogachara with strong strains of Madhyamika.

19. There does seem to be one sense in which the person might survive. In Vedantic theism, as also in the process theism of A. N. Whitehead and Charles Hartshorne, God's memory is so vivid that the person's life would be as though eternally reenacted, like a halo in a river with rapids. See, e.g., Charles Hartshorne, *Omnipotence and Other Theological Mistakes* (1984), 32–34.

20. Here is another of the many thought-experiments explored by Parfit, *Reasons and Persons* (1984). Faced with mandatory travel to Mars, by a teletransporter (as in *Star Trek*) that destroys your current body, then replicates it down to subatomic configurations at the speed of light on Mars seconds later or the conventional way by spacecraft (requiring, let us say, two years), which would you choose? I have gotten mixed results when I have questioned students on this, and Parfit reports the same, explaining that people's prior metaphysical conceptions seem to determine their intuitions: 200ff. Personally, I would go the long way. The living body is not the only factor in personal identity, but surely it gets some weight.

21. Here we shall follow primarily the classical Vedantic and tantric inheritance, though there is a Samkhya notion of a subtle body that influences tantra in particular. According to Ishvarakrishna's *Samkhya-karika* (c. 400), the *linga sharira,* the "subtle body" that is the vehicle for transmigration, is made of five subtle elements (*tan-matra*) matching the five gross elements, earth, water, fire, air, and ether (*akasha,* the medium of sound): tr. G. Larson (1979), 268–69. In everyday life, we are acquainted with these subtle elements as the sense data delivered by the five distinct sense organs, odors of subtle earth, tastes of subtle water, visions of subtle fire (*tejas*), tactile sense data of subtle air, and sounds of subtle ether. This theory moves some Yoga philosophers (in our broad sense) to think about the *kosha*s, and later the chakras, as composed of different subtle

elements. But no one seems very sure about the connections, and the Samkhya view becomes absorbed in tantric principles of manifestation.

We should also note that there is now a rather large contemporary literature on near-death and out-of-body experiences that constitute evidence for survival. Such reports are not usually tied to a yogic or occult psychology, making them all the more probative for the fact of survival but not very useful for tracing the psychological lines that matter.

22. Mention of five *koshas* or bodies first occurs in the *Taittiriya Upanishad,* c. sixth century B.C.E. (Brahmanandavalli 2ff.): see appendix A. The word *kosha* does not appear in this passage, but it does appear earlier in the Upanishad (*Taittiriya* 1.4.1), and the commentators, rightly to my mind, carry over the conception to the list of five.

The *skandha* concept appears in the Pali canon (of which, scholars surmise, there was a Sanskrit version), and is used as an organizational category by the great commentator Buddhaghosha (c. 400) and others in the southern tradition. Among early Sanskrit texts where the notion is similaly organizational is the *Abhidharma-kosha* of Vasubandhu (c. 350).

Surendranath Dasgupta brings out the importance of the notion for Buddhist psychology at the beginning of an excellent survey of the central concepts of early Buddhism, *A History of Indian Philosophy* (1922), 1:93: "We have seen that the Buddha said that there was no atman (soul). He said that when people held that they found the much spoken of soul, they really only found the five khandhas [*skandhas*] together or any one of them."

23. The idea of such canals (*nadi,* also *hita*) connecting occultly the parts of our larger self is as old as the *Brihadaranyaka* (2.1.19 and 4.2.3) and *Chandogya* (8.6.1–3 and 8.6.6) Upanishads.

24. A famous passage in the *Brihadaranyaka* uses the word *loka* twice in the sense of field of vision, not parallel universe, since the passage is talking about a living person. Verse 4.3.32 (translated in my *Classical Indian Metaphysics,* 1995, 11): "An ocean, a single seer without duality becomes he whose world (*loka*) is *brahman,* O King," Yajnavalkya instructed. "This is his supreme way. This is his supreme achievement. This is his supreme world (*loka*). This is his supreme bliss. Other beings live on just a small portion of this bliss."

The other world or worlds or vision fields are said to be accessible by means of the pranic body through which we survive death. Sleep and dreams are supposed to provide evidence supplementing the testimony of those who are "travelers" by means of yogic trance. The accessibility is underpinned by the omnipresence of Brahman, according to Vedanta, although even Advaita Vedantins also hold that a subliminal being connects with nonphysical forces and beings inhabiting the various worlds, i.e., "levels" of Brahman.

25. The Upanishads mention hells, as do Buddhist texts. In my own view, this world can be hell enough! We might also note that it is commonly proclaimed in Puranas and tantras that ours is the only world where spiritual progress (through

 yoga) is possible. Ours is the only world of soul making. Other worlds are typal in the sense that their denizens do not develop through life, death, and rebirth.

26. I know no Tibetan, though since many technical terms in Tibetan Buddhist texts are taken from Sanskrit I can see a level of interlock beyond concepts expressed in English. The two translations I have relied on are: W. E. Evans-Wentz, *The Tibetan Book of the Dead* (Oxford: Oxford University Press, 1957), and Francesca Freemantle and Chögyam Trungpa, *The Tibetan Book of the Dead* (Boulder: Shambala, 1975).

Although I cannot claim to have consulted the translation by Robert Thurman, I may say that his *The Jewel Tree of Tibet* (2005) is the best introduction to Tibetan Buddhism I know of, capturing the tradition's spirit as an "enlightenment engine." At the end, Thurman comments on his own reading and translation of the *Tibetan Book of the Dead,* making sure we see the big picture that there are no dead persons. Our consciousnesses are ever moving on to new experiences and opportunites. We are right now as much dead as anyone.

27. Probably this is not the expression in Tibetan, but it used in the Freemantle and Trungpa translation (1975), 33ff.

28. *The Tibetan Book of the Dead,* tr. Freemantle and Trungpa (1975), 72ff.

29. Some Tantric Buddhists utilize a chakric schema that is practically identical with the Shaivite pictured in figure 4C, although a system of three chakras and other variations occur, as also within Shaivism. Here is a sample usage from an old Tibetan synoptic textbook, *Fundamentals of the Buddhist Tantras,* by Mkhas Grub Rje (c. 1500), tr. F. D. Lessing and A. Wayman (1968), which links up with the Shaivite *Hatha Yoga Pradipika* in its mention of a central channel or "middle vein," *avadhuti,* as well as "four Voids," 321: "through the "gate" of being a fit vessel for that [completion of the discipline], he contemplates in piercing the "centers" (i.e., lotus or *chakra* centers of the body). Thus . . . he makes the wind [*prana*] enter, dwell, and dissolve in the middle vein" (*avadhuti*); from that the four Voids are produced."

The diversity in the numbers, etc., can be accounted for by the complexity of our occult natures and connections to pranic, mental, and spiritual worlds or continua, in my opinion. To have a yogic experience of an opening or piercing in any single chakra from any direction can be, according to contemporary accounts as well as classical texts, an overwhelming experience. It would be easy to miss further occult complexity through being absorbed in something special, it would seem.

Another way to appreciate this last point using Tibetan Buddhist conceptions and our Jaina methodology is to consider that if the "three realms," the Formless Realm, the Form Realm (with its eighteen heavens), and the Desire Realm (with its six heavens and five migrations)—see, e.g., Robert Thurman, *Essential Tibetan Buddhism* (1995)—are in any way real (i.e., if there is to be a truth here, *syat,* as would say our positive perspectivalists), and if, the way all this occult complexity relates to us is through a subtle body of centers of consciousness or chakras, then surely we should expect diversity in chakric accounts from our variously limited points of view.

30. Sir John Woodroffe (a.k.a. Arthur Avalon) translated and commented upon the *Shat-chakra-nirupana* of Purnananda Giri of the sixteenth century in *The Serpent Power* (1928), which has had enormous influence, indeed probably too much influence, through another enormously popular treatment, Mircea Eliade's *Yoga: Immortality and Freedom* (1954, 1969). Eliade erroneously and achronistically projects Purnananda's version as the paradigmatically tantric theory—as pointed out by Paul Mueller-Ortega, "On Subtle Knowledge and the Refinement of Thought" (2005), 182.

Nevertheless, there is much overlap and a mainstream conception, as articulated, e.g., by Sanjukta Gupta, whom I follow: "Tantric Sadhana: Yoga," which is a chapter in *Hindu Tantrism*, by Sanjukta Gupta, Dirk Jan Hoens, and Teun Goudriaan (1979). Gupta presents the mainstream picture, filling in details from a wide range of texts (170–79). I rely also to some extent on Hiroshi Motoyama, *Theory of the Chakras* (1981), who himself relies, in part, on Woodroffe and (to be sure) the *Shat-chakra-nirupana*.

31. Such imagery occurs throughout the literature on the "living liberated," *jivan mukta*. The Shaiva Siddhanta authors of South India seem especially "fond," as Chacko Valiaveetil puts it, "of expressing this union in love in terms of a mystical marriage" (*Liberated Life* [1980], 132). See also the papers in *Living Liberation in Hindu Thought*, ed. A. Fort and P. Mumme (1996).

32. I have informal evidence for "chakric experience is not uncommon": informal surveys among students (eyes closed) about this, also with yoga teachers whom I have, through weeks of attending their classes, felt emboldened enough to ask. Now a standard take on this kind of avowal is that it is bad karma to talk about such experience. So my guess is that no formal survey would reveal anything of interest, and that the incidence of such occurrence is actually higher than my informal surveys would indicate.

33. The notion of yogic perception is discussed in Nyaya under *Nyaya Sutra* 4.2.38, where *samadhi* is conceived as a kind of *yaugika pratyaksha*. The notion is elaborated in the later, noncommentarial literature such as the *Nyaya-manjari* by Jayanta Bhatta (c. 850). It is universally supposed among Nyaya philosophers, although Raghunatha (c. 1500) famously quips against the Vaisheshika argument for atoms that if they are seen yogically, that we should find some yogins and ask. The thesis that there is yogic perception as a knowledge source is clearly expressed also in Prashastapada (c. 500), the great Vaisheshika philosopher, *Padartha-dharma-samgraha* (tr. Jha [1982], 392ff.). For the Buddhist theory), the Yogachara Buddhist theory, that is, see Charlene McDermott, "Yogic Direct Awareness as Means of Valid Cognition in Dharmakirti and Rgyal-tshab" (1991). The Madhyamika Buddhist who rejects the projects of epistemology may be counted an exception. But he too—like the Vishishtadvaita Vedantin who holds that testimony (viz., the Upanishadic revelation) trumps yogic perception—views

 the *summum bonum* as achieved through a kind of meditation, which counts as yogic perception for our purposes here. The *Kularnava Tantra* (c. 1100) makes a particularly clear statement about the authority of yogic perception; see, in appendix D, *Kularnava* 2.87–89. And so on.

34. Descartes thought that propositions restricted in content to appearances (experiences themselves), e.g., "It looks as though I am seeing a hand"—a claim that is true whether or not it is really a hand that I am seeing—were known with certainty, infallibly. Early twentieth-century Cartesians such as Bertrand Russell and A. J. Ayer considered such propositions "basic" in the further sense that the justification for everything that we believe about the world (i.e., everything we know outside of math and logic) derives from their certainty, the certainty of basic propositions. However, it seems a person can be wrong about an appearance ("No, it really looks more like a foot"), and no one has been able successfully to specify justification-transfer rules needed to justify an "observation statement" that is about a physical object, e.g., "I *see* a *hand*," from a basic proposition, "It looks as though I am seeing a hand."

With these two cracks in the dike, a flood of further objections has sent philosophers scurrying to other positions, externalist like Nyaya, as well as to coherentism, a kind of life raft for internalists (every belief helps to justify every other in a big circle of mutual support, i.e., coherence).

35. Roderick Chisholm, *Theory of Knowledge* (1977), 76; William Alston, *Perceving God* (1991), 79.

36. Among Ian Stevenson's many books and papers, probably *Twenty Cases Suggestive of Reincarnation* (1974) is the best known and most often cited. But let me recommend in addition a study in which the main types of evidence for reincarnation are laid out in the manner of a philosopher (where Stevenson shows the importance of children's spontaneous acts): *Children Who Remember Previous Lives* (1987). There is also in particular *Unlearned Language* (1984), which presents the evidence of xenoglossy.

37. There are some pretty good philosophic engagements with the broad topic of survival—Robin Harwood, *The Survival of the Self* (1998) and R.W.K. Paterson, *Philosophy and the Belief in a Life After Death* (1995)—but these do not really wrestle with Stevenson's evidence or theories (though Paterson has three or four pages of sympathetic discussion of some of Stevenson's evidence in the midst of a broad examination of parapsychology, 180–84). Paul Edwards presents an unfair treatment in *Reincarnation* (2001), more about which at the end of the section.

There is an excellent philosophic study of some related evidence, again, not so much for reincarnation as survival: Stephen Braude, *Immortal Remains: The Evidence for Life After Death* (2003). Intentionally bracketing the spiritual theories that incorporate a view of the continuation of consciousness, Braude shows that survival or persistence, however interpreted, is the best explanantion of certain evidence. His conclusion is that certain indisputable facts push even the philosophic skeptic to admit survival as the best hypothesis.

4. REBIRTH

38. I was quite delighted to find this statement by Stevenson at the end of his *Reincarnation and Biology* ([1997], 180–81):

> Having drawn attention to the limitation of genetics and environmental influences in early life, I need now to state that I do not propose reincarnation as replacing these factors. I regard it as a third factor that may fill some of the gaps in the knowledge we presently have about human personality and, as the cases of this work suggest, about the human body also. I turn now to some of the implications of the acceptance of reincarnation as such a contributing factor.
>
> The most important consequence would be acknowledgment of the duality of mind and body. We cannot imagine reincarnation without the corollary belief that minds are associated with bodies during our familiar life, but are also independent of bodies to the extent of being fully separable from them and surviving the death of their associated body. (At some later time, they become associated with a new physical body.) In saying this I declare myself an adherent of interactionist dualism. Proponents of dualism do not deny the usefulness of brains for our everyday living, but they do deny that minds are nothing but the subjective experiences of brain activity. How minds and brains interact during life is part of the agenda for future research, but that is equally true of the claims confidently made by many neuroscientists who assert that minds are reducible to brain activity. We need not, however, be misled into mistaking claims for accomplishments.

39. See *Trends in Rebirth Research*, ed. Nimal Senanayake (2001).

40. The argument appears in the earliest stratum of Nyaya literature, the *Nyaya Sutra*, and remains intact through the centuries. Here is the version from Udayana (c. 1000) and his *Atma-tattva-viveka* (translation by me from V. Dvivedhin, 1986):

> And, if it were the body that has consciousness, then a (newborn) child would not be able for a first time to make effort (to acquire something desired or to avoid something disliked). For, without desire or aversion, effort makes no sense. And without recognition (*pratisandhana*, recognitive synthesis) of how the desired is to be acquired, desire makes no sense. Inasmuch as (under the circumstances) there would be no memory (on the part of the newborn child) of the connection that has not been experienced in the current lifetime, such recognition (*pratisandhana*) would not happen (whereas in fact the newborn desiring milk reaches for the breast of its mother). And with respect to what has been experienced in another birth, the experiencer (presuming, *ex hypothesi*, that it is the physical body), having (been cremated and) turned to ashes, there would be no remembering by another (body, that is, still supposing counterfactually that it is the body that is the locus of consciousness). Furthermore, in this very lifetime the causal relation between (*samskara*-forming)

experiences at the one end and effort (and action) at the other is definitely known. And so, in the absence of the one (experience, etc.), there is absence of the other (desire, etc.)—a proposition that is easy to grasp. (However, there is desire, etc., and so there must have been experience, etc.)

41. *YS* 3.18 is on the *siddhi* of rebirth memory. Krishna tells Arjuna in the *Gita* (4.5) that he can remember his previous births. And the common view in Buddhism is that this and other *siddhi*s are by-products of mental concentration.

42. Let me sketch the background of the philosopher-yogin, Sri Aurobindo (Ghose), 1872–1950. As Aravinda Ackroyd Ghose, he received what was called at the end of the nineteenth century a Western education. After returning to India from England in 1892, Aurobindo became first a politician and then a yogin. Author of a long work of spiritual metaphysics, *The Life Divine,* as well as of several on yoga practice, most importantly *The Synthesis of Yoga,* he was also a poet and composed an epic poem, *Savitri.* Almost all of his writing is in English, but the sources of his philosophy are mainly in Sanskrit. The young Aravinda began learning Sanskrit at Cambridge University, but on his return to India he became an avid student of classical Indian culture and, as mentioned, a politician and later a yogin with a self-avowed "silent mind."

In overview, we may say that Aurobindo uses the highbrow vocabulary of his Victorian education as well as the spiritual language of Vedanta and tantra to try to forge what he touts as a spiritual philosophy suited for our global society by being sensitive to science. How well the theory connects to biology, however, is questionable, since it is not clear that his use of the term "evolution" is scientific. But this is besides the point for our purposes, since here we concern ourselves not with the question of the connection of his views with science but with a metaphysical argument of his for reincarnation.

43. Here is a stretch of very abstract reasoning from Aurobindo, first considering and then rejecting the possibility that the One could simply assume our personalities each in turn without translife continuity, or with only, as in Buddhism and Advaita Vedanta, (illusory) karma-maintained continuity ending in dissolution of individuality in the single spiritual consciousness.

> The One Being personalised would pass through various forms of becoming at fancy or according to some law of the consequences of action, till the close came by an enlightenment, a return to Oneness, a withdrawal of the Sole and Identical from that particular individualisation. But such a cycle would have no original or final determining Truth which would give it any significance. There is nothing for which it would be necessary; it would be merely a play, a Lila. . . . [On my theory in contrast] the progressive ascent of the individual becomes a keynote of this cosmic significance, and the rebirth of the soul in the body becomes a natural and unavoidable consequence of the truth of the Becoming and its inherent law. Rebirth is an indispensable machinery for the working out of a spiritual evolution. . . .

. . . It is through the conscious individual that this recovery [i.e., self realization, spiritual enlightenment] is possible; it is in him that the evolving consciousness becomes organized and capable of awakening to its own Reality. The immense importance of the individual being, which increases as he rises in the scale, is the most remarkable and significant fact of a universe which started without consciousness and without individuality in an undifferentiated Nescience. This importance can only be justified if the Self as individual is no less real as the Self as cosmic Being or Spirit and both are powers of the Eternal. It is only so that can be explained the necessity for the growth of the individual and his discovery of himself as a condition for the discovery of a cosmic Self and Consciousness and of the supreme Reality. If we adopt this solution, this is the first result, the reality of the persistent individual; but from that first consequence the other result follows, that rebirth of some kind is no longer a possible machinery which may or may not be accepted, it becomes a necessity, an inevitable outcome of the root nature of our existence. (Aurobindo, *The Life Divine* [1973], 754–56)

44. Aurobindo, *The Life Divine* (1973), 671–78.

45. This is an old epithet used by Vedantins of all stripes that derives from several Upanishads. Aurobindo's notion of Sachchidananda departs from the Advaita understanding in a theistic and tantric direction, with the Chit portion understood as "Chit-Shakti," divine "Consciousness-Force" (to use his terms and spellings).

46. Paul Edwards, *Reincarnation: A Critical Examination* (2001), which, sadly, was published just before his death.

47. Edwards, *Reincarnation: A Critical Examination* (2001), 279.

5. Powers

1. Effort of will is implicit in the notion of *samadhi*. True, the word *samadhi* is used in the *YS* to articulate the *summum bonum* psychologically, and the metaphysics of the *YS* demands that effort be on the side of *prakriti,* our everyday intuitions be damned. But the very etymology of the word reveals a voluntarist sense. It is a noun derived from the verbal root *dha,* to put or hold, which when joined with verbal prefixes *sam* and *a* (long *ā*) to form the stem, *sam-a-dha,* as a verb is used in an active and voluntarist sense: "to place or put or hold or fix together . . . ; to compose, set right, . . . put in order; . . . to effect, cause, produce" are some of the meanings listed in the Monier-Williams *Sanskrit-English Dictionary* (1851). I would not insist upon "ability to maintain trance" to render the word in the *YS*. But this translation fits nicely with the overall voluntarism of yoga practice.

The great scholar of yoga, Mircea Eliade, coined the term "enstacy" as a translation of *samadhi*. Unlike ecstacy (standing outside oneself), enstacy (standing within) comprises an inner bliss. Others, of course, have offered alternative renderings. My view is that the word should be anglicized (as it has been already in some circles). As an interpreter, I would prefer a translation with a voluntarist spin, something along the lines of "yogic accomplishment."

2. Yogic trance, *samadhi,* has a cognitive dimension. Many of the *siddhi*s are cognitive, and *YS* 3.25 says in general that "the object of any effort is known, whether subtle, hidden, or distant, by directing on it the higher light." This connects the higher consciousness made available by yoga to the world. Furthermore, how could *samadhi* be part of what *samyama* is (control through conscious identification) and also transcend all powers? This is an outright inconsistency.

3. Throughout Hinduism, mantralike prayers—addressed to Vishnu, Kali, the elephant-headed Ganesha (*ganeshaya namah*), and so on—ask the deity to remove obstacles (*vighna*). Processes have natural flows, including, say, mastering Headstand (*shirshasana*) or writing a book, which, once the intention is set (presupposing a coherent plan), will be completed if no obstacles occur. Thus one performs *mangala,* does something auspicious, to invite the appropriate protection.

4. The word *asmita* is a synonym for *ahamkara* (egoism), which is alluded to at *Samkhya-karika* 3 and mentioned at *karika* 22 apparently as the principle of individuation; see Gerald Larson, *Classical Samkhya* (1979), which contains a translation, for these verses, 256 and 262–63.

5. Interestingly, one could also read *YS* 4.4 as proposing a teleological conception of the *purusha,* not of *prakriti* (as pronounced earlier in the text, viz., *YS* 2.21): the conscious being is impelled to embodiment. Thus we would have a conception similar to the Whiteheadean concept of God, who is always necessarily embodied.

6. Abhinava too mentions this conception of the bodhisattva; see the end of the first selection from his works in appendix D.

7. Shankara uses the metaphor of the world as "play," *lila,* "sport," without purpose, according to his commentary on *Brahma-sutra-bhashya* 2.1.34 (Georg Thibaut, trans., *The Vedanta Sutras of Badarayana* [1962], 358–59). But it is the Vaishnava preceptors, Vallabha (c. 1500) along with the yogin and saint Chaitanya of the same time, and Chaitanya's followers Rupa and Jiva Gosvami in particular who make the tasting of *rasa* in spiritual experience the leading motif of their Yoga philosophies.

On the Buddhist side, we might mention the Four Purities central to Tibetan tantrism, which as Vajrayana (lightning bolt) practices are meant to bring enlightenment in a single birth: seeing your body as the body of the deity; seeing your environment as the *mandala* (cosmic circle) of the deity; seeing your pleasures as the enjoyments of the deity; and acting only for the benefit of others.

8. Vivekananda, *The Complete Works of Swami Vivekananda,* 5:137 (letter dated 9 July 1897). The letter must have been published in an early collection since Aurobindo flags the passage in his *Synthesis of Yoga* (1973, first published 1914–1920), by quoting at length, 257–58.

9. Abhinava goes light on *kama,* sexual desire, as opposed to *krodha,* anger,

in his commentary on *Gita* 3.37, a verse that seems to imply that both are obstacles: Arvind Sharma, *The Gitartharthasangraha of Abhinavagupta* (1983), 126–26. Rupa Gosvami puts passionate love and devotion to Krishna as more important than *moksha,* liberation, which is then no longer the *summum bonum; Bhakti-rasamrita-sindhu,* tr. D. Haberman (2003).

10. See Plato, *Phaedrus* (in the standardized pagination) 245c–246b and 253c–254e; *Republic* 435b–c, 436a–d, 437b–d, and 439c–442b; and *Symposium* 209e–212b, in particular.

11. Nyaya's teleological argument is one of a host of theistic proofs put forth by Udayana (c. 1000) in his *Nyaya-kusumanjali,* ed. Goswami (1972). Of Udayana's many arguments, Gangesha (c. 1325), the new logician, writes only on the teleological in a long section of the inference chapter of his *Tattva-cinta-mani.* That section has been translated (and analyzed) by John Vattanky, *Gangesa's Philosophy of God* (1984). The simplest version runs: Earth and the like are caused (by a conscious agent, namely God), since they are (artifactlike) effects, like a pot. This and all of Udayana's arguments are ably scrutinized by Gopikamohan Bhattacharya, *Studies in Nyaya-Vaisheshika Theism* (1961). See also George Chemparathy, *An Indian Rational Theology* (1972).

12. Officially the *pramana*, the knowledge source, for the existence and nature of God is scripture, according to Vedantic theists upholding *bhakti*, who often reject rational theology as irrelevant or inconclusive. My point is, however, about the views of the practitioner that seem implicit in what she says and does. In Buddhism, the origin would of course be (divine) "emptiness" or the Buddha Mind, which is not really an origin but serves as an absolute reality and foundation of everything ("everything is empty"). In tantra, the origin is the Goddess, nature not mechanical but infused with divine consciousness.

13. This is not the only source of *bhakti.* Music and other forms of beauty and art, even philosophy, are said to provoke *bhakti,* which has several wellsprings. But though the emotion is not just for the teacher aspect of the divine, this does seem particularly important. Compare *YS* 1.26 (appendix C), which conceives of the *ishvara* as teacher—a position we shall focus on at the end of the section.

14. The word *maya* is understood by Advaitins as illusion, but this seems wrong here. The word derives from the root *ma,* to measure, delimit, and here it suggests that the special divine descent is like the overall process of creation (*sarga,* here Krishna using the verb, *srijami,* "I create [by emanating]"), where God, or Brahman, measures itself out, i.e., delimits itself, in becoming the finite universe.

15. The translation is mine. The Sanskrit is from the edition by Gokhale (1950).

16. Compare the Christian idea in "For God so loved the world that he sent his only begotten son" (John 3.16).

17. That the *Gita* is a yoga manual is recognized by tantrics such as Abhinava, who wrote an important commentary translated by Arvind Sharma (1983). The *Gita* is not to be understood as only a Vedantic text.

18. That *bhakti* brings the yogic goal is said explicity by Vyasa under *YS* 1.23, using the word.

19. The distinctiveness of the commentary attributed to Shankara—who may or may not be the eighth-century Advaitin (before he became an Advaitin)—crystallizes in the reading of this stretch of sutras on the *ishvara, YS* 1.23ff.: *The Complete Commentary by Shankara on the Yoga Sutras,* tr Trevor Leggett (1990), 107ff. Notably, Vyasa himself presents, under sutra 1.24, an argument for the existence of God (or the Lord, *ishvara*) that is much like the ontological argument put forth in the West by Bishop Anselm in the twelfth century. Nothing greater can be conceived, for if there were something greater, that would be the Lord. Shankara writes extremely long subcommentary on Vyasa's commentary on this and the next sutra, 1.25, which says that the Lord has maximal knowledge, and the two authors—especially Shankara, who considers several ways the Lord could be known—achieve a great moment in rational theology.

Vachaspati (c. 950) also writes a lot of subcommentary on this stretch of sutras, but does not go in the direction of *bhakti* and its lore or of rational theology, but rather toward Samkhya and views and accomplishments attributed to its legendary founder, Kapila. Vijnana Bhikshu (c. 1500) assimilates the *ishvara* teaching into the Vedantic Brahman teaching explicitly and straightforwardly, quoting Vedantic texts. Shankara does too though less explicitly, and quotes the *Gita*. Vachaspati's commentary is translated by J. H. Woods in *The Yoga-System of Pantanjali* (1914); Vijnana Bhikshu's by T. S. Rukmani, *Yogavarttika of Vijnanabhiksu* (1981–1989).

20. That conception, "preferred divinity," *ishta devata,* in turn, scholars call "henotheistic"; see the next note below.

21. This the "henotheistic" idea of Hinduism is traceable to the *Rig Veda* and is prominently expressed in the *Gita* as well as theistic Upanishads. From the *Rigveda Samhita,* tr. S. P. Sarasvati and S. Vidyalankar, 8 vols. (1977–1980) (I have made a few alterations):

> They have styled him Indra (the Chief of the gods), Mitra (the Friend), Varuna (the Venerable), Agni (Fire), also the celestial, great-winged Garutma; for although one, poets speak of him diversely; they say Agni, Yama (Death), and Matarishvan (Lord of breath). (*Rig Veda* 1.164.46.)

> The divine architect, the impeller of all, the multiform, has begotten and nourished a numerous projeny, since all these worlds belong to him. (*Rig Veda* 3.55.19.)

> The ten hundreds stand there as one; I have beheld the most excellent form of the gods. (*Rig Veda* 5.62.1.)

> His steady light, swifter than the mind, stationed throughout the moving world, indicates the way to happiness. All the gods are of one accord and

one intention; they proceed unobstructed according to a single will. (*Rig Veda* 6.9.5.)

The following verses from the *Gita* express the henotheistic idea transparently: 4.11, 9.23–24a, 11.15–16a, and 11.37b–38.

22. The formulation by the great Nyaya rational theologian Udayana (c. 1000) gives the example of weaving as well as of grammar. To the objection that at least some such tasks require that God be embodied, whereas God is not embodied, Udayana replies by quoting the *Gita,* verses 3.23 and 3.24: (in effect) God becomes embodied from time to time. These verses indicate the *avatara* doctrine; Krishna asserts that he must work to maintain the worlds since people everywhere (in all crafts) follow his example: *Nyaya-kusumanjali,* ed. Goswami (1972), 599. (N. S. Dravid has translated this work: *Nyaya-kusumanjali of Udayanacarya* [1996]; our argument appears on 414–15.) Gopikamohan Bhattacharya, *Studies in Nyaya–Vaisheshika Theism* (1961), 133, cites the commentary of Vardhamana (Gangesha's son, c. 1350) arguing against the further objection that a body as a locus of works is also the locus of pleasure and suffering and thus incompatible with the nature of God. Vardhamana replies that though to God there attaches no unseen force (*adrishta*) that compels embodiment, that of individuals does force God to take a body—compare *Gita* 4.7 (see appendix B).

Dan Arnold connects the Mimamsa doctrines of the eternity and unspoken character of the Veda (not spoken by any person, *apaurusheya,* including Shiva, Vishnu, and so on) to the arguments of Jerry Fodor that the view of language as convention faces the difficulty that the stipulations that form conventions ("Let 'apple' pick out apples") presuppose a language of stipulation (or whatever the generative engine): "On Semantics and *Samketa*" (2006). Fodor speculates that the brain is hard-wired in "mentalese," that there is a core language that is not conventional. In other words, not all language is learned or even invented, since there has to be a language of invention. Here from a very different angle we see the strength of the criteriological argument of Udayana.

23. The *alankara shastra,* which is concerned mainly with poetics, is historically rooted in the *Natya Shastra,* a text as early as 200 B.C.E. that is an extraordinary how-to compendium for actors, musicians, dancers, carpenters, costumers, stage managers, and (above all) authors in putting on together a spectacle (probably for several days) in which theater was at the center. In the midst of details about musical instruments and dialects is advice to authors to try to evoke *rasa*, aesthetic relishing, of the dominant or abiding human emotions, sexual feeling, mirth, grief, anger, vitality, fear, repulsion, and wonder.

In a famous verse (6.16), Bharata lists eight *rasa*s: "The erotic, comic, tragic, furious, heroic, frightening, gruesome, and the marvellous—these are the names of the eight 'relishings' known in dramatics." He goes on to define *rasa* and to detail its relation to other types of psychological state. Through these ideas, the *Natya Shastra* stands as the foundational text not only of classical Indian dramatics but also, as mentioned, of the *alamkara shastra,* the classical aesthetics and literary criticism that stretches through the very latest and best Sanskrit authors. An excellent translation in two volumes is by Manmohan Ghosh (1961–67).

24. The secrecy of the Kaula rituals and the requirements for admission are apparently meant to exclude those unable to appreciate the occult. This is the rough equivalent of the need with respect to aesthetic objects to be aesthetically prepared, to be a like-hearted, *sahridya,* member of the audience—to use Abhinava's term for the connoisseur. The uninitiated would disrupt the ceremonies, like someone laughing inappropriately during a play.

25. Har Dayal, *The Bodhisattva Doctrine in Buddhist Sanskrit Literature* (1932), 168–71. Masatoshi Nagatomi explains the view of the great Yogacara philosopher Dharmakirti of the seventh century that to reject compassion is impossible, as it is transformative. Compassion becomes, for the advanced practitioner, the inherent nature of her consciousness—in a striking use of a substantivalist metaphor—its very stuff: "*Manasa-Pratyaksha:* A Conundrum in the Buddhist *Pramana* System," included in Nagatomi, et al., *Sanskrit and Indian Studies* (1980), 246–47, including a long quotation (in English) from Dharmakirti's *Pramana-varttika,* chapter 2.

26. The Buddhist transformation theme is not only karmic but innatist. As does what we saw in chapter 4 of the *Yoga Sutra* and its *siddhi* tradition, the Buddhist tantric picture comes to include manifestation from the top, or from the inside out. Consciousness is inherently compassionate and wise, hence the six perfections of those who awaken to its intrinsic and transformative influence, in the later conceptions. Indeed, the assimilation of the perfections to yogic *siddhi*s is made explicitly along with an innatism totally consonant with that of the *YS*: see Dayal, *The Bodhisattva Doctrine in Buddhist Sanskrit Literature* (1932), 20 and 26–29, in particular. In brief, the perfections are the natural flowers of enlightened consciousness.

27. We noted a rough equivalent of the *Gita*'s karma yoga in the "giving" enjoined in early Buddhism; see chapter 3, note 43, and, again, Egge, *Religious Giving and the Invention of Karma in Theravada Buddhism* (2002). Ellison Findly argues, in *Dana: Giving and Getting in Pali Buddhism* (2003), that the emergent institution and practices of giving to monks and nuns (of various classifications) were absolutely at the center of the culture of early Buddhism. In Mahayana or northern Buddhism, it is remarkable that the first of the six perfections, *paramita,* exhibited by the perfect individual, the bodhisattva, is *dana,* giving or charity. Furthermore, in karma yoga the giving has to be directed through *bhakti,* and so the heart is arguably in the lead. The karma yoga teaching of the *Gita* crucially includes *bhakti,* as does the way of the bodhisattva. Look again at the Four Purities of Vajrayana, above, note 7.

28. Rupa Gosvamin, *Bhakti-rasamrita-sindhu,* tr. D. Haberman (2003), the first "Wave of the Southern Quadrant," verses 23–217.

29. My translation. See also (in appendix A) *Katha* 2.1.12:

That one that is difficult to know, hidden, immanent, set in the cavern (of the heart), resting in the depths. . . .

From the same Upanishad, *Katha* 4.7 (R. Hume translation, 1921):

She who rises with life (*prana*),
Aditi (Infinity), maker of divinity,
Who stands entered into the secret place [of the heart],
Who was born forth through beings—
This verily is That.

30. Swami Muktananda, *Play of Consciousness* (1978), 159.

31. See note 21 to appendix D below on the mantra *hamsa,* which is the favorite of Abhinava's Kaula tradition.

32. Purananda's *Shat-chakra-nirupana,* "Description of the Six Chakras," was translated and popularized by Sir John Woodroffe in *The Serpent Power* (1928). Hiroshi Motoyama edited and polished a few verses, including verse 26, in *Theories of the Chakras* (1981), 173: "He who meditates on this Heart Lotus becomes like the Lord of Speech. . . . This Lotus is like the celestial wishing tree, the abode and seat of Shiva. It is beautified by the Hamsa (here the Jivatma, the individual soul) which is like the steady tapering flame of a lamp in a windless place."

33. Satyananda Saraswati, *Kundalini Tantra* (1984), 164.

34. Aurobindo, *The Life Divine* (1973), book 2, part II, chapter 25, "The Triple Transformation," 889–909.

35. Like Vivekananda and Satyananda Saraswati and others, Aurobindo is often counted a neo-Vedantin because of his championing of ideas of the Upanishads. I, however, have been calling him a tantric. The lesson perhaps is that in different ways tantra permeates neo-Vedanta.

Many of Aurobindo's major works were first published serially in a journal of yoga entitled *The Arya*, 1914–1921. *The Life Divine* and *The Synthesis of Yoga* were later extensively revised. The epic poem, *Savitri,* marginally unfinished at the time of Aurobindo's death (1950), was published posthumously. Talk of a psychic element and psychic transformation occurs throughout, especially his later work, but part of a chapter near the end of *The Life Divine* (1973) is right on point: "The Triple Transformation," 889–918.

36. Aurobindo, *The Life Divine* (1973), 225.

37. Aurobindo, *The Life Divine* (1973), 893:

On this ignorant surface we become dimly aware of something that can be called a soul as distinct from mind, life, or body; we feel it not only as our mental idea or vague instinct of ourselves, but as a sensible influence in our life and character and action. A certain sensitive feeling for all that is true and good and beautiful, fine and pure and noble, a response to it, a demand for it, a pressure on mind and life to accept and formulate it in our thought, feelings, conduct, character is the most usually recognized, the most general and characteristic, though not the sole sign of the influence of this psyche.

38. Rupa Gosvamin, *Bhakti-rasamrita-sindhu,* tr. D. Haberman (2003), the second "Wave of the Southern Quadrant," verses 291–93, in particular.

39. The poem by Jayadeva, the *Gitagovinda* (c. 1150), is a fine literary example of the Vaishnava motif of divine love play. An excellent translation is by Barbara Stoler Miller, *The Love Song of the Dark Lord* (1977).

40. Yogic traditions converge on the desiderata of a healthy body and mind, freedom from destitution, availability of spiritual instruction, and sufficient leisure for practice.

41. John Rawls, *A Theory of Justice* (1971), 118–92.

42. As explained in chapter 4, this realm is continuous with others.

43. In a different context (economic strategies for development as opposed to Yoga philosophy), Amartya Sen puts forth a similar idea, a model of people as having "basic capacities"; see"Goods and People" in his *Resources, Values and Development* (1984).

44. There is sometimes a sense—following the *Gita* or another assurance—that if one is a sincere seeker then rebirth as a seeker is secure. This may be true, but there would seem to be very real possibilities of slippage (I may speak for myself), at least in a future life. So over the long run, one might, like Rawls, want the least advantaged to benefit from inequalities.

45. The Sanskrit (spelled in the indological fashion): *agnim īḷe purohitam yajñasya devam ṛtvijam / hotāram ratna-dhātamam.* For the translation, I follow the gloss given by Jagannatha Vedalankara, which is published (in Sanskrit) in two places: *Bhargo Devasya Dhimahi* (1992), 21, and *Agni-mantra-mala* (1976), 78.

46. The textual case to be made with respect to the Veda is beyond my personal competence, and I do not think that a yogic and occult interpretation has much standing among professional vedists. But even among indologists there are some who suggest such a reading, e.g., J. Gonda, *The Vision of the Vedic Poets* (1963), chapters 11 and 12 in particular. And there is no lack of scholarly support among the traditionally educated in India, for example, K.V. Kapali-Sastry, *Rig-Bhashya Bhumika* (1952), as well as Aurobindo, *Hymns to the Mystic Fire* (1973). The idea is explicitly expressed in the *Gita* (15.14) as well as in the Upanishadic theme of interiorization of the sacrifice (see the second section of chapter 3 here as well as appendix A). A particularly apt passage is *Brihadaranyaka Upanishad,* chapter 5, sections 6–9.

47. See again note 21 to appendix D on *hamsa*. The mantra, *so 'ham* (I am That), which has the advantage of being only two syllables in length, may be superior in another respect too: as pointed out in the note, it reads backwards (roughly) as "Hamsa," which is a symbol of the *jivatman*. Also, the sound *ham* (hum) is a so-called seed mantra for the throat chakra. No wonder Shankara

identifed the Upanishadic verse where it appears (*Isha* 16) as a *mahavakya*, great statement (though his stated reason is just the meaning, which he takes to be identity of self and Brahman)! Surely, moreover, we would join distinguished lineages in uttering it, a mantra that almost competes with *om* (and nothing can compete with *om*) for endorsement in yogic texts. However, the sound "nim" in *agnim* (fire) is often taken in tantric traditions to be a heart mantra, and although the word's sense may be different from that of *so 'ham*, it would be intended to pick out the same referent.

Appendix A. Select Yogic Passages from the Early Upanishads

1. I have checked all occurrences of the word *yoga* that have been flagged in indices of eight or nine translations as well as several editions and, most importantly, the concordance compiled by Colonel Jacob, *A Concordance to the Principal Upanishads and Bhagavadgita* (1891, 1963, 1082 pages). But the colonel misses a few occurrences, especially forms of the root from which *yoga* is derived, and I suspect that there are others I have not noticed (though probably not too many). Rather arbitrarily, however, I am not including the passages in which forms of the verb appear. These are more controversial occurrences of the "self-discipline" idea, and the passages translated are sufficient to make the connection between yoga and the early Upanishads.

On the basis of research and arguments by J.A.B van Buitenen, I am not including the stretch of the *Maitri Upanishad* where the usage occurs (dramatically in 6.25, where the word is used not only in the sense of self-discipline but also in that of union, *The Maitrayaniya Upanishad* [1962], 85, in particular).

2. Shankara, c. 700 C.E., the oldest Sanskrit commentator whose texts are extant, wrote on eleven Upanishads and quoted four others (see the quotation below from S. Radhakrishnan). Shankara's rival Ramanuja, c. 1050 C.E., did not write commentaries on individual Upanishads, but includes in his *Shribhashya* hundreds of sometimes long quotations from the fifteen quoted by Shankara, plus four or five in addition. On most of these, Ramanuja's follower, Rangaramanuja, c. 1600, wrote commentaries.

Sarvepalli Radhakrishnan, *The Principal Upanishads* (1953), traces the history of Western translation, making several learned comments (21): "Prince Muhammad Dara Shikoh's collection translated into Persian (1656–1657) and then into Latin by Anquetil Duperron (1801 and 1802) under the title *Oupekhat* contained about fifty. [H. T.] Colebrooke's collection contained fifty-two, and this was based on Narayana's list (c. AD 1400). The principal Upanishads are said to be ten. Shankara commented on eleven, *Isha, Kena, Katha, Prashna, Mundaka, Mandukya, Taittiriya, Aitareya, Chandogya, Brihadaranyaka*, and *Shvetashvatara*. . . . [Beyond the fifteen or so known and discussed by classical Vedantins] other Upanishads are more religious than philosophical. . . . They glorify Vedanta or Yoga or Samnyasa or extol the worship of Shiva, Shakti, or Vishnu. [Scripted is then the following footnote.]

There is, however, considerable argument about the older and more original Upanishads. Max Mueller translated the eleven quoted by Shankara together with the *Maitri*. Deussen, though he translates no less than sixty, considers that fourteen of them are original. . . . English translations of the Upanishads have appeared in the following order: Ram Mohan Roy (1832), Roer (1853) (*Bibliotheca Indica*), Max Mueller (1879–1884) (*Sacred Books of the East* . . . [and Professor Radhakrishnan continues to list eight other translations prior to his own in 1953]."

3. "Secret doctrine" is not a bad translation for the word *upanishad,* since the meaning is most literally that which is gathered from a guru in a "sitting" with student practitioners, as scholars have shown. However, "mystic doctrine" seems to me better.

The proposition that there are yogic requirements to be eligible to receive what appear to be metaphysical doctrines reverberates throughout yogic traditions, tantric traditions in particular. For example, in the *Kularnava Tantra* (*KT*) Shiva tells Devi that there is no point in telling the truth about things unless one has become ready for it by lifetimes of yogic discipline. This is a main theme of *KT* chapter 1 (see appendix D).

4. Upanishads are a genre of Sanskrit literature. The genre demands speculative philosophy, as it presupposes yoga practice. The philosophy is actually not all that difficult to interpret. The disputes among the Vedantic subschools focus mainly on Brahman and its relation to the individual consciousness, and on this topic different Upanishadic passages say different things. In my own interpretation of particular passages (and all translation involves interpretation), I generally (but not always) follow Shankara along with the elegant English of Sarvepalli Ramakrishnan, *The Principal Upanishads* (1953), who himself seems usually to follow Shankara.

5. Vedantins are not the only philosophers with reverence for the Upanishads, not the only ones to try to assimilate scripture into a web of belief also informed by sense perception and inference. For instance, Nyaya philosophers join others in the Hindu mainstream in taking liberation to be the epistemic province of the Upanishads. On this subject—not on everything—the Upanishads are the *pramana,* the knowledge source. The knowledge sources include *sruti,* scripture or revealed hearing, but only on *mukti* and, with qualifications, *dharma* is *sruti* not liable to be trumped by weightier authority, Nyaya insists. And even on the Upanishads themselves, Vedantin voices are not the only authorities. An example is the question of what type of knowledge is enjoined by the Upanishads. The great "New Logician" Gangesha (c. 1325) agreed with the Vishishtadvaita Vedantins that the Upanishadic sources do not mean propositional knowledge. In enjoining knowledge of self, something like self-perception, an immediately intuitive consciousness, is the end in mind, he says (in his *mukti-vada, Tattva-cinta-mani* II, part 2, ed. N. S. Ramanuja Tatacharya, 1999, 429–30, my translation):

> So much being said, let us take up liberation: "Verily the self is to be learned about, thought about, and made immediate in meditation [made real to

experience, *sakshatkartavya*]," is a scriptural statement (that is pertinent). And from (other) scriptural statements learning that the self is distinct from the body and the rest, we discriminate, singling out scientifically (by shastric means) the types of things that words pick out (*padartha,* the "categories"), carrying out the thinking (the *manana* enjoined), which becomes firm about it through considering the possibilities of it being understood (in a wrong way).

> And it is incorrect that (directly) from knowledge of (the fundamental) truths produced in conformity with scripture there ceases to be, for the one for whom this has become immediate, false cognition along with (perverted) dispositions, the seeds of transmigratory existence. For such is not found with such phenomena as directional confusion (on the part of someone dizzy where knowledge does not end the dizziness).

The point is, as Gangesha goes on to say, that yoga practice is also necessary, not just intellectual understanding of the Upanishads. Here we may be inspired, then, by the Nyaya interest in yoga.

6. Mircea Eliade, *Yoga Immortality and Freedom* (1954), finds first and foremost Vedic *tapas* (ascetic heat) as a concept continuous with *yoga,* 106–14. K. S. Joshi, "On the Meaning of Yoga" (1965), supports this conclusion with better citations and argument.

7. Early Vedic usages of the word *yoga* are principally yoking or joining, a pair of animals, for instance, and more abstractly any connection between two things, including even an application of a rule to an instance. See the discussion in the last section of chapter 1.

8. The *Maitri* belongs to the Maitrayaniya lineage of the *Krishna Yajur Veda*. There is no commentary by Shankara, and hardly any scholar assigns it to the oldest and principal group, partly because it gives the name Shiva to its all-in-all theistic conception of Brahman, the Absolute. In verse 4.5, it mentions the triad of classical Hinduism, Brahma, the Creator (the word is masculine in gender, as opposed to the word for the Absolute, *brahman,* which is neuter), Vishnu, and Rudra (an early name for Shiva). Max Mueller, however, argues persuasively that the language and style (a certain use of euphonic combination or *sandhi*) of the Upanishad point to an early date. See *The Upanishads* in the series edited by Mueller, *The Sacred Books of the East,* vol. 15, part 2 (1884), xlvii–xlviii. However, the *Maitri* is pretty clearly later than the advent of Buddhism.

The *Maitri* is a theistic Upanishad with a remarkable use of the word *yoga* in 6.25. However, van Buitenen (see note 1 above) has cogently argued that the passage is an interpolation. Tantric texts may deserve the credit for the new meaning of mystical union—or the *Gita* the credit for *yoga-yukta,* united (with your higher self) through yoga, an expression that occurs repeatedly.

9. See again, above, note 6. Among the most resonant passages from the *Rig Veda* employing the word *tapas* is a line from 10.129, the "Hymn of Creation," verse 4: "That One was born by force of *tapas* (ascetic heat)." This is echoed, for

 example, by *Katha* 4.6 ("the One born of old from *tapas*"). *Mundaka* 1.2.11 is a clear example where *tapas* means in general yoga practices (though it is usually translated "austerities").

10. This is to follow the recension that the Nyaya philosopher, Gangesha, apparently has, since this is what he quotes (using standard transliteration): *ātmā vā are śrotavyo mantavyo nididhyāsitavyaḥ* (*Tattvacintamani* II, part 2, ed. N. S. Ramanuja Tatacharya [1999], 396). Other recensions add the word *draṣṭavyaḥ* (is to be seen) after *are*, but almost all Vedantic as well as Nyaya philosophers remember the theme of the verse as that the self is to be learned about through hearing, thought about, and made immediate in meditation: *shravana, manana,* and *nididhyasitavya.*

11. Gangesha, for example, discusses at length libertation in connection with the *Brihadaranyaka* quotation (*Tattvacintamani* II, part 2, ed. N. S. Ramanuja Tatacharya [1999], 429ff). See note 5 above.

12. Although "immediate meditational experience" is controversial as a gloss, Gangesha apparently has an Upanishadic edition that includes the word *sakshatkara*—put before the eyes, made immediate in experience—as part of the Upanishadic text (*Tattvacintamani* II, part 2, ed. N. S. Ramanuja Tatacharya [1999], 429).

13. The Sanskrit edition I use for the following translations is *Ten Principal Upanishads* (1964), which also contains Shankara's commentary. All translations are my own. One previous English rendering more than others has guided my eye and ear: Sarvepalli Radhakrishnan, *The Principal Upanishads* (1953). I have also consulted R. Hume (1921), Sri Aurobindo, *The Upanishads* (1973), V. Roebuck (2000), and E. Easwaran (1987).

14. *Brihadaranyaka* 4.3.9–10 uses *loka* in a similar way, where there is no suggestion that the "world" seen would be other than this world we ordinarily see, though now known as the Brahman: "'An ocean, a single seer without duality becomes he whose world (*loka*) is *brahman,* O King,' Yajnavalkya instructed. 'This is his supreme way. This is his supreme achievement. This is his supreme world (*loka*). This is his supreme bliss. Other beings live on just a small portion of this bliss.'"

15. For the mainstream yogic understanding of the breaths, see Iyengar, *Light on Yoga* (1979), 45, "prana . . . which moves in the region of the heart and controls respiration; apana, which moves in the sphere of the lower abdomen and controls the function of eliminating urine and faeces; samana, which stokes the gastric fires to aid digestion; udana, which dwells in the thoracic cavity and controls the intake of air and food; and vyana, which pervades the entire body and distributes the energy derived from food and breath." Swami Satyananda, *Asana, Pranayama, Mudra, Bandha* (1996), discusses the five "airs" as part of the pranic body, providing a drawing (364–66). The notion is in the earliest Upanishads (e.g., *Brihadaranyaka* 1.5.3) as well as the *Yoga Sutra* (3.39 and 3.40).

Here is also an interesting passage from Aurobindo, *Record of Yoga* (2001), II:1462:

There are five pranas, viz.: prana, apana, samana, vyana, and udana. The movement of the prana is from the top of the body to the navel, apana from Muladhara to the navel. Prana and apana meet together near the navel and create samana. The movement of vyana is in the whole body. While samana creates bhuta from the foods, vyana distributes it into the body. The movement of udana is from the navel to the head. Its work is to carry the virya (tejas) to the head. The movement of udana is different to the Yogin. Then its movement is from the Muladhara (from where it carries the virya to the crown of the head and turns it into ojas) to the crown of the head. [All spelling following the original.]

16. *Shvetashvatara* 2.10 is echoed by *Gita* 5.11.

17. On *Shvetashvatara* 2.11, Sarvepalli Radhakrishnan (1953) quotes (translating) the *Lankavatara Sutra* of Buddhism: "In his exercise, the Yogin sees (imaginatively) the form of the sun or the moon or something looking like a lotus, or the underworld or various forms such as skyfire and the like" (721).

Appendix B. Yogic Passages in the *Bhagavad Gita*

1. The translation here is my own, as is that of all the verses to follow. The Sanskrit is taken from *The Bhagavad Gita with the Commentary of Shri Shankaracarya,* ed. Dinkar Vishnu Gokhale (1950).

2. For example, the great historian of religions and interpreter of Yoga, Mircea Eliade, *History of Religious Ideas* (1982), II:241: see above, note 43 to chapter 4, where Eliade is quoted.

3. In the classical Vedantic concept as articulated especially by Ramanuja, God is a much more powerful being than, say, according to Nyaya. But in no Vedantic theology is God free from universal laws in self-determination. The Vedantic is not the Cartesian voluntarist God who can make 5 + 7 = 13. Thus the mention of God's own yoga in *Gita* 11.8 can be interpreted as a vision of the laws and principles of manifestation.

4. *The Bhagavad Gita with the Commentary of Shri Shankaracarya,* ed. Dinkar Vishnu Gokhale, (1950). Matthew Dasti helped me choose the passages that appear to be the most relevant to yoga practice, leaving out the stretches of text more exclusively devoted to metaphysical conceptions. Among translations by others that I have consulted and that inform the effort here are, in order of my sense of helpfulness and debt: Franklin Edgerton (1952), J.A.B. van Buitenen (1981), and Barbara Stoler Miller (1986). Both Shankara and Ramanuja wrote extensive commentaries that I have consulted, using Shankara's in particular as a dictionary. I have not consulted any English translation of Shankara, but the translation and commentary on Ramanuja's *Bhashya* by J.A.B. van Buitenen, *Ramanuja on the Bhagavadgita* (1968), has been invaluable.

5. The idea of self-enlivening, *bhavana,* is crucial to the aesthetic tradition drawn on by Abhinava Gupta; see the second section of chapter 5.

6. Conscious identification and control, *samyama,* is perhaps the absolutely most important concept of the *Yoga Sutra;* see the discussion of *siddhis* as flowing from *samyama* in the first section of chapter 5.

7. Janaka is a king who is a character in the *Brihadaranyaka Upanishad* and is often mentioned as an example of a yogin who lives in the world.

8. Compare *YS* 1.12: "Restriction of fluctuations is accomplished through practice (*abhyasa*) and disinterestedness (*vairagya*)." It seems likely Patanjali knew the *Gita,* partly because *abhyasa,* practice, is vague and *vairagya,* disinterestedness, not so vague, hence an odd coupling and memorable phrase.

9. See note 3 immediately above.

Appendix C. The *Yoga Sutra*

1. Philipp Maas, *Samadhipada* (2006). Maas's apparatus includes twenty-one published editions of the *YS* as well as manuscripts in eight alphabets from different regions of India. For *YS* chapters 2 through 4, I have relied on Vimala Karnatak (ed.), *Patanjala-yoga-darsanam,* 4 vols. (1992), which follows the sub-commentaries (on Vyasa) by Vachaspati (c. 950) and Vijnanabhikshu (c. 1500).

2. Stephen Phillips, "The Conflict of Voluntarism and Dualism in the *Yoga-sutra*" (1985).

3. The word *atha,* now, is viewed within traditional circles as a ritually auspicious way to begin a text (*mangala:* see note 54 to chapter 3).

4. See note 7 to chapter 1 on *chitta.*

5. Probably what is meant is that these are five major types, not that all fluctuations of *chitta* fall into a clear subcategory. Emotions, for example, seem to be left off the list that follows.

6. This is a definition of nonveridical cognition that sounds a lot like that of Nyaya; see note 10 to chapter 3.

7. Yoga clearly involves control over desire (a form of *prana*) as well as thought and emotion. Although desire is not on the list of types of fluctuation at 1.6, *chitta* should be thought of as comprising it.

8. An alternative translation: Afterward, from perception of the *purusha,* there is lack of desire for (manifest or unmanifest) phenomena.

9. The stretch of sutras beginning here (1.23) and running through 1.28 is discussed in the second section of chapter 5 on *bhakti.*

10. The match of compassion and the painful (*duhkha*) here is in accordance with the traditional matchings of *rasa* (aesthetic relishing) with *bhava* (natural emotional state); see the second section of chapter 5.

11. Sutra 1.35 seems to say that mental silence arises from observing sense experience. Vyasa, however, gives a different spin: by concentrating on a particular sense-organ activity along with the nature of its objects in general—e.g., the tasting organ and taste in general—one gets an experience of a subtle,

prephysical evolute of nature, *prakriti*. This is important feedback, for it confirms a person's trust in yogic teachings and practices and thus helps to lead to mental silence.

12. An alternative translation for 1.37: A mind (is quiet and restrained) whose objects are no longer colored by desire.

13. The technical term, *samapatti,* has been variously translated and interpreted. Integration of the parts of the being in a yogically balanced fashion is a reading slightly different from yogic balance, with *samapatti* as yogic integration (a rendering that is true to the etymology of *sam* + *ā* + the root, *pat*).

14. The word *prajna* is employed in Mahayana Buddhism to capture the sixth and best attribute of a bodhisattva, the "perfection of wisdom and insight," *prajna-paramita.*

15. The last two sutras (1.50 and 1.51) are discussed in the book, pp. 85–86.

16. Sutra 2.5 frames the mistake—the "spiritual ignorance," *avidya*—in the reverse of the typical order in tantra. There the mistake is not to see the eternal, etc., in the noneternal, etc.

17. The notion of moral payback implicit here in 2.14 is discussed in this book at the end of chapter 3.

18. See, above, pp. 144–45, on the idea, "All is suffering."

19. This sutra (2.21) together with 2.18 presents a wonderfully teleological conception of *prakriti,* nature. Though these links between nature and the conscious being look rather like metaphysical patchwork, at least now we can understand the urge to practice yoga: it is in nature, in her essential heart .

20. Vyasa interprets 2.23 as saying that the conjunction, though misleading for the moment, leads eventually to the genuine perception of the conscious being's own powers as well as the separate powers of *prakriti*—in consonance with the optimistic, teleological outlook of 2.21 and 2.18.

21. For example, nurturing thoughts and feelings of nonharmfulness is a practice to be employed to check a feeling of wanting to injure someone.

22. According to the tantric interpretation of Swami Satyananda Saraswati (1976), this sutra (2.37) says that from mastery of this *niyama* the yogin or yogini comes to live in an atmosphere of abundance, impersonally enjoying, so to say, the wealth of the world.

23. Freed from concern for wealth, you are relaxed enough to remember—by way of triggering *samskaras* formed in previous births—activities in previous lives, including what it was you did that is key to your present personality and station in life. Thus this sutra does not have to be read theistically. The theistic interpretation—here I follow Swami Satyananda (1976)—has it that, cleansed of personal interests, you can discern God's reason for giving you the current birth along with your individual *dharma,* what you should try to do or be.

24. Sutra 2.45 is discussed in the second section of chapter 5.

25. 2.46 is the famous sutra on asana. The point seems to be that whereas it is perhaps not so hard to do an asana and make it firm and steady if you put in

 the effort, mastery entails the ability to do it effortlessly, easily, with pleasure (*sukha*).

26. Possibly, in accordance with modern tantra, the last part of the sutra (2.47) encourages, in certain asanas, meditation on *kundalini,* the serpent power, the shakti in the lowest of the seven centers, chakras, according to the occult physiology.

27. Sutra 2.52 echoes *Isha Upanishad,* verse 15: "The face of Truth is covered with a golden lid."

28. The classical commentators take sutra 3.3 to indicate a transcendence of subject/object consciousness. But it may mean an utter absorption in an object with no self-consciousness. See, above, notes 1 and 2 to chapter 5, on *samadhi.*

29. An alternative translation for sutra 3.6 following Vyasa: The yoga of conscious identification (*samyama*) is to be developed in stages.

30. In other words, *samyama* is intrinsic to, though perhaps not fully developed in, the practices of nonharmfulness, cleanliness, asanas, and so on, according to sutra 3.7. B.K.S. Iyengar makes much of a mutual entailment of all the limbs (or in a weaker version, mutual support), in his *Tree of Yoga* (2002) and elsewhere. The limbs are not stages, in this view, but rather to be practiced simultaneously.

31. For instance, a person might constantly concentrate on *om* to the point that a moment of perishing consciousness and a moment of arising consciousness would have exactly the same content, presumably for long periods.

32. Properties and moments of change of property fall into discrete units—it seems to be assumed here in accordance with Buddhists and others. States of mind, perceptions, rememberings, etc., are momentary. However, the changes would occur in *chitta,* mind stuff. This and the last sutra (3.14 and 3.15) are metaphysical statements, combining the picture of the mind as a kind of substance with that of a serial nature for mental occurrences.

33. Sutra 3.17 seems to endorse the philosophic task of differentiating the likes of use and mention, sense and reference, object and view, or word, meaning, and reference. But how, then, could the *siddhi* be credible? (None of my philosophy colleagues has it.)

34. An additional sutra does not appear in most published editions I have seen, and Karnak (1992) does not include it. But there is no harm in looking at it in a note:

> 3.21′. etena śabdâdy-antar-dhānam uktam.
>
> By this (by the information in 3.21) is explained the disappearance of sound and so on.

As the representations of Maas, *Samadhipada* (2006) make plain, sutras in manuscripts were often written entirely embedded within the commentary by Vyasa. And here indeed Vyasa uses almost the very words of 3.21' in his commentary on 3.21.

35. Vyasa explains that the "cosmic becoming," or "universe," mentioned in sutra 3.26 consists of seven worlds, or planes of being, ranging from our world of earth (*bhu*) to the three worlds of the Brahman along with three intermediate worlds.

36. The interpretation of this *siddhi* as intellectual knowledge, as expertise in astronomy, is implausible. The implausibility urges us to find a metaphor. Unfortunately, there is no consensus about what occult phenomena may be meant. And it is interesting that usually long-winded Vyasa has practically nothing to say about this sutra (3.27) or the next, and we are left wondering what kind of knowledge, *jnana,* is intended.

37. The last three sutras (3.29–31), and perhaps the next, appear to express the tantric occult physiology of chakras and energy canals. Vyasa talks, however, about elements one interior to another, suggesting cylinders, as in the sheath or *kosha* theory.

38. Counter to the mainstream, I think the word *pratibhad* (3.33) is an adjective, qualifying an understood *samyamat.*

39. Sutra 3.36 makes a strange use of the word *varta* (normally "news," not "smelling"), but I follow Vyasa in completing the list.

40. Georg Feuerstein, *The Yoga-sutra of Patanjali* (1979) thinks—contrary to Vyasa—that sutra 3.38 may be referring to an astral or subtle body as opposed to the physical body. Swami Satyananda, *Four Chapters on Freedom* (1976) says this is a very advanced *siddhi* that should not be tried at home.

The conceptual problem is that *chitta* is individuated by *purusha*: one *chitta,* one individual conscious being, that is to say, one mind, one *purusha.* And each mind has its own body, one would think. But this sutra says otherwise. Bodies can be controlled by alien *chitta,* which here seems less thought and emotion than a kind of psychic energy.

41. See note 15 to appendix A on the five breaths or *prana*s.

42. Ether is the medium of sound, according to mainstream classical Indian physics. There are also other conceptions, as noted, some of which relate the elements and subtle elements of Samkhya to *kosha*s and chakras.

43. Feuerstein, *The Yoga-sutra of Patanjali* (1979), 118, cites the *Mahabharata* (12.318.7) for assigning the *siddhi*s in general to the subtle or pranic body as opposed to the physical.

Vyasa provides the list of eight: shrinking, expansion, lightness or levitation, extension (wide occult reach), freedom of preference, general mastery, creativity, and wish-fulfillment. See also, in appendix E, my comments under verse 3.8 of the *Hatha Yoga Pradipika* for a slightly different list from King Bhoja (c. 1050) and the *HYP* commentator, Brahmananda (nineteenth century).

44. Sutra 3.48 is not to be interpreted as promising omnipotence but presumably mastery over one's own *prakriti,* although it does say *pradhana,* which means the principal or root.

45. Other translators and interpreters take sutra 3.53 to refer to differentiating material things of the same type, two pots, for instance. However, since two

 pots cannot be in the same place (at the same time), a better reading seems to be that the discrimination is to be between consciousness and nature—which do occupy, so to say, the same place at the same time, at least in the sattvafication of nature. This interpretation also accords better with the topic of the immediately preceding and following sutras.

46. The stretch of sutras opening the fourth book, 4.1–4, is discussed in the first section of chapter 5.

47. All voluntary action has *chitta,* mind, as the *purusha*'s instrument or intermediary. People are numerous, acting in diverse ways, but an action on anyone's part involves *chitta,* which is of a single type for everyone. As remarked, some have translated *chitta* as mind stuff (e.g., J. H. Woods). In Samkhya, and sometimes in Vedanta too, it is considered a kind of subtle matter. It is the receptacle or locus of *samskara,* mental dispositions, such as skills, memories, and habits.

It is my view that it is pretty consistently treated by Patanjali as a third basic kind of existent, especially here in the fourth chapter, along with consciousness (*purusha*) and nature (*prakriti*). Of course, the official position is to make it part of *prakriti.*

48. The implication sutra 4.7 seems to make is that the yogin is free of karmic payback, but perhaps the idea is a little more elaborate. The yogin's karma could be of such a universal or harmonious order that it invites no payback, as in the theme of the *Gita.* In any case, the sutra does not deny that the yogin acts and thereby makes karma.

49. This is the first time the word *vasana* has been used. Previously, the theory of karma had been couched in terms of *samskara,* mental dispositions. The suggestion seems to be that *vasana*—like Ducasse's talents and deep dispositions that could bridge lifetimes (see chapter 4)—are translife *samskara,* whereas at least some *samskara* perish with the death of the body.

50. Here (4.10) we get an idea of connection, albeit obscure, between mental dispositions and desire, or, as say the commentators, desire to live, *ashisha* (*āśiṣa*). The next sutra (4.11) says that it is a causal connection, and Vyasa and his followers try to spell it out more precisely. I speculate that Patanjali sees the eternity of the *purusha* projected into nature as a desire to continue forever in one's current identity. Vijnanabhiksu constructs an argument about the permanence of *chitta,* the substratum of desire and mental dispositions. It echoes Udayana's argument for rebirth, reviewed in chapter 4.

Sutra 4.10 echoes Buddhist teaching. Compare the Second Noble Truth: "Suffering comes from desire (which has no beginning)." It's as though near one's core, though not part of one's genuine essence, there is a desire component, perhaps common with all life. The sutra also reinforces Vedantic readings and the Vedantic tendency to see *chitta* as a form of *prana* (breath, life energy), a universal vital substance to which desire is natural.

51. This claim of causal relationship mirrors the structure and interrelationship of the Four Noble Truths: "Eliminate desire, and suffering, its fruit, will be eliminated." Vyasa's reading, through the notion of *alambana,* dependence (of *x*

on *y*), does express this structure as 4.11's main point. But the terms of the relationship, which he understands to be determined by content, are not for him in either case subconscious mechanisms but rather consequences of action understood hedonically, in terms of pleasure and pain; Vyasa's "six-spoked wheel of existence," which really has only five spokes, similarly parallels and contrasts with the famous twelve-spoked wheel of early Buddhism, the *bhava chakra*. It runs: 1) from virtue, pleasure, and from vice, pain; 2) from pleasure, attachment/attraction, and from pain, aversion; 3) action (to acquire what attracts or to avoid that to which one is averse); 4) consequences of action (in benefits to others or injury); 5) virtue and vice—and so on, around again. The Buddhist wheel includes death and rebirth.

52. This and the following two sutras, the triad 4.12–14, address the metaphysics of time from a Samkhya perspective.

Vyasa takes a straightforward interpretive route, proposing a realism about past and future that is severely qualified. The past and the future do not exist in the same way as the present. The future exists as "to be manifest" and the past as "having been experienced." Nevertheless, we, and especially yogins, have knowledge of things past and future, and so there must be truth makers (facts of the matter) grounding the knowledge.

53. Vyasa interprets the subtle (*sukshma*) in sutra 4.13 as applying to the past and the future, which is generic, unmanifest, or potential. Nature, which is composed of the three strands, *sattva, rajas,* and *tamas*, is the font of all possibility. Indeed, in a sense all particulars preexist (or postexist) in that they are true potentials within *prakriti,* combinations of the strands. This is the doctrine of *sat-karya vada*, the "preexistence of the effect," which is aired at length in the subcommentaries.

The point from the perspective of yogic practice is apparently to have a view that would give us a sense of nature as a whole—including the three times—and that would lead us to indifference to particular happenings. This in turn, would be, in Patanjali's conception, a step toward utter transcendence.

54. Sutra 4.15 begins a stretch of text that is, in my opinion, Patanjali's best philosophizing, best stretch, that is to say, of argumentation concerning mind and consciousness. The most compelling arguments of the entire *YS* occur here.

Counter to the Samkhya theme of seeing everything as like everything else in being a transformation of *prakriti,* the passage opens with the current sutra establishing "mind" (*chitta*) as—let us say, to make the point clear—belonging to a distinct category. *Chitta* is different from worldly things, as well as different from consciousness. Patanjali's philosophy has been mislabeled a dualism. For all intents and purposes, it posits a triplicity of consciousness, mind, and object. Note, furthermore, that minds are paired with *purusha*s, with individual conscious beings: one *purusha,* one *chitta*. Of course, *chitta* is also colored and variously determined by objects and natural processes.

In terms, then, of the three categories, Patanjali's yoga could be characterized as the bringing of the *chitta* under the control of the *purusha,* free from the influence of *prakriti*. The mind becomes an instrument like the hand, which one can hold still or move purposefully, not like a neighbor's radio, over which one has no control.

55. Objects exist independently of cognition. The question at the end of the sutra (4.16) helps us to see this quickly—whatever be the arguments of idealists, Buddhists and others, who would convince us that objects are mind dependent. The *fluctuations* of our *chitta*, i.e., what objects are to us, are, of course "mind dependent," being composed of *chitta* and shaped—I would say in opposition to the standard interpretation of Patanjali—in part by the individual conscious being (who practices yoga and *samyama* in particular). The world is common to everyone, though I have my individual *chitta* and you yours, with mine conforming (to some extent) to my volition and yours to your volition.

56. B.K.S. Iyengar, *Light on the Yoga Sutras of Pantanjali* (1976), suggests this interpretation of 4.17, which is different from Vyasa's. Another possibility for the "according to" phrase is: "depending on the coloring conferred." This would continue what appears to be engagement with Buddhist idealism. One concedes the "grain of truth" in the opponent's position: our individual expectations and conditioning determine, as you Buddhists insist, what objects are for us differently from what they are for others—and it all comes out determined in the best way when we practice yoga (or the Eightfold Path of the Buddha). Here we all agree. But let us not concede the essential, namely, here, the view of objects as real and external to *chitta*.

57. Each individual knows his or her own mind and is capable of controlling it, not other minds. At least, normally this would be the case. Knowledge of one's own mind as embracing fluctuations over time proves the enduringness of oneself as the knower.

This argument is standardly used against Buddhists who would deny the separate existence of a self, as discussed in chapter 4. Only a self that endures is capable of the knowledge that we have of our minds fluctuating in one way at one time and in another way at another, or, in a different conception, has memory of cognizing something earlier. Memory dispositions, *samskara,* formed by previous experience are triggered and cause remembering. In the *YS*'s conception, the individual who has knowledge of certain fluctuations occurring at a certain time and of others occurring at other times is one and the same, that is to say, unchanging.

There would seem to be, on this view, no possibility of unconscious mental fluctuations. The tie between the *purusha* and its *chitta* seems implausibly tight. But again, the yogic point would be that the individual can take control.

58. Here again (4.19) Patanjali sides with classical realists, Nyaya philosophers, and others, against Buddhist idealists (and Advaitins and others): cognitions are *not* self-luminous since they are themselves known. Cognitions are instruments of a self's knowledge of the world, according to Nyaya, and themselves have intentionality—or a content, an object-directedness—evidenced in terms of the things known. But cognitions (*jnana*) can be cognized as cognitions,

through apperception, *anuvyayasaya*, an after-cognition, in Nyaya. Patanjali appears to have similar views about *chitta*. Here Nyaya's cognitions are fluctuations of *chitta*. So since *chitta* is perceived, it is not self-luminous.

59. In the context of the classical arguments, nonsimultaneity of self- and object-cognition—sometimes presented as phenomological fact—buttresses the view of cognition as other-illumined, *para-prakasha*. Here (4.20) the point seems to hook up with the supposition that the *purusha* is required for the mind to be known. Two sutras below (4.22), it is claimed that the *chitta*, the mind, *can* know simultaneously the *purusha* and the world, under certain conditions.

It is tempting to read 4.20 as presenting a battle over the directedness of *chitta*, whether to cognize self *or* world. Thus it would show the true dualism of the old Yoga worldview, to choose world or self. I take it that part of the "tantric turn" is to deny that the yogin cannot know the world at the same time as the self is known. However, that idea seems already present with the message of 4.23, which is then a "tantric" sutra, like many in *YS* chapter 3. The right reading here seems to be that the *chitta* cannot cognize both itself and the world at the same time, not that it cannot reflect the *purusha* and cognize itself at the same time (as asserted in 4.23).

60. A unitary *purusha* is required to know *chitta*, not one cognition after another, as, for instance, Nyaya holds. Here Patanjali sides with Nyaya's adversaries who advocate the self-illumination thesis. Such a regress argument against "other-illuminationism" is often repeated in philosophic texts as a mainstay of "self-illuminationism."

The point here (4.21), then, seems to be to insist that the mind is a unitary substance subject to fluctations, as opposed to a stream of individual cognitions occurring one after the other. Note that the Buddhist schools share with Nyaya the picture of cognition as serial. Patanjali takes a different view, which he supposes allows him, but not Nyaya, to avoid the regress objection.

Consciousness rests with the self; it is intrinsic. The conscious being grasps mentality in a single swoop, so to say, past, present, and future fluctuations not yet manifest. It does not grasp *chitta* by means of other *chitta*. Otherwise, there would be an insuperable gap. An unbridgeable gap would also open were we to think of *chitta* as incapable of cognizing itself. The pertinent background assumption seems to be that the *purusha* uses *chitta* when it is no longer moved by the world, to self-cognize and to reflect the *purusha*'s spiritual reality.

Remembering too would be impossible on the serial view, which sees cognition as fleeting. One could not simultaneously know that one is remembering something or other and actually remember the something or other, nor, again, could one remember perceiving it.

61. The first word of this sutra (4.22) is *chiti*, power of consciousness, not *chitta*, mind. Perhaps it should be thought to designate the *purusha*, but I have translated it as I understand it, namely, as *chitta* or a form that the mind can take. The word recurs in the very last sutra, 4.34.

Different readings are offered by the classical commentators and, as might be expected, by modern interpreters. Vijnanabhikshu, for example, finds here a double reflection theory: the reflection of the *purusha* in the mind doubles back such that the mind as seemingly conscious is located in the *purusha,* who is, then, the knower. Vachaspati interprets the sutra in line with his view that the higher mind (*buddhi*) is the knower in everyday knowledge, not the *purusha.*

My reading is in line with the following sutra, 4.23, which says explicitly that the *chitta* is capable of knowing both the *purusha* and the world. Here, it seems to me, we have either the breakdown of the metaphysical dualism of *purusha* and *prakriti* as classically interpreted or a psychological bridge concept, actually both.

Practicewise, the sutra makes entire sense. One tries to still the mind in order, within the mind, to know the self.

62. This sutra (4.24) continues the argument against the philosophers of other schools. In Western philosophy, Immanuel Kant is famous for supposing that the mind synthesizes impressions and thoughts in concepts, with the unity of the deepest organizational concepts provided by the unity of the self. That is to say, the unity that makes thought possible is the "transcendental unity of apperception." Kant's idea is not too removed, it seems to me, from Patanjali's here. The *chitta* unifies the information of the senses, in part by absorbing the information stored in *samskara* (formed in the current life) and indeed that of the deep activators than span lifetimes, *vasana.*

63. In this fourth chapter it is at this point, sutra 4.25, that Patanjali turns away from the holistic goal of transformation to the other-worldliness of *kaivalya.* Note that the sutra can be read as indicating a process, suggesting that a yogin who sees the distinction would naturally *want* no part of nature. And that idea would be compatible with the idea of another yogin, the tantrini, let us call her, who would *not* abandon embodied existence. Mahayana Buddhism sees the choice as between becoming a "solitary buddha" (*pratyeka buddha*) and a bodhisattva.

64. It is the *chitta* that is the beneficiary of yoga practice, according to the conception here (4.26).

65. Various theories have been offered, none obviously superior to the rest, about why the state is called Cloud of Dharma. I would like to say, with a touch of sarcasm, that it is because *dharma* is clouded, that is, duty abandoned along with the world in a kind of self-indulgence of expectation of self-bliss.

66. Sutra 4.31 may be read as an argument in favor of world abandonment. There remains little of interest once one has had a taste of self-absorption. This could be right.

67. Apparently, the individual nature of the yogin, that portion of *prakriti* making up his body and mind (and whatever subtle bodies too, presumably), would decompose into the generic elements or principles (*tattva*) into which nature can be analyzed. No longer would there be individual embodiment and continuity of karma across lives.

68. This sutra (4.33) seems to say—partly by the pragmatics of its placement near the end of the text—that just before passing into the state of utter self-

absorption known as *kaivalya,* aloneness (an aloneness of contemplation of contemplation, so to say), the yogin can see the process propelling him to the *summum bonum*. If this is right, I should like to emphasize that such a person could not report his or her experience, since reporting requires use of mental and bodily instruments. Thus this sutra is speculation.

69. The use of the word *chiti* here (4.34) for the *purusha*'s power of consciousness suggests reading *chiti* at 4.22 (see above) in the same way, namely, as a conscious power inherent to the conscious being and as distinct from *chitta*. However, I stand by my rendering of 4.22, taking the usages to be different.

Appendix D. Selections from (Tantric) Kashmiri Shaivite Texts

1. Teun Goudriaan and Sanjukta Gupta, *Hindu Tantric and Shakta Literature* (1981), present the history of indological study of Hindu tantra along with the broad divisions of tantric literature (1–31).

2. David White, *The Alchemical Body* (1996), 335ff.

3. This is a summary judgment that Professor Sanderson has made in many venues. See, in particular, the discussion in "Shaivism and the Tantric Traditions," in *The World's Religions,* ed. S. Sutherland, et al. (1988), 679–80.

4. Edwin Gerow, "Abhinava's Aesthetics as a Speculative Paradigm" (1994), 186–87.

5. Indologists use the metaphor of "streams" of Shaivism, among which are Trika, Krama, and Kaula, which are streams of both practices/rituals and philosophy, whereas Pratyabhijna and Spanda are only philosophies. These five "systems," if you will, are brought together by Abhinava, although before him they have different Agamas that do not, apparently, have the same views.

Trika gets its name from a "triad" of Agamas taken to be most important in convergence with philosophic or theological ideas, the "triad" of Shiva, Shakti, and their union, and other symbols or sets with three members; Krama from the psychological thesis that spiritual progress to enlightenment is a matter of a "sequence" of steps; and Kaula, of course, the "family" of seekers, though the word can mean the entire universe and has other connotations too (see note 12 below). Pandey, *Abhinavagupta* (1963), 594–97, identifies different meanings of *kula,* and, on 295–96 and 597–603, different meanings of *trika*.

It seems that the Kaula comes to be the preferred name for the umbrella of unification Abhinava achieves—like a stream that becomes a mighty river after converging with other streams, which then could be known by the other names, like the lower Mississippi thought of as the continuation of the Missouri.

6. According to Somadeva Vasudeva, who has translated and explained large portions of the *Malini-vijayottara Tantra,* Abhinava does not occupy himself very much with yoga because he takes this and other Tantras clearly to spell out the necessary practices. There is no need for him to detail them again; see *The Yoga of the Malinivijayottaratantra* (2004), 146.

7. The four, which Abhinava takes from various Agamas, are: the "nonway," *anupaya*, for those whose immersion in the self is effortless, without practice prerequisites; the "way of Shambhu (Shiva)," *shambhavopaya,* for those from whom the effort needed is minimal; the "way of the Shakti worshipper (*shakta*)," *shaktopaya,* for those whose practice is to be mainly through the mind, involving meditation, *japa* (mantra repetition, in particular *so 'ham*), and *tarka* (spiritual reasoning: see below); and the "way of the minute," *anavopaya,* for those whose natures are coarser, requiring more of the traditional disciplines of asana, *pranayama,* and so on. The four are not really separate paths but rather form a continuum starting with the fourth. See K. C. Pandey, *Abhinavagupta* (1963), 314–15, who cites Abhinava's *Tantraloka*. Some of these terms—*anupaya,* etc.—have slightly different meanings with other authors and texts. See, e.g., Navjivan Rastogi, *The Krama Tantricism of Kashmir* (1979), 4–17.

Surprisingly, Abhinava says *tarka* (spiritual reasoning) is the most important "limb" (*anga*) of yoga, more important than any and all of the eight listed by Patanjali. Thus *tarka* is not (as with Nyaya) counterfactual reasoning meant to undermine an opponent's position or to strengthen one's own but rather something like Kant's transcendental reasoning. That is to say, *tarka* is able to reveal the conditions of the possibility of our experience, which are, in brief, the *tattva*s or "principles" of Shiva/Shakti's manifestation. Its importance derives from its ability to correct the dualistic misimpressions derived from sense perception, specifically that objects are discrete entities with nothing unifying them and that we as individuals are their perceivers.

Taken together, Abhinava's criticism of the "eight-limbed yoga" (*ashtanga yoga*) of Patanjali and his advocacy of *tarka* show that for him the mind matters. Mental silence, *chitta-vritti-nirodha* (*YS* 1.2), is only a step along the path. It is to be interpreted as the ability to turn off mental chatter at will. The ability clearly does not preclude *tarka,* which we might render as "metaphysical reasoning." See Paul Mueller-Ortega, "On Subtle Knowledge and the Refinement of Thought" (2005).

8. This is the main thesis of dozens of essays collected in *Poet-Saints of India,* ed. M. Sivaramkrishna and S. Roy (1996).

9. K. C. Pandey (1963) has to date presented the most comprehensive study in English. Much of the text has been translated into Italian; see Raniero Gnoli, *Tantraloka* (1980).

10. Pandey, *Abhinavagupta* (1963), 549. See also Pandey's appendix B, 909–42.

11. Goudriaan and Gupta, *Hindu Tantric and Shakta Literature* (1981), 95.

12. Sir John Woodroffe (a.k.a. Arthur Avalon) composed a sketchy summary that includes translations of a few remarkable verses. He is also the general editor of a series of tantric texts in Sanskrit, including our *Kularnava Tantra,* which was edited by Taranatha Vidyaratna and published in Madras in 1916. That text, along with Woodroffe's introduction in English and an eloquent summary by M. P. Pandit in English (more than a hundred pages in length and highly

recommendable), was published in 1965, and the book has been reprinted several times since. It is listed as Arthur Avalon, *Kularnava Tantra* (1965). The Sanskrit I follow is from this edition.

Advanced teacher of Anusara Yoga Christina Sell flagged the *Kularnava Tantra* (*KT*) for me. She also transcribed a first draft of a translation that we made together.

M. P. Pandit's summary is not only eloquent but also quite extensive, sometimes following the text closely. In addition, true translations of some portions of the *Kularnava Tantra* have appeared. The chapters on the guru, 12 and 13, have been translated in part by André Padoux, "The Tantric Guru," in David White, ed., *Tantra in Practice* (2000), 41–51. This same book contains translations by Douglas Brooks, "The Ocean of the Heart: Selections from the *Kularnava Tantra*," 347–60. Brooks translates about 80 verses drawn from almost all of the text's 17 chapters (there are approximately 125 verses per chapter).

Brooks's introduction to Kaula philosophy in *Tantra in Practice,* which is given in connection with the verses he renders, is the best I have seen, penetrating, concise, and comprehensive. Unfortunately, however, Brooks mistranslates the word *kula* as "heart." This is at best a metaphorical sense that is not at all evident unless a lot of Shaiva philosophy is explained. The word *kula* means ordinarily "family" or any group closely connected through emotional or other bonds. A related meaning is the body, the "family" of limbs, and a third everything, the "family" of the universe.

Georg Feuerstein has translated chapter 9, on yoga, 134 verses, with an occasional explanatory comment: *The Yoga Tradition* (1998), 369–79. Feuerstein anglicizes the Sanskrit *kula,* treating it as a proper name. This practice would be fine if we were told the word's range of meanings, the name's connotations. Gudrun Buhnemann has translated chapter 15, on the "preliminary ritual," *puras-charana,* in *Ritual and Speculation in Early Tantrism: Essays in Honor of André Padoux,* ed. T. Goudriaan (1992), 61–106. What Buhnemann describes as a "free translation" of the entire text by Ram Kumar Rai has been published, but I have, unfortunately, not been able to secure it. Goudriaan and Gupta, *Hindu Tantric and Shakta Literature,* also translate (elegantly) a few verses (93 and 94).

13. Chapter 3 of the *KT* takes up a traditional division of Tantras and Agamas into four, matching the four directions, adding a fifth, the Urddhva Amnaya, "Upper Road of the High Tradition"—a vertical axis distinct from the four horizontal directions. The five issue from the five mouths of Shiva, all leading to enlightenment but with the "Upper Road" as the best (3.19).

14. Presumably, Shiva refers here (2.3) to the "yoginis" who are said to have stood at the center of especially the early Kaula rituals.

15. As explained (note 13), from each of Shiva's five mouths comes a different scriptural tradition. An alternative reading of 2.5 says "firmly established from mouth to mouth." God (Shiva/Devi) is, nevertheless, here too implied as the founding Guru, the World Teacher, who stands at the head of the lineage, as (S) he does of all teaching of crafts. (See the second section of chapter 5.)

16. Although the Shaivite is mentioned separately, the Right-handed, Left-handed, and Siddhanta are usually considered forms or streams of Shaivism. Siddhanta Agamas are dualist, borrowing from Samkhya with less alteration than in other systems or streams. The Right-handed, M. P. Pandit writes (Avalon 1965:30), is "the path where karma, bhakti, and jnana are *skilfully* harmonized and synthecized" (italics in the original). The Left-handed is a path of transgression or reversal from "outward-directed" energies (*pravritti*) to the "inward" (*nivritti*), also according to Pandit (30–31).

17. An alternative reading of 2.9: it comes as a gift directly from Shiva.

18. This is to accept the alternative reading given by Vidyaratna in a footnote to 2.23 from one of his manuscripts.

19. There are three denominative verbs (verbs made from nouns) in this verse, all in the reflexive mode, *atmane-pade* (becomes), as opposed to the transitive or irreflexive, *parasmai-pade* (acts on). To preserve the construction in English, we might say, anglicizing *bhoga,* which means "enjoyment": "On the Way of the Family, bhoga yogas, being-tripped-up dances, and life heavens, O Queen" (*bhogo yogāyate sākṣāt pātakaṃ sukṛtāyate / mokṣāyate ca saṃsāraḥ kuladharme kulêśvari*).

20. Here in honor of all Anusara teachers let me translate (with transliteration in the standard form) one more verse. Chapter 14, verse 38 is responsible, I am told, for the "Anusara" name: "*śakti-pātânusāreṇa śiṣyo 'nugraham arhati / yatra na śaktir na patati tatra siddhir na jāyate.*"

> The student, the disciple becomes worthy and capable of Grace by *aligning with* (*anusāra*) the descent (or reception, literally, "fall") of Shakti (divine energy). Where Shakti is not descending (alternatively, where the guru's initiation has not been received), no perfection (*siddhi*) is born.

An alternative translation is provided by Brooks, "The Ocean of the Heart: Selections from the *Kularnava Tantra,*" 359. Brooks does not give, as I have, occult ambience to "descent of Shakti," interpreting *śakti-pāta* as amounting to initiation and the grace received from the guru in the ceremony. The text is probably meant to be taken also in that sense. And the overall context of chapter 14 is against me. Nevertheless, double meaning is a virtue of the verses of *KT* as it is for poetry in general. The *KT* is elegant poetry, exhibiting all the tropes loved by aestheticians, including, to be sure, *shlesha,* the pun or double entendre. Unfortunately in English there is no way to render double meaning except by the artificial means of parentheses (no phrase in English means both descent of Shakti and initiation). Note that M. P. Pandit (Woodroffe 1965:104) in his summary reads the phrase pretty much the same way I do (or, I should say, I follow him): "The disciple receives the Grace according to the impact of the Shakti, *shakti-pata;* where there is no impact of *shakti,* there is no fulfillment."

21. Here are the first and third verses from Paul Mueller-Ortega's translation of Abhinava's *Anubhava-nivedana-stotra,* "The Song of Praise Intended to

Communicate the Direct Experience of the Absolute," which has a total of four verses; from David White, ed., *Tantra in Practice* (2000), 585–86.

> 1. The accomplished Tantric yogin, whose mind and breath have been dissolved through complete immersion in the innermost object of perception, the supreme goal of yoga—such a yogin then abides with a silenced but open vision, the pupils of the eyes unmoving. Though he [is seen to] gaze still on the outer world, in truth his vision assuredly does not rest on its [apparent outwardness]. This is the seal of Shambhu—the shambhava mudra, the Shaiva "seal" of unitary consciousness, the performing of the ultimate "stance" of Shiva's illumination.
>
> This state of true and ultimate mystical vision, O Divine Master, is produced only because of your potent and illuminating grace. This is the domain of Shambhu, the gracious Lord, the true state of reality which is beyond the experience of . . . the fullness [of the conditions of ordinary awareness] as well as beyond even the [extraordinary] void states [of advanced Tantric meditation]. . . .
>
> 3. In that state, whatsoever words may emerge from the mouth of such a yogin are, indeed, transcendentally charged mantras. The aggregate form of the body—within which the experience of pleasure and pain are constantly arising—that very bodily form [of the illuminated yogin] is nevertheless the mudra or seal that reveals [the experience of the Absolute].
>
> The spontaneous and natural flow of the breath [which produces the natural mantric sound *hamsa* continuously]—that, indeed, is the extraordinary and highest yoga itself. Having directly experienced the unparalleled splendor, the illuminating glory of the divine shakti, in truth, what will then not reveal itself to me?

A word about the mantra, *hamsa,* which has both a literal and a figurative meaning as well as a distinct, double meaning when its two syllables are taken in reverse order, *sa* and *ham.* By attraction from the "Great Statement" of the *Isha Upanishad,* viz., *so 'ham,* its second or double meaning is: "I am He (the Conscious Being in the Sun and everywhere, the Absolute, the Brahman)." The mantra *so 'ham* has extraordinary resonance. It is the climax of the Upanishad, while the short *Isha,* which has only eighteen verses, comes first in traditional Vedantic collections (in both Advaita and theistic lineages). Then, there is the primary meaning of the word, *hamsa,* which is the Siberian crane—as I surmise on the basis of the evidence (against several divergent translation conventions, "goose," "swan," "eagle," etc., partly because this bird, unlike the other candidates, flies over the Himalayas to summer in the north while wintering in India). Thus the secondary meaning, connected beautifully to the first, is the transmigrating individual, *jivatman* (see the beginning of the third section of chapter 5). Repeating this mantra thousands of times, the seeker hears *so 'ham* equally with the generic name of his individual soul—the mantra is Abhinava's favorite as well as glorified in numerous Kula texts, e.g., *Kularnava Tantra,* chapter 3, almost the whole of which is devoted to praising its virtues.

The text of the hymn I translate is from K. C. Pandey, *Abhinavagupta* (1963), 952–53 (placed immediately before the *Anubhava-nivedana-stotra*).

22. Lilian Silburn, *Hymnes de Abhinava* (1970), 37–47 and 85–97. My only criticism of the commentary, which runs several pages in inspired prose, is that the professor takes perhaps too much opportunity to elaborate Abhinava's monistic philosophy. Some ideas of Silburn's have the barest *point d'appui* in the poem's actual words. Her comments are nevertheless usually insightful and informative.

23. Here and in the next verse, in-breath and out-breath are only meant in part (Silburn's translation is in error here, 87). In breathing in, pranic energy flows up. In breathing out, pranic energy in the form called *apana,* down-breath energy, moves down. Air may in the first case be going in and down, but the pranic energy rises; similarly with out-breath, that is, the energy pushes down. The divinities are stationed in the *prana,* in the first two of five types (see note 15 to appendix A). This suggests endorsement of *pranayama* as a yogic method, but see again note 7 to this appendix.

The two energies are the portals for entry into the occult domain, where our ordinary faculties and activities become material for offerings by the various divinities to Shiva/Shakti (as Silburn points out).

24. The word *vimarsha,* translated here "self-consciousness," means more broadly "reflection," as in the mental effort required to make an inference. One "reflects" upon seeing smoke that wherever is smoke there is fire, and that thus there must be fire here too. With Abhinava and his predecessors in Pratyabhijna (Recognition) philosophy and the *Spanda-karika* ("Verses on the [Divine] Vibration [Creative of the Universe]"), the word is used for the process of self-realization, or self-immersion, where there is a recognition that comprehends both the universal/transcendent ("That") and the individual/immanent ("This"): "That is This."

The word *lila,* "play," has Advaita and more broadly monist reverberations: see note 7 to chapter 5, above. Brahman self-manifests for the purpose of novel delight. Everything contributes to *ananda* from the right perspective.

The use of the masculine "Bhairava" so often together with the feminine "Bhairavi" suggests the figure of the Ardha-narishvara, Half-Female God, depicted in statues as divided at midline into, on the statue's right, a divine male torso, etc., and, on the left, a divine female.

25. One may wonder whereto in our bodies are there references? The answer: certitude and rational intelligence. These are divinities in our body consisting of higher mind, to use the theory of the *kosha*s; see figure 4A.

26. Here we see explicitly expressed the thesis that pride and egoism—so

vilified in yogic traditions—are a force of divine manifestation, offered to the Ultimate by—we might note—the most tolerant and indulgent of the divinities, the Mother, Shambhavi, the Kind. Abhinava makes explicit which deity reigns in which region of the divine lotus in a couple of verses such as this one. For the other identifications, I rely on Silburn (1970).

27. The Sanskrit word translated "imagined possibilities" is *vikalpa,* imagination in the technical sense of not being about the present or past but rather the future. But these are really thoughts that present life "options," so to say, the imagined possibilities of getting what we want and avoiding what we want to avoid that our chattering minds occupy themselves with daily.

28. The six philosophies are those that are Vedic in lineage and, let us say, religious practice, though all hardly regard the Veda in the same way: Mimamsa, Vedanta, Nyaya, Vaisheshika, Samkhya, and Yoga. The thirty-six categories are of Shiva/Shakti and their manifestation according to the Trika school (which Abhinava infuses into his overall Kaula). The expression translated "proprietor of the field," *kshetra pati,* echoes the *Gita,* chapter 13.

29. J. L. Masson and M. V. Patwardhan, *Santarasa* (1969). The Sanskrit text that I translate appears on 115–17, and Masson's and Patwardhan's translation on 130–35.

30. There is no need to amend and read, following Masson and Patwardhan (note 5, p. 130), *vishayasyaiva* for *vishayasyeva.* The point is that unlike sensory objects, the self is also subject, and so the self is object "as it were" (*iva*).

31. This is not to accept Masson and Patwardhan's emending to *yoga*, "in connection with," from *ayoga,* "not in connection with."

32. Masson and Patwardhan say (note 3, p. 132) that they cannot understand the reason for the citation. But this is easy. The *Yoga Sutra* claim is that *samadhi* as an experience leaves "traces," *samskara*, the mental dispositions we have so often discussed. But these that lead to spiritual tranquility are special traces, special dispositions, in that they push one to *shanti* and further experience of *samadhi.* Sly Abhinava has referred us to a transformational theory of the *YS* that stands in tension with its official dualism: the mystical state has worldly consequences.

Appendix E. Selections from the *Hatha Yoga Pradipika*

1. George Briggs, *Gorakhnath and the Kanphata Yogis* (1938), provides novel-worthy descriptions of yogins in this tradition coupled with textual background. Finding descriptions of what he views as a similar lineage in the early epic the *Ramayana* and elsewhere, Briggs argues that the lineage may be very old indeed. There is, he judges, evidence for similar yoga practice in Vedic times in a hymn about a *muni* (sage/mage) with wild hair, as suggested also by a few other scholars, as he points out (210–12).

2. *The Hathayogapradipika* of Svatmarama, with the commentary *Jyotsna* of

 Brahmananda, ed. and trans. A. A. Ramanathan and S. V. Subrahmanya Sastri (1972), and *Hathayogapradipika,* trans. Swami Muktabodhananda (1993).

3. Asanas are named and some briefly described. For details, I recommend *Light on Yoga* by B.K.S. Iyengar and the publications of the Bihar School of Yoga—including the *HYP* translation and commentary already mentioned—but also especially Swami Satyananda Saraswati, *Asana Pranayama Mudra Bandha.* Precise physical instructions are given over dozens of pages.

4. Wind is fourth in its subtlety, air being known by touch and sound, whereas ether, the fifth element, *akasha,* is known only by sound, earth by all five sense modalities, water by four, and *tejas,* the fiery element, by three.

5. See note 25 to chapter 1 for a comment on verse 2.46 in the context of a yoga class.

6. See note 43 to appendix C for Vyasa's list of eight *siddhi*s in his commentary on *YS* 3.45. King Bhoja (c. 1050) has a practically identical list as the one here in his *Rajamartanda* commentary, which is an independent commentary on the *YS* (not a subcommentary on Vyasa), also under 3.45, although instead of *prapti,* cognition at a distance, Bhoja has *kama-vasaya,* dwelling wherever desired; Dhundhiraj Sastri, ed. (1930, 1982), 158.

7. Ramanathan and Subramanya Sastri, eds., *The Hathayogapradipika* of Svatmarama (1972), Brahmananda's commentary, 75 (in the Sanskrit page-numbering).

8. Ramanathan and Subramanya Sastri, eds., *The Hathayogapradipika* of Svatmarama (1972), 85, the English quotation. Brahmananda's complaint runs on 181–85 in the separate Sanskrit page numbering.

Bibliography

Alper, Harvey, ed. *Understanding Mantras*. Albany: State University of New York Press, 1989.

Alston, William. *Perceiving God: The Epistemology of Religious Experience*. Ithaca, N.Y.: Cornell University Press, 1991.

Anacker, Stefan. *Seven Works of Vasubandhu*. Delhi: Motilal Banarsidass, 1984.

Arnold, Dan. "On Semantics and *Samketa:* Thoughts on a Neglected Problem with Buddhist *Apoha* Doctrine." *Journal of Indian Philosophy* 34 (October 2006): 415–78.

Apuleius. *The Golden Ass*. Trans. Robert Graves. New York: Farrar, Straus & Giroux, 1951.

Augustine. *Of True Religion*. Trans. J.H.S. Burleigh. Chicago: Regnery, 1959.

Aurobindo, Sri. *The Future Poetry*. Sri Aurobindo Birth Centenary Library, vol. 9. Pondicherry: Sri Aurobindo Ashram Trust, 1973.

——. *Hymns to the Mystic Fire*. Sri Aurobindo Birth Centenary Library, vol. 11. Pondicherry: Sri Aurobindo Ashram Trust, 1973.

——. *The Life Divine*. Sri Aurobindo Birth Centenary Library, vols. 18 and 19. Pondicherry: Sri Aurobindo Ashram Trust, 1973.

——. *Record of Yoga*. 2 vols. Pondicherry: Sri Aurobindo Ashram Trust, 2001.

——. *Savitri*. Sri Aurobindo Birth Centenary Library, vols. 28 and 29. Pondicherry: Sri Aurobindo Ashram Trust, 1973.

——. *The Synthesis of Yoga*. Sri Aurobindo Birth Centenary Library, vols. 20 and 21. Pondicherry: Sri Aurobindo Ashram Trust, 1973.

——. *The Upanishads*. Sri Aurobindo Birth Centenary Library, vol. 12. Pondicherry: Sri Aurobindo Ashram Trust, 1973.

Avalon, Arthur (Sir John Woodroffe), ed. *Kularnava Tantra*. Summarized by M. P. Pandit; Sanskrit text ed. Taranatha Vidyaratha. Delhi: Motilal Banarsidass, 1965.

——. *Shakti and Shakta*. New York: Dover, 1978.

Basham, A. L. *The Wonder That Was India*. New York: Grove Press, 1954.

Bennigson, Thomas. "Is Relativism Really Self-Refuting?" *Philosophical Studies* 94, no. 3 (June 1999): 211–35.

Benson, Herbert. *The Mind/Body Effect*. New York: Berkeley Books, 1980.

Bharati, Aghehananda. *Ochre Robe*. Santa Barbara, Calif.: Ross-Erikson, 1988.

——. *The Tantric Tradition*. 1965; reprint, Garden City, N.Y.: Anchor, 1970.

Bhat, M. S. *Vedic Tantrism: A Study of Rgvidhana of Saunaka with Text and Translation*. Delhi: Motilal Banarsidass, 1987.

Bhatta, Mammata. *Kavya-Prakasa*. Trans. S. N. Ghoshal Sastri. Varanasi: Chowkhamba Sanskrit Office, 1973.

Bhattacharya, Gopinath. *Tarka-samgraha by Annambhatta*. Calcutta: Progressive, 1976.

Bhattacharyya, Gopikamohan. *Studies in Nyaya-Vaisheshika Theism*. Calcutta: Sanskrit College, 1961.

Bhattacharyya, K. C. *Search for the Absolute in Neo-Vedanta*. Ed. George B. Burch. Honolulu: University Press of Hawaii, 1976.

——. *Studies in Philosophy*. Ed. Gopinath Bhattacharyya. 2 vols. Calcutta: Progressive, 1956, 1958.

Blofeld, John. *The Tantric Mysticism of Tibet*. New York: E. P. Dutton, 1970.

Bodas, Rajaram, ed. *Patanjalayogadarsana,* with the *Tattva-Vaisaradi* of Vacaspati Mishra. Bombay Sanskrit and Prakrit Series, no. 46. Bombay: Government Central Press, 1917.

Braude, Stephen. *First-Person Plural: Multiple Personality and the Philosophy of Mind*. New York: Routledge, 1991.

——. *Immortal Remains: The Evidence for Life After Death*. Lanham, Md.: Rowman and Littlefield, 2003.

Briggs, George. *Gorakhnath and the Kanphata Yogis*. Delhi: Motilal Banarsidass, 1938.

Bronkhorst, Johannes. *Karma and Teleology*. Tokyo: International Institute for Buddhist Studies of the International College for Advanced Buddhist Studies, 2000.

Brooks, Douglas Renfrew. *Auspicious Wisdom: The Texts and Traditions of Srividya Sakta Tantricism in South India*. Albany: State University of New York Press, 1992.

——. "The Ocean of the Heart: Selections from the *Kularnava Tantra*." In *Tantra in Practice,* ed. D. White. Princeton, N.J.: Princeton University Press, 2000.

——. *The Secret of the Three Cities*. Chicago and London: University of Chicago Press, 1990.

Brown, Cheever Mackenzie. *The Triumph of the Goddess: The Canonical Mod-*

els and Theological Visions of the Devi-Bhagavata Purana. Albany: State University of New York Press, 1990.

Brunner, Hélène. "The Place of Yoga in the Saivagamas." In *Pandit N. R. Bhatt Felicitation Volume*. Delhi: Motilal Banarsidass, 1994.

Buhnemann, Gudrun, ed. *Ritual and Speculation in Early Tantrism: Essays in Honor of André Padoux*. Albany: State University of New York Press, 1992.

Buitenen, J.A.B. van. *The Bhagavad Gita in the Mahabharata*. Chicago: University of Chicago Press, 1981.

——. "Dharma and Moksa." *Philosophy East and West* 7 (1957): 33–40.

——. *The Mahabharata, Books I–V*. 3 vols. Chicago: University of Chicago Press, 1973–1978.

——. *The Maitrayaniya Upanisad*. The Hague: Mouton, 1962.

——. *Ramanuja on the Bhagavadgita*. Delhi: Motilal Banarsidass, 1968.

——, tr. *Ramanuja's Vedarthasangraha*. Poona, India: Deccan College Postgraduate and Research Institute, 1956.

Chakrabarti, Arindam. "I Touch What I Saw." *Philosophy and Phenomenological Research* 52, no. 1 (March 1992): 103–16.

——. "Is Liberation (Moksa) Pleasant?" *Philosophy East and West* 33 (1983): 167–82.

——. "Telling as Letting Know." In *Knowing from Words*, ed. A. Chakrabarti and B. K. Matilal. Dordrecht: Kluwer Academic, 1994.

Chalmers, David. *The Conscious Mind*. New York: Oxford University Press, 1996.

Chappel, Christopher Key, ed. *Jainism and Ecology*. Cambridge, Mass.: Harvard Center for World Religions, 2002.

——. *Karma and Creativity*. Albany: State University of New York Press, 1986.

——. *Nonviolence to Animals, Earth and Self in Asian Traditions*. Albany: State University of New York Press, 1993.

——. "Reading Patanjali Without Vyasa: A Critique of Four *Yoga Sutra* Passages." *Journal of the American Academy of Religion* 62, no. 1 (1994): 85–105.

Chappel, Christopher Key and Yogi Ananda Viraj (Eugene P. Kelley Jr.). *The Yoga Sutras of Patanjali: An Analysis of the Sanskrit with Accompanying English Translation*. Delhi: Sri Satguru Publications, 1990.

Chatterjee, K. N. *Vijnapti-matrata-siddhi* (Vasubandhu's *Vimshatika* and *Trimshika* along with Sthiramati's Sanskrit commentary, translated with the Sanskrit text). Varanasi: Kishor Vidya Niketan, 1980.

Chemparathy, George. *An Indian Rational Theology*. Vienna: Indologische Institut der Universität Wien, 1972.

Chisholm, Roderick. *Theory of Knowledge*. 2nd ed. Englewood Cliffs, N.J.: Prentice Hall, 1977.

Cosby, Kate and Andrew Skilton, trans. *Santideva, The Bodhicaryatara*. Oxford: Oxford University Press, 1996.

Coulter, H. David. *Anatomy of Hatha Yoga*. Honesdale, Pa.: Body and Breath, 2001.

Coward, Howard. *Bhartrihari*. Boston: Twayne, 1976.

Curtiss, Susan. *Genie: A Psycholinguistic Study of a Modern-Day "Wild Child."* New York: Academic Press, 1977.

Danielou, Alain. *Shiva and Dionysus: The Religion of Nature and Eros*. Trans. K. F. Hurry. New York: Inner Traditions International, 1984.

——. *Yoga: The Method of Re-Integration*. London: Christopher Johnson, 1949.

Dasgupta, Surendranath. *A History of Indian Philosophy*. 5 vols. Cambridge: Cambridge University Press, 1922–1955.

——. *The Study of Patanjali*. Calcutta: University of Calcutta, 1920.

——. *Yoga as Philosophy and Religion*. London: Kegan Paul, 1924.

——. *Yoga Philosophy in Relation to Other Systems of Indian Thought*. Calcutta: University of Calcutta, 1930.

Dayal, Har. *The Bodhisattva Doctrine in Buddhist Sanskrit Literature*. 1932; reprint, Delhi: Motilal Banarsidass, 1970.

Deussen, Paul. *The Philosophy of the Upanisads*. Trans. A. S. Geden. New York: Dover, 1966.

——. *Sixty Upanisads of the Veda*. 2 vols. Trans. V. M. Bedekar and G. B. Palsule. Delhi: Motilal Banarsidass, 1980.

Deutsch, Eliot. *Advaita Vedanta*. Honolulu: University Press of Hawaii, 1969.

Doniger, Wendy, with Brian K. Smith. *The Laws of Manu*. London: Penguin, 1991.

Dravid, N. S. *Nyaya-kusumanjali of Udayanacarya*. New Delhi: Indian Council of Philosophical Research, 1996.

Ducasse, C. J. *A Critical Examination of the Belief in a Life After Death*. Springfield, Ill.: Charles Thomas, 1961.

——. *Nature, Mind, and Death*. La Salle, Ill.: Open Court, 1951.

Dundas, Paul. *The Jainas*. London: Routledge, 1992.

Dupuche, John R. *Abhinava: The Kula Ritual*. Delhi: Motilal Banarsidass, 2003.

Dvivedhin, Vindhyesvariprasada and Lakshmana Sastri Dravida, eds. (Udayana's) *Atmatattvaviveka*. Calcutta: Asiatic Society, 1986.

Dyczkowski, Mark S.G. *The Doctrine of Vibration: An Analysis of the Doctrines and Practices of Kashmir Saivism*. Albany: State University of New York Press, 1987.

Easwaran, Eknath. *The Upanishads*. Petaluma, Calif.: Nilgiri Press, 1987.

Edgerton, Franklin. *The Bhagavad Gita*. Cambridge, Mass.: Harvard University Press, 1952.

Edwards, Paul. *Reincarnation: A Critical Examination*. Amherst, N.Y.: Prometheus, 2001.

Egge, James R. *Religious Giving and the Invention of Karma in Theravada Buddhism*. Richmond, Surrey: Curzon, 2002.

Eliade, Mircea. *A History of Religious Ideas*. Vols. 1 and 2. Trans. W. R. Trask. Chicago: University of Chicago Press, 1978, 1982.

——. *Patanjali and Yoga*. New York: Schocken, 1975.
——. *Yoga: Immortality and Freedom*. Trans. W. Trask. Princeton, N.J.: Princeton University Press, 1973.
Emavardhana, Tipawadee and Christopher D. Tori. "Changes in Self-Concept, Ego Defense Mechanisms, and Religiosity Following Seven-Day Vipassana Meditation Retreats." *Journal for the Scientific Study of Religion* 36, no. 2 (June 1997): 194–207.
Evans-Wentz, W. Y. *The Tibetan Book of the Great Liberation*. London: Oxford University Press, 1968.
Feuerstein, Georg. *The Philosophy of Classical Yoga*. Rochester, Vt.: Inner Traditions International, 1996.
——. *The Shambhala Encyclopedia of Yoga*. Boston: Shambhala, 1997.
——. *The Yoga Tradition*. Prescott, Ariz.: Hohm Press, 1998.
——. *The Yoga Sutra of Patanjali*. Rochester, Vt.: Inner Traditions, 1979.
Findly, Ellison. *Dana: Giving and Getting in Pali Buddhism*. Delhi: Motilal Banarsidass, 2003.
Fodor, Jerry A. *A Theory of Content and Other Essays*. Cambridge, Mass.: MIT Press, 1990.
Fort, Andrew O. and Patricia Y. Mumme, eds. *Living Liberation in Hindu Thought*. Albany: State University of New York, 1996.
Frankfurt, Harry G. "Freedom of the Will and the Concept of a Person." *Journal of Philosophy* 68, no. 1 (1971): 5–20.
Frawley, David. *The Creative Vision of the Early Upanishads*. Madras, India: Rajsri Printers, 1982.
——. *Tantric Yoga and the Wisdom Goddesses*. Salt Lake City, Utah: Passage Press, 1994.
——. *Wisdom of the Ancient Seers: Mantras of the Rig Veda*. Salt Lake City, Utah: Passage Press, 1992.
Ganeri, Jonardon. "Cross-Modality and the Self." *Philosophy and Phenomenological Research* (October 2000).
Garfield, Jay. *The Fundamental Wisdom of the Middle Way: Nagarjuna's Mulamadhyamika-karika*. New York: Oxford University Press, 1995.
Gerow, Edwin. "Abhinava's Aesthetics as a Speculative Paradigm." *Journal of the American Oriental Society* 114, no. 2 (1994): 186–208.
Ghosh, Manmohan. *Natya-sastra*. 2 vols. Calcutta: Manisha Granthalaya, 1961–67.
Gnoli, Raniero. *The Aesthetic Experience According to Abhinava Gupta*. Chowkhamba Sanskrit Studies, vol. 62. Varanasi: Chowkhamba Sanskrit Series Office, 1968.
——. *Tantraloka*. Torino: Unione Tipografico-Editrice Torinese, 1980.
Gokhale, Dinkar Vishnu, ed. *The Bhagavad Gita with the Commentary of Shankaracharya*. Poona Oriental Series 1. Pune: Oriental Book Agency, 1950.
Gonda, Jan. *The Vision of the Vedic Poets*. The Hague: Mouton, 1963.
——. "Why Are *Ahimsa* and Similar Concepts Often Expressed in a Negative

Form?" In *Four Studies in the Language of the Veda*, 95–117. The Hague: Mouton, 1959.

Gopal, K. S., S. Laksamanan, and S. Batmanabane. "A Study of the Effect of Bandhas in Pranayama on Pulse Rate, Heart Rate, Blood Pressure and Pulse Pressure." *Medicine and Surgery* 14, no. 10 (1974): 5–8.

Goswami, Mahaprabhulal, ed. *Nyayakusumanjali* (of Udayana). Mithila Institute Ancient Texts Series 23. Darbhanga: Mithila Institute, 1972.

Goudriaan, Teun, ed. *Ritual and Speculation in Early Tantrism: Essays in Honor of André Padoux*. Albany: State University of New York Press, 1992.

Goudriaan, Teun and Sanjukta Gupta. *Hindu Tantric and Sakta Literature*. Wiesbaden: Otto Harrassawitz, 1981.

Graham, Peter. "Liberal Fundamentalism and Its Rivals." In *The Epistemology of Testimony,* ed. J. Lackey and E. Sosa. New York: Oxford University Press, 2006.

Grassmann, Hermann Gunther. *Worterbuch zum Rig-Veda*. Leipsig: F. A. Brockhaus, 1873.

Gupta, Bina. *The Disinterested Witness*. Evanston, Ill.: Northwestern University Press, 1998.

——. *Perceiving in Advaita Vedanta*. Lewisburg, Pa.: Bucknell University Press, 1991.

Gupta, Sanjukta, Dirk Jan Hoens, and Teun Goudriaan. *Hindu Tantrism*. Leiden: Brill, 1979.

Haberman, David L., trans. *The Bhakti-rasamrta-sindhu of Rupa Gosvamin*. New Delhi: Indira Gandhi Centre for the Arts, 2003.

Halbfass, Wilhelm. *India and Europe: An Essay in Understanding*. Albany: State University of New York Press, 1988.

——. "Karma, *Apurva,* and 'Natural' Causes." In *Karma and Rebirth in Classical Indian Traditions,* ed. Wendy Doniger O'Flaherty, 268–302. Berkeley: University of California Press, 1980.

——. *On Being and What There Is: Classical Vaisesika and the History of Indian Ontology*. Albany: State University of New York Press, 1992.

——. *Studies in Kumarila and Sankara*. Reinbek: Inge Wezler, 1983.

Hartshorne, Charles. *Omnipotence and Other Theological Mistakes*. Albany: State University of New York Press, 1984.

Harwood, Robin. *The Survival of the Self*. Aldershot: Ashgate, 1998.

Hauer, Jakob Wilhelm. *Der Yoga: Ein indischer Weg zum Selbst*. Stuttgart: Kohlhammer, 1958.

Hawley, John Stratton. *Krishna, the Butter Thief*. Princeton, N.J.: Princeton University Press, 1983.

Hayes, Richard P. *Dignaga on the Interpretation of Signs*. Dordrecht: Kluwar, 1987.

Herzberger, Radhika. *Bhartrhari and the Buddhists*. Dordrecht: D. Reidel, 1986.

Hick, John. *Evil and the God of Love*. New York: Harper & Row, 1966.

Hiltebeitel, Alf. *The Ritual of Battle: Krishna in the Mahabharata*. Albany: State University of New York Press, 1990.
Hiriyanna, M. *Indian Conception of Values*. Mysore: Kavyalaya Publishers, 1975.
Hopkins, Edward Washburn. *The Religions of India*. 2nd ed. 1885; reprint, New Delhi: Munshiram Manoharlal, 1970.
——. "Yoga-technique in the Great Epic." *Journal of the American Oriental Society* 12, no. 2 (1901): 333–79.
Hume, David. *A Treatise of Human Nature*. Oxford: Oxford University Press, 1888.
Hume, Robert, trans. *The Thirteen Principal Upanishads*. Oxford: Oxford University Press, 1921.
Iyengar, B.K.S. *Light on Pranayama*. New York: Crossroad, 1987.
——. *Light on the Yoga Sutras of Patanjali*. London: Aquarian/Thorsons, 1993.
——. *Light on Yoga*. Rev. ed. New York: Schocken, 1979.
——. *Tree of Yoga*. Boston: Shambhala, 2002.
Jacob, Colonel G. A. *A Concordance to the Principal Upanishads and Bhagavadgita*. 1891; reprint, Delhi: Motilal Banarsidass, 1963.
Jaini, Padmanabh S. *The Jaina Path of Purification*. Delhi: Motilal Banarsidass, 1979.
James, William. "Does Consciousness Exist?" *Essays in Radical Empiricism*. New York: Longmans, Green, 1912.
——. *The Varieties of Religious Experience*. 1902; reprint, New York: Penguin, 1982.
Janacek, Adolf. "The Methodical Principle in Yoga According to Patanjali's Yoga Sutras." *Archiv Orientalni* 19 (1951): 514–67.
——. "To the Problems of Indian Philosophical Texts." *Archiv Orientalni* 27 (1959): 463–75.
——. "The 'Voluntaristic' Type of Yoga in Patanjali's Yoga Sutras." *Archiv Orientalni* 22 (1954): 69–87.
Jha, Ganganatha. *The Prabhakara School of Purva Mimamsa*. Delhi: Motilal Banarsidass, 1978.
——. *Purva-Mimamsa in Its Sources*. Varanasi: Benaras Hindu University Press, 1964.
Joshi, K. S. "The Concept of Saiyama in Patanjali's Yoga Sutra." *Yoga-Mimamsa* 8, no. 2 (1965): 1–18.
——. "On the Meaning of Yoga." *Philosophy East and West* 15, no. 1 (January 1965): 53–64.
Kafka, Franz. *The Metamorphosis and Other Stories*. Trans. J. Neugroschel. New York: Charles Scribner's Sons, 1993.
Kant, Immanuel. *Critique of Pure Reason*. Trans. Norman Kemp Smith. New York: St. Martin's Press, 1965.
——. *Groundwork of the Metaphysics of Morals*. Trans. H. J. Paton. New York: Harper & Row, 1964.

Kapali-Sastry, K. V. *Rig-Bhashya Bhumika*. Pondicherry: M. P. Pandit, 1952.

Karnatak, Vimala. *Patanjala-yoga-darsanam*. 4 vols. Varanasi: Banaras Hindu University, 1992.

Keith, Arthur B. *The Religion and Philosophy of the Veda and Upanishads*. Harvard Oriental Series, vols. 31–32. Cambridge, Mass.: Harvard University Press, 1925–26.

Kinsley, David. *Hindu Goddesses: Visions of the Divine Feminine in the Hindu Religious Tradition*. Berkeley and Los Angeles: University of California Press, 1986.

——. *Tantric Visions of the Divine Feminine: The Ten Mahavidyas*. Berkeley: University of California Press, 1997.

Kothari, L. K., A. Bordia, and O. P. Gupta. "Studies on a Yogi During an Eight-Day Confinement in a Sealed Underground Pit." *Indian Journal of Medical Residence* 61, no. 11 (November 1973): 1645–50.

Kraftsow, Gary. *Yoga for Transformation*. New York: Penguin, 2002.

——. *Yoga for Wellness*. New York: Penguin, 1999.

Kramrisch, Stella. *The Presence of Siva*. Princeton, N.J.: Princeton University Press, 1981.

Krishna, Gopi. *The Awakening of Kundalini*. New York: E. P. Dutton, 1975.

——. *The Real Nature of Mystical Experience*. New York: New Concepts, 1978.

Krishnamurti, J. *Talks and Dialogues*. 1968; reprint, New York: Avon, 1970.

Kumar, Muni Mahendra, trans. *Ayaro Acarangasutra*. New Delhi: Jain Vishva Bharati, 1981.

Kuvalayananda, Swami and S. A. Shukla, eds. *Goraksasatakam*. Bombay: Kaivalyadhama S.M.Y.M. Samiti, 1858.

Lackey, J. and E. Sosa, eds. *The Epistemology of Testimony*. New York: Oxford University Press, 2006.

Larson, Gerald James. *Classical Samkhya*. Delhi: Motilal Banarsidass, 1969.

Larson, Gerald James and Ram Shankar Bhattacharya, eds. *Samkhya*. In *Encyclopedia of Indian Philosophies*, ed. Karl Potter, vol. 4. Delhi: Motilal Banarsidass, 1987.

Leggett, Trevor, trans. *The Complete Commentary by Sankara on the Yoga Sutras*. London: Kegan Paul, 1990.

Levine, Michael P. *Pantheism: A Non-theistic Concept of Deity*. New York: Routledge, 1994.

Lindtner, Christian. *Nagarjuniana*. Delhi: Motilal Banarsidass, 1986.

Lorenzen, David. "Kapalikas and Kalamukhas: Two Lost Shaivite Sects." In *Yoga: The Indian Tradition,* ed. Ian Whicher and David Carpenter. New York: RoutledgeCurzon, 2003.

Maas, Philipp André. *Samadhipada*. Aachen: Shaker, 2006.

Macdonnell, A. A. *Vedic Mythology*. 2 vols. 1912; reprint, Varanasi: Indological Book House, 1963.

MacInerney, Charles. *Shavasana, the Art of Relaxation*. Audio cassette. Austin, Tex.: Charles MacInerney, 1995.

Mahadevan, T.M.P. *The Philosophy of Beauty*. Bombay: Bharatiya Vidya Bhavan, 1969.

Masson, J. L. and M. V. Patwardhan. *Santarasa*. Poona: Bhandarkar Oriental Research Institute, 1969.

Matilal, Bimal Krishna. *Epistemology, Logic, and Grammar in Indian Philosophical Analysis*. The Hague: Mouton, 1971.

——. "The Jaina Contribution to Logic." In *The Character of Logic in India*, ed. Jonardon Ganeri and Heeraman Tiwari, 127–39. Albany: State University of New York Press, 1998.

——. *Perception: An Essay on Classical Indian Theories of Knowledge*. Oxford: Clarendon Press, 1986.

Matilal, Bimal Krishna, ed. *Moral Dilemmas in the Mahabharata*. Delhi: Motilal Banarsidass, 1989.

Mayeda, Sengaku. *A Thousand Teachings* (an annotated translation of Shankara's *Upadeshasahasri*). Tokyo: University of Tokyo, 1979.

McDermott, Charlene. "Yogic Direct Awareness as Means of Valid Cognition in Dharmakirti and Rgyal-tshab." In *Mahayana Buddhist Meditation,* ed. Minoru Kiyota. 1978; reprint, Delhi: Motilal Banarsidass, 1991.

Miller, Barbara Stoler. *The Bhagavad-Gita*. New York: Columbia University Press, 1986.

——. *Love Song of the Dark Lord: Jayadeva's Gitagovinda*. New York: Columbia University Press, 1977.

Misra, Sri Narayana, ed. *Patanjalayogadarsana,* with Vyasa's *Bhasya,* Vacaspati Misra's *Tattva-Vaisaradi* and Vijnana Bhiksu's *Yoga-Varttika*. Varanasi: Chowkhamba, 1971.

Mkhas Grub Rje. *Fundamentals of the Buddhist Tantras*. Trans. F. D. Lessing and A. Wayman. The Hague: Mouton, 1968.

Mohanty, J. N. *Classical Indian Philosophy*. Lanham, Md.: Rowman and Littlefield, 2000.

Monier-Williams, Monier. *Sanskrit-English Dictionary*. London: W. H. Allen, 1851.

Moody, Raymond. A., Jr. *Life After Life*. Covington, Ga.: Mockingbird, 1975.

Motoyama, Hiroshi. *Theories of the Chakras*. Wheaton, Ill.: Theosophical Publishing House, 1981.

Mueller, Max, ed. and trans. *The Upanishads: The Sacred Books of the East*, vol. 15, part 2. 1884; reprint, Delhi: Motilal Banarsidass, 1965.

Mueller-Ortega, Paul. "On Subtle Knowledge and the Refinement of Thought." In *Theory and Practice of Yoga*, ed. Knut A. Jacobsen. Koninklijke: Brill, 2005.

Mueller-Ortega, Paul, trans. "Abhinava's *Anubhava-nivedana-stotra*, 'The Song of Praise Intended to Communicate the Direct Experience of the Absolute.'" In *Tantra in Practice,* ed. David White. Princeton, N.J.: Princeton University Press, 2000.

Muktabodhananda, Swami, trans. *Hathayogapradipika*. 2nd ed. Munger: Bihar School of Yoga, 1993.

Muktananda, Swami. *Play of Consciousness (Chitshakti Vilas)*. San Francisco: Harper & Row, 1978.

Murphy, Michael. *The Future of the Body*. Los Angeles: J. P. Tarcher, 1992.

Murphy, Michael and Steven Donovan. *The Physical and Psychological Effects of Meditation: A Review of Contemporary Research with a Comprehensive Bibliography 1931–1996*. Ed. and intro. Eugene Taylor. Sausalito, Calif.: Institute of Noetic Sciences, 1997.

Murty, K. Satchidananda. *Reason and Revelation in Advaita Vedanta*. 1959; reprint, Delhi: Motilal Banarsidass, 1974.

Nagatomi, Masatoshi. "*Manasa-Pratyaksha:* A Conundrum in the Buddhist *Pramana* System." In *Sanskrit and Indian Studies: Essays in Honor of Daniel H.H. Ingalls,* ed. Nagatomi et al. Dordrecht: D. Reidel, 1980.

Nikhilananda, Swami, trans. *The Gospel of Sri Ramakrishna*. (Conversations recorded in Bengali by Mahendranath Gupta.) New York: Ramakrishna-Vivekananda Center, 1942.

Nozick, Robert. *Philosophical Explanations*. Cambridge, Mass.: Harvard University Press, 1981.

Nyanamol, Bhikku, trans. *The Path of Purification* (Buddhaghosha's *Visuddhimagga*). 2 vols. Boulder: Shambala, 1976.

O'Flaherty, Wendy Doniger, ed. *Karma and Rebirth in Classical Indian Traditions*. Berkeley: University of California Press, 1980.

——. *The Origins of Evil in Hindu Mythology*. Berkeley and Los Angeles: University of California Press, 1976.

Padoux, André. "The Tantric Guru." In *Tantra in Practice,* ed. David White. Princeton, N.J.: Princeton University Press, 2000.

Pandey, K. C. *Abhinavagupta*. Rev. ed. Varanasi: Chowkhamba, 1963.

Parfit, Derek. *Reasons and Persons*. Oxford: Clarendon Press, 1984.

Paterson, R.W.K. *Philosophy and the Belief in a Life After Death*. New York: St. Martin's Press, 1995.

Patton, Laurie. "Nature Romanticism and Sacrifice in Rgvedic Interpretations." In *Hinduism and Ecology,* ed. Christopher Key Chappel and Mary Evelyn Tucker, 39–58. Cambridge, Mass.: Harvard Center for World Religions, 2002.

Peers, E. Allison, trans. *The Autobiography of St. Teresa of Avila*. Garden City, N.Y.: Doubleday, 1960.

Pensa, Corrado. "On the Purification Concept in Indian Tradition, with Special Regard to Yoga." *East and West* 19 (1969): 194–228.

Phillips, Stephen H. *Classical Indian Metaphysics*. Chicago: Open Court, 1995. Indian edition, Delhi: Motilal Banarsidass, 1997.

——. "The Conflict of Voluntarism and Dualism in the *Yogasutra*." *Journal of Indian Philosophy* 13, no. 4 (December 1985): 399–414.

——. "Gangesha on *Mukti*." Paper presented at South Asia Seminar, University of Chicago, 2006.

——. "Mystic Analogizing and the 'Peculiarly Mystical.'" In *Mysticism and Language,* ed. Steven Katz, 123–42. New York: Oxford University Press, 1992.

Phillips, Stephen H. and N. S. Ramanuja Tatacharya. *Epistemology of Perception.* (Gangesha's *Tattva-cinta-mani, pratyaksha-khanda,* introduction, translation, and commentary.) New York: American Institute of Buddhist Studies, 2004.

Plato. *Collected Dialogues.* Ed. Edith Hamilton and Huntington Cairns. Bolligen Series 71. Princeton, N.J.: Princeton University Press, 2005.

Potter, Karl H. *Encyclopedia of Indian Philosophies* 2nd ed. Vol. 1: *Bibliography.* Delhi: Motilal Banarsidass, 1983.

——. "The Karma Theory and Its Interpretation in Some Indian Philosophical Systems." In *Karma and Rebirth in Classical Indian Traditions,* ed. Wendy Doniger O'Flaherty 241–67. Berkeley: University of California Press, 1980.

——. "The Naturalistic Principle of Karma." *Philosophy East and West* 14 (1964): 39–50.

Prasad, Jwala. "The Date of the Yoga Sutras." *Journal of the Royal Asiatic Society* 84 (1930): 365–75.

Prasad, Rajendra. "The Concept of Moksa." *Philosophy and Phenomenological Research* 31 (1971): 381–93.

Prasada Rama, trans. *The Yoga Sutras of Patanjali with the Commentary of Vyasa and the Gloss of Vacaspati Misra.* Vol. 4 of *The Sacred Books of the Hindus,* ed. B. D. Basu. Allahabad: Panini Office, 1912.

Prashastapada. *Padartha-dharma-samgraha.* Trans. Ganganatha Jha. Varanasi: Chaukhambha Orientalia, 1982.

Price, H. H. *Belief.* New York: Humanities Press, 1969.

Priest, Graham. *Beyond the Limits of Thought.* Oxford: Clarendon, 2002.

Priest, Graham and Jay Garfield. "Nagarjuna and the Limits of Thought." In *Beyond the Limits of Thought,* ed. Graham Priest. Oxford: Clarendon, 2002.

Proudfoot, I. *Ahimsa and a Mahabharata Story.* Canberra: Australian National University, 1987.

Quarnström, Olle, trans. *The Yogasastra of Hemacandra.* Harvard Oriental Series 61. Cambridge, Mass.: Harvard University Press, 2002.

Radhakrishnan, Sarvepalli. *An Idealist View of Life.* 2nd ed. London: George Allen & Unwin, 1937.

——. *The Principal Upanishads.* London: George Allen & Unwin, 1953.

Ramanathan, A. A. and S. V. Subrahmanya Sastri, eds. and trans. *The Hathayogapradipika of Svatmarama,* with the commentary *Jyotsna* of Brahmananda. Madras: Adyar Library, 1972.

Ramanuja Tatacharya, N. S., ed. *Tattvacintamani* of Gangesha. Vol. 2, part 2. Tirupati: Kendriya Sanskrit Vidyapeetha, 1999.

Rastogi, Navjivan. *The Krama Tantricism of Kashmir.* Delhi: Motilal Banarsidass, 1979.

Rawls, John. *A Theory of Justice.* Cambridge, Mass.: Harvard University Press, 1971.

Renou, Louis. "Etude Védiques: *Yoga.*" *Journal Asiatique* 241, no. 1 (1953): 177–80.

——. *Religions of Ancient India.* 1953; reprint, New York: Schocken, 1968.
Roebuck, Valerie. *The Upanisads.* New York: Penguin, 2000.
Rogo, D. Scott. *Parapsychology: A Century of Inquiry.* New York: Taplinger, 1975.
Rosch, Eleanor. "Is Wisdom in the Brain?" *American Psychological Society* 10, no. 3 (May 1999): 222–23.
Ross, W. D. *The Right and the Good.* 1930; reprint, Oxford: Clarendon, 2002.
Ruegg, David. *The Literature of the Madhyamaka School of Philosophy in India.* Wiesbaden: Harrassowitz, 1981.
Rukmani, T. S. *Yogavarttika of Vijnanabhikshu.* 4 vols. Delhi: Munshiram Manorhalal, 1981–1989.
Sanderson, A. "Shaivism and the Tantric Traditions." In *The World's Religions,* ed. S. Sutherland, et al. Boston: G. K. Hall, 1988.
Sarasvati, Swami Satya Prakash and Satyakam Vidyalankar, trans. *Rigveda Samhita.* 8 vols. New Delhi: Veda Pratishthana, 1977–1980.
Sastri, Mahadeva A., ed. and trans. *The Yoga Upanisads with the Commentary of Sri Upanisad-Brahma-Yogin.* Adyar Library Series 6. Madras: Adyar Library and Research Centre, 1920.
Satyananda Saraswati, Swami. *Asana Pranayama Mudra Bandha.* Munger: Bihar School of Yoga, 1989.
——. *Four Chapters on Freedom.* Munger: Bihar School of Yoga, 1976.
——. *Kundalini Tantra.* Munger: Bihar School of Yoga, 1996.
——. *A Systematic Course in the Ancient Tantric Techniques of Yoga and Kriya.* 2nd ed. Munger: Bihar School of Yoga, 1989.
Schmidt, Hanns-Peter. "The Origin of *Ahimsa.*" In *Mélanges d'Indianism à la mémoire de Louis Renou,* 625–55. Paris: Boccard, 1968.
Schubring, Walter. *The Doctrine of the Jainas.* Trans. Wolfgang Beeurlen. Delhi: Motilal Banarsidass, 1962.
Schweizer, Paul. "Mind/Consciousness Dualism in Samkhya-Yoga Philosophy." *Philosophy and Phenomenological Research* 53 (1993): 845–59.
Sen, Amartya. *Resources, Values and Development.* Cambridge, Mass.: Harvard University Press, 1984.
Senanayake, Nimal, ed. *Trends in Rebirth Research.* Ratmalana: Sarvodaya Vishva Lekha, 2001.
Shankara. *Ten Principal Upanishads* (with the commentary of Shankara). Delhi: Motilal Banarsidass, 1964.
——. *Upadesasahasri.* Ed. and trans. Swami Jagadananda. Madras: Sri Ramakrishna Math, 1970.
Sharma, Arvind. *The Gitartharthasangraha of Abhinavagupta.* Leiden: Brill, 1983.
——. *A Jaina Perspective on Philosophy of Religion.* Delhi: Motilal Banarsidass, 2001.
Shastri, Dhundhiraja, ed. *Patanjalayogadarsana,* with the *Raja-Martanda* of Bhoja Raja, *Pradipika of Bhavaganesa, Vrtti* of Nagoji Bhatta, *Mani-Prabha* of Ra-

mananda Yati, *Pada Candrika* of Ananta-Deva Pandit, and *Yoga-Sudhakara* of Sadasivendra Sarasvati. Varanasi: Chowkhamba, 1930.

Shastri, J. L., ed. *Upanisat-Samgrahah*. Delhi: Motilal Banarsidass, 1970.

Sheik, Anees, ed. *Handbook of Therapeutic Imagery Techniques*. Amityville, N.Y.: Baywood, 2002.

Silburn, Lilian. *Hymnes de Abhinava*. Paris: Institut de Civilisation Indienne, 1970.

——. *Kundalini: The Energy of the Depths*. Albany: State University of New York Press, 1988.

——. *Le Vijnana Bhairava*. Paris: Editions E. De Boccard, 1961.

Singh, Jaideva. *Pratyabhijinahrdayam: The Secret of Self-Recognition*. Rev. ed. Delhi: Motilal Banasidass, 1980.

——. *Siva Sutras: The Yoga of Supreme Identity*. Delhi: Motilal Banarsidass, 1979.

——. *Spanda-Karikas: The Divine Creative Pulsation*. Delhi: Motilal Banarsidass, 1980.

——. *The Yoga of Delight, Wonder, and Astonishment*. Albany: State University of New York Press, 1991.

Sivaramkrishna, M. and Sumita Roy. *Poet-Saints of India*. New Delhi: Sterling, 1996.

Smythies, John R. and John Beloff, eds. *The Case for Dualism*. Charlottesville: University Press of Virginia, 1989.

Speyer, J. S., trans. *Jataka-Mala* (Garland of Birth Stories). In *Sacred Books of the Buddhists*, ed. Max Mueller, vol. 1. London: Oxford University Press Warehouse, 1895.

Sridhar, M. K. and Purushottama Bilimoria. "Animal Ethics and Ecology in Classical India—Reflections on a Moral Theory." In *Indian Ethics*, ed. Purushottama Bilimoria, Joseph Prabhu, and Renuka Sharma, I:297–327. Aldershot: Ashgate, 2007.

Stanescu, D. C., B. Nemery, C. Veriter, and C. Marechal. "Patterns of Breathing and Ventilatory Response to CO_2 in Subjects Practicing Hatha-Yoga." *Clinical Respiratory Psychology* 16, no. 5 (1980).

Stcherbatsky, Theodor. *The Central Conception of Buddhism*. London: Royal Asiatic Society, 1923.

Stevenson, Ian. *Children Who Remember Previous Lives*. Charlottesville: University Press of Virginia, 1987.

——. *Twenty Cases Suggestive of Reincarnation*. 2nd ed. Charlottesville: University Press of Virginia, 1974.

——. *Where Reincarnation and Biology Intersect*. Westport, Conn.: Praeger, 1997.

——. *Unlearned Language: New Studies in Xenoglossy*. Charlottesville: University Press of Virginia, 1984.

Tagare, G. V., trans. *Bhagavata Purana*. 4 vols. Delhi: Motilal Banarsidass, 1978.

Taimni, I. K. *The Science of Yoga*. Adyar, Madras, India and Wheaton, Ill.: Theosophical Publishing House, 1961.

Tarkatirtha, A. M., Taranatha Nyayatarkatirtha, and H. K. Tarkatirtha, eds.

Nyaya-darsanam (*Nyaya-sutra* with four commentaries, the *Nyaya-sutra-bhasya* of Vatsyayana, the *Nyaya-sutra-varttika* of Uddyotakara, the *Nyaya-sutra-varttika-tatparyatika* of Vacaspati Misra, and the *Vrtti* of Visvanatha). Calcutta Sanskrit Series 18. 1936–44; reprint, New Delhi, Munshiram Manoharlal, 1985.

Teresa, Saint, of Avila. *The Complete Works*. Trans. E. Allison Peers. London: Sheed and Ward, 1972.

Thibaut, Georg, trans. *The Vedanta Sutras of Badarayana*. With Shankara's commentary. New York: Dover, 1962.

——. *Vedanta Sutras with Ramanuja's Commentary*. In *The Sacred Books of the East,* ed. M. Mueller, vol. 48. Oxford: Oxford University Press, 1904.

Thurman, Robert. *Essential Tibetan Buddhism*. New York: HarperCollins, 1995.

——. *The Jewel Tree of Tibet*. New York: Free Press, 2005.

Tola, Fernando and Carmen Dragonetti. *The Yoga Sutras of Patanjali: On Concentration of Mind*. Trans. K. D. Prithipaul. Delhi: Motilal Banarsidass, 1961.

Tripurari, Swami B. V. *Aesthetic Vedanta: The Sacred Path of Passionate Love*. Eugene, Ore.: Mandala, 1996.

——. *Jiva Goswami's Tattva-Sandarbha: Sacred India's Philosophy of Ecstasy*. Eugene, Ore.: Clarion Call, 1995.

Trungpa, Chogyam. *Cutting Through Spiritual Materialism*. Boulder and London: Shambhala, 1973.

——. *The Myth of Freedom*. Berkeley, Calif.: Shambala, 1976.

Tucci, Guiseppe. *The Religions of Tibet*. Berkeley and Los Angeles: University of California Press, 1980.

——. *The Theory and Practice of the Mandala*. London: Rider, 1971.

Tye, Michael. *Ten Problems of Consciousness*. Cambridge, Mass.: MIT Press, 1995.

Udapa, K. N., R. H. Singh, and R. A. Yadav. "Studies on the Effect of Some Yogic Breathing Exercises (Pranayams) in Normal Persons." *Indian Journal of Medical Research* 63 (August 1975): 1062–65.

Valiaveetil, Chacko. *Liberated Life*. Madurai: Arun Anandar College Dialogue Series, 1980.

Vasudeva, Somadeva. *The Yoga of the Malini-vijayottaratantra*. Pondicherry, India: Institut Français de Pondichéry, 2004.

Vattanky, John. *Gangesa's Philosophy of God*. Madras: Adyar, 1984.

Vedalankara, Jagannatha. *Agni-mantra-mala*. Pondicherry: Sri Aurobindo Society, 1976.

——. *Bhargo Devasya Dhimahi*. Pondicherry: Sri Aurobindo International Centre for Education, 1992.

Vidyasagara, Jibananda, ed. *Yoga Sutra*. 3rd ed. Calcutta: Bacaspatya, 1940.

Vivekananda, Swami. *The Complete Works of Swami Vivekananda*. 8 vols. Calcutta: Advaita Ashrama, 1977.

Vonnegut, Kurt, Jr. *Cat's Cradle*. New York: Delacorte, 1963.

Walli, Koshelya. *Ahimsa in Indian Thought*. Varanasi: Bharata Manisha, 1974.
Walsh, Roger. "The Consciousness Disciplines and the Behaviorial Sciences." *American Journal of Psychiatry* 137 (June 1980): 663–73.
Warren, Henry Clarke. *Buddhism in Translations*. 1896; reprint, New York: Atheneum, 1973.
Wenger, M. A. and B. K. Bagchi. "Studies of Autonomic Functions in Practitioners of Yoga in India." *Behaviorial Science* 6 (1977): 312–23.
Werner, Karel. *Yoga and Indian Philosophy*. New Delhi: Motilal Banarsidass, 1977.
Whicher, Ian. *The Integrity of the Yoga Darsana*. Albany: State University of New York Press, 1998.
Whicher, Ian and David Carpenter, eds. *Yoga: The Indian Tradition*. New York: RoutledgeCurzon, 2003.
White, David. *The Alchemical Body*. Chicago: University of Chicago Press, 1996.
——. "Ceci n'est pas un Yogi: Reconsidering the Early History of Yoga in India." Paper presented at South Asia Seminar, University of Texas at Austin, 2007.
——. "Yoga in Early Hindu Tantra." In *Yoga: The Indian Tradition,* ed. Ian Whicher and David Carpenter. New York: RoutledgeCurzon, 2003.
White, David, ed. *Tantra in Practice*. Princeton, N.J.: Princeton University Press, 2000.
Whitehead, Alfred North. *Process and Reality*. 1929; reprint, New York: Macmillan, 1969.
Wilkins, Charles, trans. *Fables and Proverbs from the Sanskrit* (the *Hitopadesha*). 1886; reprint, Gainesville, Fla.: Scholars' Facsimiles and Reprints, 1968.
Williams, Bernard. "The Self and the Future." *Philosophical Review* 79, no. 2 (1970): 161–80.
Williams, Paul. *The Reflexive Nature of Awareness: A Tibetan Madhyamaka Defence*. Richmond, Surrey: Curzon, 1998.
Wilson, Stephen R. "In Pursuit of Energy: Spiritual Growth in a Yoga Ashram." *Journal of Humanistic Psychology* 22, no. 1 (Winter 1992): 43–55.
Wittgenstein, Ludwig. *Philosophical Investigations*. Trans. G.E.M. Anscomb. New York: Macmillan, 1953.
Woodroffe, Sir John (Arthur Avalon). *The Garland of Letters*. 7th ed. Madras, India: Ganesh, 1979.
——. *The Serpent Power.* 3rd ed. Madras: Ganesh, 1928.
——. *Sakti and Sakta*. 1913; reprint, Madras: Ganesh, 1969.
Woods, James Haughton, trans. *The Yoga System of Patanjali*. Harvard Oriental Series, vol. 17. Cambridge, Mass.: Harvard University Press, 1914.
——. "The Yoga Sutras of Patanjali as Illustrated by the Commentary Entitled 'The Jewel's Lustre' or Maniprabha." *Journal of the American Oriental Society* 34 (1914): 1–114.

Index

For Sanskrit words and anglicizations, see also the glossary.

B
132
.46
P48
2009